MURDER AND ASSASSINATION

MURDER AND ASSASSINATION

• • •

by ALBERT ELLIS, Ph.D., and
JOHN M. GULLO, M.A.

Lyle Stuart, Inc., New York, N. Y.

Library of Congress Catalog Number: 72–94454

Published by Lyle Stuart, Inc.
Manufactured in the United States of America

Dedicated to Janet and Sylvia

Table of Contents

Chapter

MURDER AND ASSASSINATION

Chapter 1

Introduction

It is difficult to think of a more important topic today than anger and violence and its major subheadings: murder and assassination. Men have always been violent and they have always killed, but never before in human history with such ease, such technological facilitation, and such actual and potential destruction. As Arthur Schlesinger, Jr., has shown, we in America have a long tradition of violence: "We began, after all, as a people who killed red men and enslaved black men. . . . Nor did we confine our violence to red men and black men. We gained our freedom, after all, through revolution. The first century after independence were years of incessant violence—wars, slave insurrections, Indian fighting, urban riots, murders, duels, beatings. Members of Congress went armed to the Senate and House." But this kind of rage and murder is bland compared to the human consequences of pitting man against man today.

As Norman Cousins indicates, "Violence in our world is interconnected. It is chain reactive. It runs from the small to the large and back again, from a half-crazed individual with a handgun to space armadas with explosives that can incinerate whole cities, from men who have contempt for law to nations that refuse even to consider the establishment of law in the world."

In a book edited by Nigel Calder called *Unless Peace Comes: A Scientific Forecast of New Weapons,* several authorities show exactly what will happen if man does not soon find some way to curb his tendencies toward individual and mass murder. As Daniel S. Greenberg notes in a review of this book, "The inventory of forthcoming horrors detailed in this volume is long and ghastly:

chemical and biological weapons of fiendish efficacy, battlefield robots of great power and near indestructibility, computerization of decision-making—with an accompanying possibility that great value may be assigned to preemptive military action in response to machine-made forecasts of imminent attack."

In the United States alone, which is presumably one of the more law-abiding countries of the world, the incidence of homicide and other crimes of violence is enormous. H. A. Rusk noted that "reported crimes of violence—murder, rape, felonious assault and robbery—increased by 16 percent last year. The toll included 7,600 persons shot to death and 4,400 who died from beatings and stabbings." In addition, a number of unreported killings occur, because a good many gangland victims and other murdered individuals are "missing" but never found; much crime, even in a large city like New York, goes unreported; and a good many actual murders, such as those occurring when parents beat their children to death, are claimed to be the result of other causes.

A recent report from the Federal Bureau of Investigation showed that the crime rate in the United States rose 148 percent during the past decade. At the start of the 1970's nearly five million known crimes were committed a year, or the number of crimes for each 100,000 people was 2,471, a 10.6 percent increase over the 1968 rate and a 148 percent increase over 1960. In the New York metropolitan area the crime rate was 4,731, almost double the national rate. A total of 555,000 crimes was reported in the area. Violent crimes numbered 95,873, including 1,105 cases of murder or nonnegligent manslaughter and 2,277 forcible rapes per year. Another report indicated, early in 1971, that major crimes in New York City increased 7.4 percent for the preceding year over the rate for the year before that. During this period, there were 1,028 cases of murder and nonnegligent manslaughter in the New York area for the first eleven months of 1970, as compared to 954 cases for the equivalent period the year before. This was an increase of 7.8 percent. In the nation as a whole, crime during the year increased 11 percent.

So confused are our attitudes toward violence that even the definition of the term is at times in doubt. In the sizable and penetrating volume, *Violence in America*, which they edited, Graham and Gurr state that " 'violence' is narrowly defined here as behavior designed to inflict physical injury to people or damage to property. Collectively, and individually, we may regard specific acts of violence as good, bad, or neutral, depending on who engages in it and against whom." But other definers are more precise. Thus, Schlesinger states: "It is important to distinguish collective from individual violence—the work of mobs from the work of murderers; for the motive and the effect can be very different. There can, of course, be murder by a mob. But not all mobs aim at murder."

The vast majority of murders and assassinations, such as those which we will examine in this book, are not committed for humanitarian motives or for political liberation. They may, in spite of the delusions of their plotters and planners, actually do some good. Occasionally, they may even do more good than harm. But by and large they are pretty senseless and achieve few of the goals their perpetrators aim for.

Murder and assassination, moreover, usually lead toward a feeling of collective powerlessness rather than to one of greater social control. As Charles Frankel wrote after the murder of Robert F. Kennedy: "This assassination, after all that has preceded it, after all that has happened to the Kennedys, can make us feel not personal helplessness and defeat but the collective helplessness of all of us. In the first moments and days after the news came in, it must have made countless people feel that there is nothing to count on, nothing secure enough to make anything difficult worth doing."

One of the main reasons for our writing this book is to help further an understanding of murder and assassination, so that we will not feel so hopeless in their wake, so that we may do something to minimize them in the future, and so that we may better understand the general destructive aspects of aggression and violence and thereby come a little closer to staving off racial conflict, cold and hot international strife, possible atomic holocaust, and other threats to human survival.

The study of murder and assassination has largely been neglected over the years. There are many popular articles and books on the subject, but most are concerned only with describing the gory details of sensational slayings. There has been no definitive attempt to explain the psychology of murderers and assassins. Material on the treatment of killers and the prevention of homicidal acts is almost nonexistent in the entire popular and scientific literature.

The authors of this book became keenly interested in the psychological aspects of murder for two important reasons. First of all, both have had first-hand contact with several murderers. The senior author, Albert Ellis, served as Chief Psychologist of the New Jersey State Diagnostic Center and subsequently as Chief Psychologist of the New Jersey State Department of Institutions and Agencies. In both positions, he interviewed and examined a number of convicted slayers, including several who were waiting to be executed in the death house at the State Prison in Trenton and a number of mothers who had killed their children and who were incarcerated in the New Jersey State Prison for Women. The junior author, John M. Gullo, was Senior Psychologist at the Illinois State Hospital at Jacksonville for several years and has interviewed and treated several murderers in the course of his professional life.

Secondly, both authors have been employing, during the last few years, a new system of psychotherapy—rational-emotive therapy—which fully accepts the challenge of working with all kinds of individuals, including such difficult and disturbed persons as psychopaths, borderline psychotics, and psychotics. They have consequently been interested in using rational-emotive therapy with murderers and, in both a supervisory and a therapeutic capacity, have been conducting some experimentation along these lines. One of the results of their experimentation is the inclusion in this book of a verbatim typescript of excerpts from actual treatment sessions with a convicted murderess, who seems to have been considerably helped, and quite possibly "cured," by the use of rational-emotive psychotherapy.

Although this book necessarily cannot cover all the significant psychological aspects of murder and assassination, it is an attempt to understand what leads men to violence and killing, how they can be helped to overcome murderous tendencies, and what can be done to minimize the occurrence of mayhem and homicide in the near and distant future.

Almost every day brings new reports of a rise in the general homicide rate, of a high army officer who is being tried on charges of mass murder, of an obviously psychotic individual who has wantonly slaughtered several innocent victims, or of some other dramatic incident of murder or assassination. How can this cruelty be stopped? Through, we hope, the kind of understanding and treatment that is suggested in the concluding chapters of this book.

Albert Ellis, Ph.D.
New York City

John M. Gullo, M.A.
Springfield, Illinois

Chapter 2

Case Histories of Murderers

That the individual who commits mass murder is either temporarily or permanently psychotic is fairly evident in most cases; for why else would he engage in a whole series of homicides? This kind of diagnosis, however, while logically clear, is essentially circular thinking: The mere fact that a person kills several others, even for no ostensible reason, does not prove that he is severely emotionally aberrated. Other confirming evidence from his life history is needed to sustain such a diagnosis.

Such evidence is usually easily available. As J. B. Martin notes, a study of his life will generally show that "a psychiatrist he visited voluntarily a few years ago will find in his records routine notes: 'loveless childhood,' 'severe anxiety and tension,' 'low affect,' 'seems flat,' 'relates poorly to authority figures,' 'feels inadequate,' 'paranoid trends.' "

More concrete evidence can be found in Dr. James M. Reinhardt's book, *The Psychology of Strange Killers.* Reinhardt examines the lives of seven multiple killers in detail. Some of the most significant findings are these:

1. Robert Bruhm, a nineteen-year-old ranch worker, without provocation shot Mrs. Sands, a young pregnant mother and wife of his employer, her ten-year-old daughter, and her seven-year-old brother. Only the seven-year-old survived. As a child, Bob set fires and urinated in the corner of the bathroom, in bed, in a washbowl, and on a sack of rabbit food. He was a chronic runaway; was depressed, restless, moody. Viewing grisly movies kept him disquiet for hours and sometimes recurringly for days. A psychiatrist who examined him testified that his "excessive use of autism is a phe-

nomenon common among schizoid personalities and also among frankly schizophrenic patients. . . . The patient makes numerous statements which cannot in themselves be called psychotic and yet I think that conservatively speaking they are indicative of a peculiar insensitivity to social situations. . . . This man is not a good candidate for psychotherapy." Reinhardt states: "My interview with Robert Bruhm, together with a review of the mass of material bearing upon his personal history, lead me to no other conclusion than that Robert Bruhm had broken with objective reality at the time of the fatal episode."

2. Nancy Hazel Doss was given a life sentence in the Women's Division of the Oklahoma State Prison for the murder of Samuel Doss, her fifth husband. She also seems to have murdered, by the use of arsenic, three prior husbands, two of her sisters, two of her children, one of her grandchildren, and her aged mother. She catered to most of her body needs immediately, no matter what the consequences were; she "talked to the Lord"; she couldn't tolerate the vulgar talk of the other women when she was in prison; she could not stand a man who bored her and had to get him quickly out of the way; she was direly in need of one lover after another, and just as soon as she disposed of one she was off with a new one; she kept dwelling in her mind on the past and on "things wondrous and not of this world"; "she said that she '. . . didn't like to poison nobody . . . even if he wasn't no good . . .' yet the 'feelin' ' that a husband was about to 'pass on' gave her a strangely serene delight. Her imagination played upon the extraordinary events moving up along her path." As Reinhardt sums up: "Image by image Nancy Hazel saw a 'gay swain who smelled of cologne.' One by one she married a 'vulgar male who smelled of sweat and manure.' One by one she killed them. She did not kill them all, but she did what she could with what she had."

3. Kenneth I. Dudley and his wife, Irene Gwyn, left Syracuse, New York, in July, 1958, with six children. When they were arrested in Virginia in February, 1961, only one child—a little girl, less than three years of age—was still alive, while the others had died of neglect, physical torment, and malnutrition (although their parents had eaten regularly). They were disposed of without cere-

mony in various states along the roads they traveled. The lifeless bodies of these children were left in the old automobile, driven by the Dudleys, for varying lengths of time. Previously, Kenneth Dudley served a sentence of one year in jail for the improper burial of another child. Whenever people who noted the plight of the children wanted to help them, the Dudleys stopped their efforts. Kenneth Dudley told authorities that he burned one of his daughters' hands over a gas stove and that he burned some of his other children with a cigarette lighter on their genitals because they would not tell him when they needed to go to the bathroom. Mrs. Dudley reported that her husband didn't care how he hit the children or where; that if they didn't speak exactly right he made them go without food; that he forced them to lie down all the time and be covered when they were motoring through the state of Arizona, "even though it was warm and they sweated awful"; that he forced them to "sit in a chair all day, with their heads down, so they'd learn not to be nosy, so to speak. They couldn't go out and play and mealtime was awful." After their apprehension, Kenneth Dudley unsuccessfully tried to commit suicide. Reinhardt found Mrs. Dudley to be not entirely unmaternal, but "she exhibited signs of masochism. I believe that she was bound to her cruel man by fear and an undefined masochistic desire."

4. Between December 1, 1957, and January 29, 1958, Charles Starkweather killed eleven people, including the parents of his girl friend, Carol Fugate, who accompanied him on his rampage, and their two-year-old daughter. Starkweather stated, "I always wanted to be a criminal." He showed no real remorse at any time; he viewed almost all those he killed as symbolic of the people who had blocked his way to a kind of naked glory. He was ashamed of his bowed legs and red hair, and had many thoughts of suicide. He hated almost everyone and frequently thought of perpetrating violence. For two years he had been obsessed with a delusion that death had him "marked," and he seemed preoccupied with thoughts of dying. Much of his habitual behavior was paranoiac. On the day after his first murder, when the police broadcast appeals for help in capturing him, he brazenly went to a used-clothing store and bought ten dollars' worth of clothes with money he had stolen from his victim. Sometimes, he told Reinhardt, his head

seemed too large for his brain—it got tilted and lost its direction, he couldn't get it set right, and when he did he never felt sure it would stay right. When he was about to be executed, there was a sound of thunder, which he thought was a warning to the people who were about to take his life.

5. Charles Noel Brown was sentenced to hang for murder in Council Bluffs, Iowa, for killing two men. He said he thought he had put five bullets into a man in Minneapolis, and had killed "maybe another" man elsewhere. He was not sure how many he had murdered, all told. His whole life was one of stealing, shooting, and running away. He never related well to the world. In spite of his confession of two murders, he wanted to believe that he "didn't kill anyone"—"Yes, I shot at people"—but he hoped that it was not his "bullet that killed somebody." Charles kept getting into fights, "always with niggers." He couldn't get interested in anything steady. He forged checks and ran away when they bounced. He had difficulty recalling a moment of serenity in his entire life. He lived in a dream world; believed that the "evil" hand of fate was going to get him; and felt that the one inevitable way of warding off this evil fate was to steal and shoot.

6. James B. Watson was sentenced to life imprisonment in California after confessing to fourteen bigamous marriages, seven of which he ended by killing his wives. How many other women he killed is unknown. In his early thirties he failed in business and felt so disgraced that he disappeared from the town where he was working. He then resorted to fraud, was indicted, and fled to Canada. He did well in business for a while, but then "I went all to pieces. . . . I had a complete nervous breakdown. My joints didn't hurt but there would be places above and below my knee that would hurt when I put my foot down and it wasn't swollen at all. Just run down completely." He had an impulse, for no good reason, to murder one of his legitimate wives, but "I was able to resist." He killed some of his other wives on a similar impulse. Although the police in Washington, after the body of one of his wives was found, had a perfect description of him, and were looking for him and the car, "I run around in Washington with that car for two months when I saw they said they was checking all the cars."

Of killing one of his wives, he stated: "We were out to the lake and discussing something and just seemed like an impulse came over me and I hit the girl without provocation. . . . We were both sitting and something came up and I just got up and took a medium-sized rock. Something just seemed to say, 'Do it.' And when it is done something would seem to say, 'Well, it is all right.' "

He reported: "All I felt after a killing seemed largely in each instance some kind of relief, yet inexplainable. The sensation experienced was a sensation of ease as if I had been relieved. Instead of remorse I had passive satisfaction or passive pleasure. I had no sexual sensation at the time but maybe for a day or so afterwards feeling more that way than normal. The greater sexual desires shortly after was from memory of the killing. Sometimes I have looked at the body in a way of satisfaction, a kind of pleasure. Yet there was no reason why I should do that because I had seen the same person in the married relations."

Watson never held a job long, never constructed or followed through a career plan of action. He felt no woman had ever really loved him, in spite of his many marriages. He regarded womankind as the "root of evil." He admitted experiencing an urge to violate sexually the bodies of his victims, and in at least one instance, a victim's body was sexually mutilated. His whole life, Reinhardt notes, "was a continuum of failure upon failure; emptiness upon emptiness, and the process was irreversible."

7. Melvin Davis Rees was convicted in Baltimore and in Spotsylvania, Virginia, of killing Mr. and Mrs. Carroll Jackson and their two young daughters, Susan and Janet. Rees was suspected also of killing at least three other young women and molesting several others. Mrs. Jackson had apparently been subjected to prolonged sexual cruelties, then beaten and strangled with a stocking. Although an intelligent individual and a competent musician, Rees had strange ideas about the supernatural and the hereafter; he was always irritated about something; he acted superior; according to one of his acquaintances, he "was always 'sick'. . . . He appeared friendly and mild most of the time, but some of the wild things he said made me wonder. . . ." He was furiously jealous of his main girl friend and easily suffered hurt pride. He

lost the capacity for regular sex consummation and became obsessed with taking, subduing, and possessing an absolutely innocent, helpless victim. Dr. Benjamin Karpman, merely by reading the newspaper reports on Rees, noted that "mental illness undoubtedly enters the case."

Another book that has several accounts of multiple murder is *The Fine Art of Murder,* compiled by Walter B. Gibson. The authors in Gibson's anthology report two instances where the murderer was convicted for slaying two or more victims and where sufficient information was known about his personal history to determine how disturbed he was. A brief summary of these cases follows:

1. Herbert Asbury reports on Herman W. Mudgett (better known as Henry H. Holmes), who was hanged in 1896 for the murder of one of his accomplices in a bizarre insurance fraud. He was thought by the police and press to have murdered from thirty to several hundred individuals. Mudgett was a forger, a bigamist, a swindler; and "a murderer who maintained a fantastic 'castle' equipped with trapdoors, secret stairways, sound-proof rooms, torture chambers lined with sheet iron and asbestos, a crematory, vats of corrosive acids and quicklime, and apparatus with which he articulated the skeletons of several of his victims and prepared them for sale to medical schools." He had a delusional theory "that the human body, by proper manipulation, could be stretched to twice its normal length, and held that universal application of the process would produce a race of giants." He was clearly psychopathic or psychotic.

2. Archie McFedries delineates the case of Bela Kiss, a resident of Czinkota, Hungary, during the second decade of the twentieth century. Kiss seems to have killed at least twenty-three ladies and one gentleman before he went off to serve in World War I. He was a devout believer in astrology, and noted to the village constable, Adolph Trauber, "The planets guide me through life, as a compass guides a sailor." After he had killed one of his wives, but had managed to do away with her with no suspicion falling on him, he was found in his dark, cold house, reduced to skin and bones and fitfully sobbing. When asked what was the matter, he replied, "I am to die by starvation. The stars have willed it." When

he escaped to the French Foreign Legion, after his many murders were committed and he had never been called to account for them, he "would regale his comrades with stories of how he had made a career of garrotting the ladies." Although he was clever in plotting his crimes, escaping detection, and going scot-free, his life was filled with senseless deeds, some of which put him into needless jeopardy.

Miriam Allen de Ford, in her book *Murderers Sane and Mad,* also has several instances of multiple murder. Where the facts are available, all the plural killers again seem to be exceptionally disturbed individuals:

1. Louise Peete was gassed in San Quentin in April, 1947, for two murders; and "indirectly, she also caused the death of at least one other person, and perhaps of three besides him." We learn that Louise "was an incorrigible liar, and in nothing more than in her age." She "never made up a small story when a big one would do." Even after she was apprehended for murder, "indubitably she was able to persuade herself, for the moment at least, of the truth of every one of her falsehoods. Listen to her as she waited for her trial for the murder of Denton: 'I am able to preserve an attitude of calm because I am innocent. I have no visions of a murdered man to shake my nerves; no torments of remorse to disturb my sleep. There are other women in this jail who are charged with the murder of men. Some cannot sleep. Perhaps their minds mirror death agonies. I have seen them pace the floor and wring their hands. I have felt tremendous sympathy for them. My heart has been wrung with the wish that I could help them. At the same time I have thanked God that I am not tormented as they are.' Can anyone doubt that the very sound of these words transformed Louise Peete—while she spoke—into the noble, wronged, innocent creature she described herself as being?"

2. William George Heirens was sentenced in Chicago in 1946 to three consecutive life sentences for three murders, besides being given one to twenty years, or one year to life, on twenty-six separate burglary and assault charges. He concentrated on stealing women's clothing and lingerie. When he murdered Frances Brown, he left a large seminal stain on her bed (though he did not rape her) and scrawled on her bureau mirror with lipstick: "For

heaven's sake catch me before I kill more. I cannot control myself." He had a burglary record dating back to age fourteen. He made up a phantom companion, George, and actually seemed to believe that George had committed some of his crimes. Although not a homosexual, he found women repulsive and obtained erotic gratification in stealing and wearing women's undergarments. He apparently blacked out in the course of some of his crimes and murders. He attempted suicide by hanging when he was in jail. He fought with the police when he was caught because he wanted them to kill him: "I knew there was something wrong with me. I hoped I could overcome it." Dr. Foster Kennedy, a psychiatrist who examined him, found that he had "partial amnesia" during the commission of his crimes; and two psychiatrists who testified at his trial found him to be "a sexual psychopath with maniacal tendencies."

3. John Reginald Halliday Christie was hanged in London on July 15, 1953, for having murdered at least six women. He supposedly raped his victims at the moment of or immediately after death. "Psychologically few men have ever been so thoroughly and incurably abnormal." As a result of his grandfather's dying when he was a child, "Death thereafter fascinated and enthralled him. He fell in love with it. Dormant for many years, that emotional twist was always there, and in the end it overwhelmed him." He was afflicted several times with what seemed to be psychosomatic ailments. He served time for theft and assault (including hitting one of his landladies over the head with a baseball bat). He condemned himself for his deeds and would have confessed to many crimes he did not commit if encouraged to do so. He was found to be, by a psychiatrist, "sexually immature," and obtained sex satisfaction only with a completely unresponsive partner—"which meant in the end a partner either unconscious or dead." His family doctor recommended psychiatric treatment for him. At his trial, psychiatrists referred to him as suffering from "gross hysteria," as "a hysterical personality," and as "abnormal and conceited, an inadequate personality." F. E. Camps tells us that Christie pleaded, as classically happens with many murderers, "everything went black" when he committed some of his crimes.

Camps reported on another multiple murderer, George Joseph Smith, who committed bigamy eight times and murder three times. Smith suffered from "over-confidence which appears to develop a feeling of omnipotence whereby the very ingenuity and care, which were the basis of previous success, give way to behaviour which, unless blessed with unbelievable luck, must end in suspicion." He repeated bigamy and murder by the same method each time; and "he not only used his own name on several occasions but very rarely concealed his interest in the financial worth of his brides." He first came to police attention at the age of nineteen, when he was convicted of larceny. Soon after he was released (in 1891), he was in jail for larceny again. He killed one of his wives only three days after she had signed a will in his favor. The more successful he was, the bolder and more rash were his crimes.

R. E. L. Masters and Eduard Lea include the cases of several multiple murderers in their book, *Sex Crimes in History.* Wherever enough data were known, these killers turned out to be highly disturbed. For example:

1. Countess Elisabeth Bathory of Hungary seems to have murdered as many as six hundred—yes, six hundred—girls in order to bathe in their blood to keep herself young and beautiful. Many of her victims were cruelly tortured. She was found to be insane and placed in protective custody, walled into a room in her own castle, for life. She seems to have known that her castle, which was filled with corpses and other evidence of her murders, was about to be raided, but made no effort to prevent the raid or to escape. Instead, she wrote a strange document invoking the Devil and beseeching him to send her ninety-nine cats to tear out the hearts of the King of Hungary, of Prime Minister Thurzo, and of other officials she believed were preparing to take action against her.

2. Gilles de Rais, often known as the original Bluebeard (though Comorre the Cursed was actually the first bearer of this name), was a Marshal of France who murdered some eight hundred boys. He became so enraged by the capture and burning of his friend, Joan of Arc, that he left his wife, refused thereafter to have intercourse with any woman, and began to spite God by his career of crime and sacrilege. He cut the throats of many of his child victims, violated them, drank their blood, and then would

fall into a comalike slumber. He not only tortured his victims but had the heads of these children "stuck on upright rods. A professional beautician, a member of his entourage, would then be called in, and the child's hair would be exquisitely curled, its lips and cheeks rouged, and so on. When enough heads were accumulated and thus prepared, Gilles would hold a kind of beauty contest, with everyone voting on which head was the most beautiful—after which the 'winner' might again be put to necrophilous use."

3. Nero, famed for fiddling while Rome burned, was extremely cruel and vicious; made a game of attacking men on their way home from dinner and dropping their bodies down sewers; stole from shops; got into numerous fights; had himself released from a den dressed in the skins of wild animals, and attacked the genitals of men and women who stood bound to stakes. He had innumerable people killed, including his own mother, Agrippina. "To mention but two more of his atrocities: he once made human torches of captive Christians, and used them to light up a garden party; and at the Games, during the public ravishing of virgins, he additionally entertained those nearby by imitating the virgins' anguished cries." He died by his own hand at the age of thirty-two.

4. Heliogabalus, another Roman emperor, had many young boys slaughtered, mutilated, and their phalli presented to him. He then tossed them on a blazing pyre as a sacrifice to his namesake, the god Elagabalus. He also caused many senators to be killed. He acted as a girl, tried to get himself castrated, and "would visit brothels, reveal his identity, evict the prostitutes, and himself fulfill the requirements of the arriving customers as best he was able." He had himself "married" to several men, including the slave, Hieracles. "He conceived the fantastic idea of abdicating in favor of the slave, who would become emperor, while he, Heliogabalus, would reign at Hieracles' side as empress." Not being able to take such shenanigans even on the part of an emperor, his rebellious subjects murdered him and tossed his body into the river.

5. Vacher the Ripper committed more murders than the more famous Jack the Ripper (who was never captured), since he slew at least eleven victims and probably twice that number. As a boy, "he amused himself by torturing and killing animals, and was obviously attracted to all that was cruel and destructive." On

March 20, 1894, he launched his career of murder "by strangling a twenty-one-year-old girl, cutting her throat, trampling on her abdomen, tearing pieces of flesh from her breasts, and, finally, violating her corpse." He attributed his actions to "irresistible impulse" and "temporary insanity." He had spent some time in a mental hospital before his crimes occurred.

6. Vincent Verzeni committed two murders and attempted several more, usually including vampirism. He started experiencing sexual pleasure at the age of twelve when wringing the necks of chickens. He said of himself: "I had an unspeakable delight in strangling women, experiencing during the act erections and real sexual pleasure. The feeling of pleasure while strangling them was much greater than that which I experienced while masturbating. I took great delight in drinking [Johanna] Motta's blood."

7. Albert Fish killed and ate between eight and fifteen children and drank their blood. He also castrated a number of boys. He was found by examining psychiatrists to be "a coprophage, or eater of excrements; a pedophile and a nymphophile; a masochist, who inserted needles into his body and flagellated himself with a paddle studded with nails; and, as mentioned, a sadist, vampire, cannibal, and lust-murderer. . . . He experienced hallucinations and a messianic delusion, proclaiming himself to be the Christ and an instrument of God's vengeance upon a sinful and depraved humanity. . . . Fish was manifestly psychotic."

8. John George Haigh was executed in August, 1949, for slaying nine people and drinking their blood. He was a religious fanatic who acted on an injunction he found in the Old Testament: "to drink water out of thine own cistern and running waters out of thine own well." He interpreted dreaming and waking "signs" to mean that his religious ardor was a drain upon his vital energies and that these might be replenished by the consumption of blood. He was obviously psychotic or seriously neurotic.

9. Peter Kurten, a resident of Dusseldorf in 1899, was found guilty of nine murders and seven attempted murders. When he was thirteen or fourteen he strangled a squirrel and experienced orgasm as a result of this sadistic act. He engaged in many acts of bestiality and, since that gave him little satisfaction, "He then began to torture animals rather than having intercourse with

them, stabbing pigs and sheep and experiencing orgasm." He throttled several of his human victims while having coitus with them; it was the sight of their blood that brought on his orgasm. "Kurten described himself, Dr. [Karl] Berg concurring, as a psychopath and a megalomaniac. To the end, he was unable to experience any sort of remorse for his crimes—or to say that he would not, if freed, at once commit others." In prison, he became thoroughly embittered against what he regarded as an unjust and oppressive society. "About his own execution, Kurten had expressed some curiosity. Would he, he enquired of Dr. Berg, after his head had been chopped off, still be able to hear, at least for a moment, the sound of his own blood gushing from the stump of his neck? That would be, he remarked, the pleasure to end all pleasures."

10. Neville Heath was executed in 1946 in England for the murder of five or more females. "Where his more serious offenses were concerned, he not only whipped and beat his female victims, but mutilated them with knives and with his teeth: biting the nipples from the breasts, tearing at the vagina with a knife or, in one case, a poker, and otherwise mutilating the bodies, all while the victims remained conscious and suffering. He admitted pausing frequently during his 'work' to enjoy the agonies of those he tortured; and where whipping was concerned, he recommended an interlude for this purpose of at least sixty seconds following each descent of the lash." He was manifestly psychotic.

G. Redston and K. F. Crossen relate the stories of a number of multiple murderers, most of them members of the Mafia and other American underworld groups. They give virtually no details on the personal or emotional lives of any of these gangsters, except Mickey Cohen, who is said to have been implicated in the murder of many of his "friends" and business associates. They note that in Cohen's case "it was estimated that he was spending at least $300,000 a year on personal living. In the process of achieving this success, Mickey began to show traits that had never been reported before. He began to wash his hands every few minutes, even interrupting a conversation or a meal to go through this ceremony, began to take showers that lasted more than an hour and could only be taken after the bathroom was thoroughly cleaned, and he developed a passion for emptying ash trays. . . .

Mickey developed another facet of his personality in those early years. While most gangsters shunned publicity, he not only courted it but often made it. There are not many photographs of leading criminals, and many of those are of men shielding their faces, but there are probably hundreds of Cohen."

Truman Capote gives a detailed history of the case of Richard Eugene Hickock and Perry Edward Smith, two Kansas killers who murdered Mr. and Mrs. Herbert W. Clutter and their young son and daughter. From Capote's story we learn that Dick Hickock had severe feelings of inadequacy about the physical injuries he had received in a car collision when he was nineteen years of age; that in spite of his lifelong history of crime and murder he considered himself perfectly normal; that he was a pedophiliac who mainly went to the Clutter house with Smith in order to rape their fifteen-year-old virgin daughter; and that he went on long drinking binges, as a result of which he neglected his business, started passing bad checks, and became a steady thief.

In spite of his severe disturbance, Hickock was relatively sane compared to Perry Smith. The latter also had severe feelings of inadequacy about physical injuries received in a motorcycle wreck. Although very bright, he was superstitious about having anything to do with nuns. As a child, he consistently wet the bed, cried in his sleep, and slid into a fury. He was very moody and was prone to "sudden cold fevers that burned and chilled." He had delusions of killing a Negro named King in his youth. He had a long history of arrests, starting in his eighth year. He confessed to having "many violent outbursts of anger while I served time in Japan and Korea." He had thoughts of suicide when incarcerated with Hickock for his crimes. In prison, he undulated all one summer "between half-awake stupors and sickly, sweat-drenched sleep. Voices roared through his head; one voice persistently asked him, 'Where is Jesus? Where?' And once he woke up shouting, 'The bird is Jesus! The bird is Jesus!' " Dr. W. Mitchell Jones, a psychiatrist at Larned State Hospital in Kansas, who had professionally examined Smith, felt that he showed "definite signs of severe mental illness." Dr. Joseph Satten of the Menninger Clinic held that when Smith attacked Mr. Clutter he was under a mental eclipse, deep inside a schizophrenic darkness.

Jack Altman and Dr. Marvin Ziporyn found many indications of severe emotional disturbance in Richard Speck, who killed eight nurses in Chicago on the night of July 13, 1966. Ziporyn, who was prison psychiatrist at the Cook County Jail while Speck was incarcerated there, and who spent many hours talking to him formally and informally, noted that (1) he was captured after the murders mainly because of a bloody suicide attempt; (2) he was addicted to alcohol, sodium amytal, and sodium seconal; (3) "he was emotionally unstable, impulsive, depressive"; (4) he was subject to violent rages, from childhood onward; (5) he had suffered a number of head injuries over the years and was probably brain damaged; (6) he had "developed an all-pervading suspicion of women, particularly in his sexual relations with them and when they displayed sexual looseness"; (7) he had been arrested thirty-six times, mostly for drunk and disorderly charges; (8) he was diagnosed by a specially appointed psychiatric panel as "sociopathic personality, anti-social behavior, with alcoholism"; (9) he entertained paranoid ideas of being persecuted by other prisoners when he was in jail.

Karl Menninger, in *The Crime of Punishment,* reports two cases of multiple murderers. In the first case, a twenty-four-year-old ex-Coast Guard member who was working in a drive-in restaurant became so angry when his mother decided to take a prolonged visit with his half sister that he manufactured a time bomb, put it in a valise, and dispatched it with her on the airplane in which she was departing. When it blew up, she and everyone else on the plane were killed. Menninger's colleagues examined this mass killer and found that, as a youth, he had beaten a cow to death—because it kicked him, he said. At another time, he set fire to a garage to get revenge on a salesman who owned a car that was kept in it; and "in spite of his superficially acceptable social adjustment he had always been psychologically abnormal and socially maladjusted. He possessed a low toleration for frustration and discipline, with egocentricity of a high degree, severely impaired judgment capacity, and a poor work record. He had previously exhibited antisocial behavior of various sorts, which had not led to treatment. . . . He was undoubtedly irrational, illogical, psychopathic, sociopathic, disorganized, and schizophrenic."

Menninger also briefly reports on the case of Robert Smith, aged eighteen, who on November 13, 1966, killed four women and a little girl in a beauty parlor in Mesa, Arizona. Smith was influenced by reading about the Richard Speck murders, which had occurred a few months before. When apprehended he stated: "I just wanted to get myself a name. I wanted to be known." He said that he had been planning a mass murder ever since his parents gave him a gun three months before for target practice.

D. L. Champion presents details on several multiple killers, and each case includes evidence that they were severely emotionally disturbed. Some of his cases we have already discussed. The others include:

1. Winnie Ruth Judd, in October, 1931, killed Agnes Anne LeRoi and Hedvig Samuelson, two women with whom she was probably involved in lesbian relations, and had their bloody bodies transported in trunks from Phoenix to Los Angeles, where she intended to dispose of them. When she was sixteen, she pretended that she was pregnant, swore out a warrant against a man who had never touched her sexually, and ran away from home. She wrote to her husband: "More than once I've told my neighbors that I was going to have a baby. When I was in Phoenix, I told a number of people that I was the mother of a little boy. I even showed some baby snapshots of you and said you were my son." She "suffered from a deep personality split." Dr. George W. Stevens, a noted psychiatrist, testifed that Winnie Ruth suffered from "dementia praecox." Dr. Edward Huntington Williams, another psychiatrist, said: "She did not know right from wrong or she would have taken far more intelligent means of disposing of the bodies." Dr. Clifford Wright "claimed that Winnie Ruth suffered from a glandular ailment that precluded her thinking like a normal person. Moreover, she was immature in both mind and body." After her conviction, Warden A. G. Walker of the Arizona State Prison insisted that a sanity board examine her, and the board "branded Winnie Ruth a madwoman. The writ directing her execution was voided, and she was ordered to spend the rest of her natural life in the Arizona State Hospital for the Insane at Phoenix."

2. Ian Brady and Myra Hindley were convicted in England

of killing three children and were probably implicated in the slaying and torture of at least a half dozen more youngsters over a five-year period. They tape-recorded one of their crimes: "The tape was unique. It recorded the minute details of the perverted rape, torture, and death of a twelve-year-old girl. Her agonized cries were interspersed with profane injunctions and ecstatic moans from the Torquemadas who slowly killed her. . . . The agonized cries, the pleading, the rattle of death itself, was the point of it all. Listening to the awful sound of a human being *in extremis* was, to Brady and his mistress, a far more powerful aphrodisiac than cantharides." All her life Myra hated work, and devoted herself to semiprostitutional activities. Brady was a petty thief and a "roller of queers." He was inordinately vain and most careful to present his left profile to strangers. Both were clearly emotionally disturbed.

3. Charles Joseph Whitman, on a broiling hot day of August 1, 1966, started sniping at passers-by from a perch high on top of the University of Texas tower in Austin, and soon had murdered sixteen men and women and wounded thirty-one. Earlier that same year, in March, he was so disturbed over his parents' separation that he visited Dr. Maurice Dean Heatley, a university psychiatrist. Dr. Heatley found him to be mentally disturbed and set another appointment for the following week; but Whitman did not keep it. Whitman loved his wife and mother and killed them "to spare them embarrassment for the mass murder he was about to perpetrate." He wrote: "I hate my father with a mortal passion. And I can't stand the pressures on me. I'm going to fight it out alone." When an autopsy was performed on him, after he was shot by a police officer, a small benign tumor was found in his brain. There is considerable evidence that Whitman was seriously disturbed all his life and that at certain times he was in a state of frenzy. In an article on the many faces of murder, Bruce Porter included one of the letters Whitman left the night before his mass shooting spree:

"I don't really understand myself these days. I am supposed to be an average reasonable and intelligent young man. However, lately (I can't recall when it started) I have been a victim of many unusual and irrational thoughts. These thoughts constantly recur, and it requires a tremendous mental effort to concentrate on useful and progressive tasks." After killing his mother the next day, Whitman wrote: "I have just taken my mother's life. I am very upset over having done it. However, I feel that if there is a heaven she is definitely there now. And if there is no life after, I have relieved her of her suffering here on earth. The intense hatred I feel for my father is beyond description."

Robert Wolf, in an editorial in *Rational Living,* points out that Whitman was the kind of person who felt it necessary to include in his last-hour survival kit—along with food and ammunition—a deodorant; that, although he and his wife worked at common jobs to make both ends meet, he felt it necessary to drive a new Chevrolet Impala; that he was a perfectionist who became quite tense about taking tests and that he was upset over two serious quizzes that he was scheduled to take on the day of the massacre. Hilda Mosse notes that he "was evidently suffering from delusions. If the psychiatrist to whom Whitman went before the murders, complaining of uncontrollable violent impulses, had discerned delusions, the murders might have been prevented."

One of the most infamous multiple murderers of all time was Albert deSalvo, the Boston Strangler, who killed at least thirteen women between June 14, 1962, and January 4, 1964, and who committed innumerable other robberies and assaults. G. Frank wrote a lengthy volume on DeSalvo; it is apparent from his research that the Boston Strangler was basically psychotic. As a child of twelve he snatched purses and committed other robberies. All through his life, until he was finally committed to Bridgewater State Hospital in Massachusetts, he engaged in many attempts at breaking and entering, assault and battery, and various kinds of sex offenses.

At DeSalvo's trial, Drs. Mezer and Tartakoff testified that he suffered from a committable mental disease, which the former described as "chronic undifferentiated schizophrenia." Dr. Tartakoff called him a "sociopath with dangerous tendencies . . . an individual who from early life has shown deviations from what are usually considered normal patterns of behavior, thinking, and emotional reactions." Dr. Amos Robey said he suffered from "schizophrenic reaction, chronic undifferentiated type" and that he "also has very extensive signs of sexual deviation."

Charles Franklin examines the characters of many of what he calls "the world's worst murderers," including Peter Kurten, John Reginald Halliday Christie, Neville George Clevely Heath, John George Haigh, and Bela Kiss, whose crimes we have already surveyed. He gives voluminous details on the patterns of severe emotional disturbance which almost all the killers in his book exhibited; and he comes to the unequivocal conclusion that "the worst murderers in the world are always psychopaths." Some additional multiple murderers that he reports upon are these:

1. The famous French murderer, Landru, was said by the London police to have murdered three hundred women, but this was probably an exaggeration. He was finally convicted of eleven killings and of swindling his victims of their life savings. When apprehended, he stubbornly refused to talk, although he admitted having known the eleven women he was accused of murdering. "What happened to these women? Landru refused to say. He refused, in fact, to discuss the matter at all, maintaining that it was far too delicate a subject for a vulgar police inquiry. This was an attitude he in all seriousness adopted. He was outraged, affronted, and would not disclose any information of matters which he maintained were entirely private and were between the ladies and himself. He had been the subject of their confidences, he said, and to reveal them was unthinkable. How could the police be so lacking in taste as to institute this unjustified intrusion into matters which were entirely private and confidential?

"Previous medical reports had indicated that Landru had suffered from some hereditary mental disturbances, but when the medical experts examined him now they found him sane and responsible. He was no doubt what we would now call a psychopath."

F. A. Mackenzie noted: "He had the gift of silence and aloofness. He was essentially mean and greedy beyond measure. Like Frederick Guy Browne, the English murderer, he could not bear to throw the possessions of his victims away, even tell-tale things that would convict him if found. He hoarded the linen, the papers and the dresses of the women he killed."

When, at his trial, many grief-stricken mothers and sisters testified that it was impossible to believe their loved ones would not have written if they had been alive (as Landru claimed they still were), Mackenzie reports: " 'The court is deeply moved by their tears,' wrote one spectator. 'Landru alone remains unmoved. It is his great callousness that is so striking in this remarkable criminal.' " States Franklin: "Landru described his activities as 'pursuing studies in feminine psychology.' 'The women went where their destinies called them,' he remarked with characteristic lack of feeling."

2. Dr. Marcel Petiot probably murdered sixty-three people, most of them Jewish refugees whom he pretended to help escape from the Nazis in the early 1940's. He seems to have murdered mostly for money and literally became a millionaire by his nefarious deeds. "Born at Auxerre in 1897, son of a minor postal clerk, he displayed early sadistic tendencies, practising unpleasantly upon helpless animals and children smaller than himself. As a boy he was known as 'that little monster Petiot.' . . . In 1916 he was working in a casualty clearing station, enjoying the sights and sounds of his fearsomely wounded fellow warriors, and stealing morphia on the side which he peddled to drug addicts in Dijon. He spent some months in a mental asylum during the war and he was diagnosed as suffering from 'war psychosis.' " He completely escaped from the police net that was out for him but then foolishly, out of vanity, appeared in the French victory parade, after World War II, "in French officer's uniform complete with phoney medals." He was consequently captured and convicted.

3. Raymond Fernandez and Martha Beck, the famous "lonely hearts killers," murdered four women whom they swindled after Raymond got them to fall in love with him. Raymond was convicted as a youth for chicken stealing and was adjudged a juvenile delinquent. Later, "he worked his passage across the Atlantic in an oil-tanker and during the voyage he suffered a severe injury by being struck on the head by a falling hatch. He was later discharged from a hospital in Curacao with a deep indentation on the front part of his head, and most of his hair gone. This injury, as was later observed in the post-mortem, left a long scar across the tissue of his brain, and completely changed his personality.

The injury turned him to crime and murder. . . . His friends said he was a different man. Even his voice was different. He became obsessed with Black Magic and believed he had a sinister power over women, and he began a systematic swindling of them through matrimonial advertisements and Lonely Hearts clubs. . . .

"So hypnotized was Martha by the love life which Raymond held in prospect for her, that she gave up everything, her useful job, her children, in order to be with him. With little hesitation she joined him in his mean and contemptible business of swindling lonely women. They went into the Lonely Hearts racket, she posing as his sister. But the trouble started with Martha's fierce jealousy. It was this jealousy which really led to the murders. Martha went to any lengths to prevent Raymond making love to his 'brides,' even going to the extent of sharing the same bed with them. . . . The second victim was sixty-six-year-old Janet Fay, a silly, romantically-sentimental woman eager for any man, and easily snared by Raymond. Having realized all her assets, she went with them to New York, where an infuriated Martha battered her to death after the usual jealous scene. . . . Two hours before the execution Fernandez sent a message to Martha saying he would like to shout his love for her to the whole world. When she got this message she said: 'Now that I know that Raymond loves me, I can go to my death with bursting joy.' "

4. Anna Maria Schonleben was executed in Bavaria in 1811 after poisoning more than eighty people, several of whom died. She was an extreme toxicomaniac who "suffered extremely from this strange psychological disturbance. The very sight of poison made her tremble with excitement and desire—desire to use it upon someone, anyone in fact. An intelligent woman, she said when sentenced to death that her death would be a fortunate thing for mankind for she lived for poison alone. . . . In poison she had discovered an instrument which gave her great power over people's lives and which satisfied her craving for revenge against mankind at whose hands she considered she had suffered."

5. Billy Palmer caused the biggest murder sensation of mid-Victorian England by poisoning some fourteen people. Born in 1824 to a wealthy family, he "went to Rugeley Grammar School

where he displayed the usual unpleasantries which are always reported in retrospect about murderers by those who knew them in their youth, such as torturing animals and cruelties to children." Apprenticed to a firm of Liverpool chemists, he was discharged for theft. While studying to be a physician, "Palmer became enamored with poisons. He began to dabble with them in such a suspicious manner that the hospital authorities barred him from the dispensary in the strongest possible terms." He was a lazy student, notorious for his inveterate gambling and dishonesty. He quite probably poisoned two of his illegitimate and four of his legitimate children. To collect on an insurance policy, he also poisoned his brother, Walter.

6. Neill Cream was a physician who used strychnine to murder several women before he was convicted for the slaying of Matilda Clover. Many authorities, including the writer Edmund Pearson, looked upon him as a "moral monster" or a "lunatic," particularly because his actions were so self-incriminating. As Franklin notes: "He could not leave his murders alone once he had committed them. He wrote self-incriminatory letters and even got in touch with the authorities demanding post-mortems on his victims. No other murderer has so ardently courted the hangman." He got into trouble early in life: "Cream made early experiments in crime and during his college days he got the reputation for being something of an arsonist. He tried unsuccessfully to swindle insurance companies thereby. . . . He dabbled in blackmail, and his reputation became so unsavoury that he left for the United States, setting up in Chicago as a practising abortionist. . . . Cream was now a drug addict and took large quantities of morphia and cocaine. He suffered from continual headaches, probably migraine, which brought about insomnia."

7. George Joseph Smith murdered three successive wives in their baths. Born to respectable parents in Bethnal Green, London, in 1872, "he turned to petty crime at an early age." After murdering and collecting insurance money on two wives, "the extraordinary thing was that he appeared to believe that he could get away with it indefinitely. It would have occurred to any normal person that brides dying in their baths in this fashion constituted unusual occurrences which would be sure to attract attention. But

Smith was not a reasonable person. He had the true psychopath's detachment from the world and belief in his right to do as he wished, regardless of society at large." He behaved badly at his own trial: "Smith had already created a bad impression by his violent outbursts during the police-court proceedings, and as the trial progressed—it lasted nine days—he resumed these outbursts, reviling and abusing the witnesses, and refusing to listen to his counsel's appeals for his silence."

8. Peter Manuel, born in New York in 1927 of working-class Scottish parents who had just emigrated there, committed at least nine wanton murders. His family returned to Scotland in the early 1930's. "Just before the war they were in Coventry, where young Peter Manuel embarked upon his career of crime in his early teens. Burglary, probation, housebreaking, approved school, robbery with indecent assault, Borstal, more burglary, finally prison, was the pattern of his thorough apprenticeship in crime. Thirteen times he escaped from custody, and at the age of sixteen he had the distinction of having it said about him by an experienced probation officer that he had never known a boy with a worse record. Years of violent crime followed. This young rebel without a cause characterized his robberies by vicious and unprovoked assaults upon his victims. . . . Manuel was not in any way a womanizer. In fact he was shy with women and did not associate with them much. This feeling of sexual inadequacy led him to commit indecent assaults and rapes. . . . With a score of nine certain murders, Manuel takes his place well up among the world's multiple killers. It is very probable that killing gave him some sexual satisfaction. Most of his victims were women and he had a habit of removing some part of their most intimate clothing. He had a craving for the limelight and a great desire to be feared."

9. James Hanratty may be deemed a multiple murderer, even though he only killed Michael Gregsten, whom he kidnaped along with his sweetheart, Valerie Storie. But he shot Miss Storie five times in the neck, close to her spinal cord, and only by a near-miracle did she live. He left home at fifteen, being unable to get on with either of his parents. "He had a fall from his bicycle which apparently caused a certain amount of amnesia. A few months later he was wandering about Brighton sleeping on the beach and

doing odd jobs for lorry drivers. He was later found unconscious in a Brighton street and taken to St. Francis Hospital, Haywards Heath, with a suspected brain haemorrhage. A craniotomy revealed no haemorrhage, but the consultant psychiatrist diagnosed him as a mental defective. Hanratty was discovered to be completely illiterate and lacking in mental or emotional development. . . . The great criminal's undistinguished career as a burglar was temporarily interrupted by a visit to the Borstal Section of Wormwood Scrubs, where an equally unsuccessful attempt to commit suicide landed him in the prison hospital. There he was recognized as a potential psychopath." After shooting Gregsten, Hanratty raped Miss Storie in the back seat of Gregsten's car, while his victim bled to death in the front seat. Later, believing both to be dead, he called the police, who had no reason to suspect him at that time, to say he was worried about being under suspicion for the murder. His call alerted the police to connecting him with the double shooting.

10. Donald Hume killed his business partner, Stanley Setty, and after spending eight years in jail for this killing he staged an unsuccessful bank raid in Zurich, shooting a cashier and a taxi driver and killing the latter. As a teen-ager, "he showed the typical psychopathic tendencies of restlessness, chronic lying, fantasy-building and being unable to settle into society." After a stint in the Royal Air Force, "for a while he did well in the black market and various illegal rackets. He posed as an R.A.F. officer and went around swindling R.A.F. stations. For this he was bound over." When he went into partnership with Setty, "he was soon doing a nice business in selling forged petrol coupons and stealing cars." In an argument, Setty called him "a bastard," which made him think of a hated parrot in his childhood home who used to call out "Bastards! Bastards!" at the children. This so incensed him that he stabbed Setty to death and felt exhilarated as he watched the life run from him "like water down a drain." After being released from prison for this murder, he published, in the *Sunday Pictorial,* a lurid confessional story, "I KILLED SETTY AND GOT AWAY WITH MURDER."

Giles Playfair and Derrick Sington, in their book *Crime, Punishment and Cure,* examine Hume's case in detail and find that he was seriously disturbed from age fourteen; that he had "a paranoid streak in him, which made him incapable of forming lasting relationships. He had an obsessive hatred of his mother, which was reflected in his basic attitude towards all women."

Nine years before he killed Setty he was treated at an R.A.F. hospital for cerebral meningitis and diagnosed as someone suffering from a severe psychopathic condition. A year later he was committed for masquerading as an R.A.F. pilot officer, after having been invalided out of the R.A.F. and remanded to Borstal for a month's mental observation. He had a consistent history of grandiosity and self-aggrandizement. Before his second murder, he behaved so abnormally with his girlfriend, Trudi Sommer, including having weeping fits, that she realized he was headed for an emotional breakdown. He threatened suicide, confessed to a false story of having been a spy during World War II, also falsely claimed to have written several books. She coaxed him into giving her a revolver with which he was going to kill himself. She stated: "After that, I couldn't look him in the eyes any more. I thought he was mad. His eyes looked terrible."

His attempt to rob a bank in Zurich was exceptionally ill-planned; and when, in the course of his attempted robbery, he wantonly killed a taxi driver, Arthur Maag, he first was "struck dumb" when his captors tried to question him and then lied for the sake of lying and told some foolish stories to the Swiss police. Although the psychiatrist at his second trial did not call him "insane," he did say that Hume was clearly a "psychopath." Playfair and Sington call him definitely "psychotic."

Gladys D. Shultz includes several cases of murder in her book on sex criminals, including the case of Winston Moseley, a multiple murderer. To quote Miss Shultz: "In a sensational New York City case of 1964, Winston Moseley stabbed to death and sexually molested a woman within full view of thirty-eight of her neighbors, watching from upper-story windows. Pleading not guilty by reason of insanity, the man confessed in open court to the sex murders of another woman and a young girl—all three of his victims were unknown to him—out of an uncontrollable urge to kill as well as to rape. Two psychiatrists testified for the defense that Moseley was a schizophrenic with catatonic reactions beyond his control . . . and incapable of stopping himself once he got the urge to kill 'and thus was unable to distinguish right from wrong.' "

Leonard Gribble, in his book *Such Women Are Deadly,* chronicles the homicidal actions of twelve murderesses. In addition to cases discussed elsewhere in this book, he includes those of several multiple slayers; and in each instance where the facts on their psychological dispositions are available, they appear to be highly disturbed. Thus, Gribble reports on the following instances:

1. Augusta Fairfield Fullam, in collaboration with her lover, Lieutenant Henry Lovell William Clark, poisoned her husband, Edward, and then helped arrange the murder of Mrs. Clark. She was crazy enough to send Lieutenant Clark over four hundred letters, most of them full of endearments and extravagant promises of future delight, and many of them seriously concerned with the problem of doing away with their respective mates. In one of her letters she quite typically wrote: "Oh, my darling, it seems too much to hope that before long the last barrier that separates us will be removed and you will be mine and I will be yours till the last. The thought is ecstasy; but at times my heart is full of fears. What if we fail! It would be too cruel! We must succeed. And what if we are discovered? This is too horrible a thought; and yet it often comes to me like a nightmare. God surely will not allow us to fail. He would not keep us apart, since we love each other so truly."

Since, at the time of writing this letter, Augusta was systematically feeding her husband arsenic, it is hard to disagree with Gribble's conclusion that she "could have been teetering on the brink of an emotional abyss." Gribble does not feel that she was irrational to the point of being insane. Technically, perhaps not; but, considering that even after the murder of her husband, she continued to send Clark as many as two or three letters a day urging him to dispose of his wife, she seems to have been at least in the borderline psychotic range.

2. In the 1870's in Brighton, England, Christiana Edmund fell madly in love with an attractive and popular physician, Dr. Beard, wormed her way into his family circle, and without any en-

couragement whatever from him fed his wife some chocolates loaded with strychnine and almost killed her. Then, to turn suspicion away from herself, she poisoned several boxes of chocolate and returned them to the candy store from which they had been purchased and she sent a good many boxes of poisoned fruits, flowers, and cake to various Brighton residents. As a result of her activities, a number of people in town became seriously ill and a four-year-old child, Sidney Albert Baker, died. She foolishly drew suspicion on herself by offering a public reward for information that would lead to the arrest of the mysterious dispenser of poison. After conviction, she lived for more than thirty years in Broadmoor prison, "convinced that she was a great lady being kept in confinement by powerful enemies because she knew their dire secrets." Her mother testified at her trial that there was a history of violent insanity on both sides of the family.

3. Grete Beier, born in 1885 the daughter of a burgomaster of a town in Saxony, murdered three of her own children. " 'I killed them all as soon as they were born,' she told the shocked court in a cold voice empty of any emotion. 'We didn't want children. We wanted to enjoy ourselves.' " She stole from her father and planned to murder a nosy family maid who informed on her. She poisoned and shot one of her lovers, an engineer named Pressler, in order to inherit money from him. Grete showed criminal tendencies while still a schoolgirl and proved impossible for her governesses to manage. She stole money from her father when in her teens and spent it to help her appearance and entice older men to support her. She kept up a long-term liaison with a forger, Herr Merker, and allowed him to pimp for her. In conjunction with Merker, whom she supplied with a copy of her father's signature, she withdrew every pfennig from her father's bank account. Although she told the priest who officiated at her execution that she repented, she does not actually seem to have regretted her many crimes or shown remorse for the depredations against people, including her close relatives, that she continually committed.

4. Jeanne Weber, a Breton, born of poor parents in the Côtes du Nord, compulsively strangled at least nine children, including her own son, Marcel, and tried to kill several others. She "was often morose as a child. She seemed to spend hours content with

the fancies and fantasies of her own thoughts." Once she left her home, at the age of fourteen, to work as a maid in the house of a local family of good standing, she never returned to the family roof, even for a visit. She took to heavy drinking shortly after her marriage to Marcel Weber and "appeared sunk in deep melancholia." Her family members thought she was insane; and two brain specialists, Dr. Wallon and Dr. Dupre, testified in court that she suffered from "nervous upsets and hysteria." After her third trial for murder, "she was found guilty but insane and transferred to the asylum for the criminally insane at Mareville, where she was kept closely confined in a cell-like room fitted with iron bars. Her physical and mental condition deteriorated from the moment of her incarceration. She was found several times in the throes of a seizure, clutching at imaginary throats while she gasped for air. During these violent attacks she foamed at the mouth and wailed with terrible intensity. One morning she was found stretched in death. She had her fingers securely locked around her own throat. The lust for death by strangling had finally destroyed her as she had destroyed her young victims."

One of the most infamous killers of all time was "Jack the Ripper," who seems to have murdered and neatly carved up the corpses of at least five bedraggled London whores. From the self-incriminating letters he wrote to the police and the newspapers at the time of his multiple-murderous activities in 1888, it seemed apparent that he was severely emotionally disturbed. But he was never apprehended and examined, and only enormous amounts of conjecture could be made about who he was and what motivated him to commit his senseless crimes.

Recent evidence, presented by Dr. Thomas E. A. Stowell, a ninety-three-year-old fellow of the Royal College, who studied under the English royal family's physician, Sir William Gull, indicates that Jack the Ripper was probably Albert Victor Christian Edward, Duke of Clarence and Avondale, grandson of Queen Victoria and heir to the throne of England. Stowell, in an article in *The Criminologist,* a magazine devoted to police work and forensic medicine, says that he has known for fifty years that Edward was Sir William's patient during and after his presumably murderous forays. As Paul O'Neil reports in *Life* magazine, "Eddy" exhibited a "paranoid extravagance of dress"; he was subject to progressive physical and mental deterioration after he contracted syphilis in his late teens; he was caught in a male brothel during a police raid when he was twenty-four and resigned his commission in the 10th Hussars; and when the police bagged him after his fourth murder he was confined to a private mental hospital in the Home Counties.

Whether or not it will ever be known, for certain, that Jack the Ripper was the Duke of Clarence and Avondale, it appears likely that the two were the same and that the Duke was indeed an individual with severe emotional aberrations.

Miriam Allen de Ford tells the story of Bonnie Parker and Clyde Barrow, who were famous enough in their day and who in recent years have been almost reincarnated in the film, *Bonnie and Clyde.* These bank robbers, together with various accomplices, probably murdered thirteen victims before they were shot to death by police officers. Clyde, according to Miss DeFord, was "an undersized, 'snake-eyed' youth, effeminate and at least a latent homosexual, a cold-blooded egoist to whom other people were either instruments he could use or obstacles to be shot out of his path. . . . People who knew him in childhood said that he enjoyed wringing a chicken's neck just short of death and watching its agony, or sometimes breaking a bird's wings and laughing at its attempts to fly."

By the time he was twenty, he had engaged in numerous robberies and safe-crackings, many of them with his brother, Buck. In spite of the great risk of returning to his native state, Texas, he insisted on doing so. "Hardly less than Bonnie, Clyde was mother-fixated. All through their last wild two years, they both kept darting back, at any risk, for fleeting visits with their families. They never went too far away to be able to get back soon." He violently hated Sheriff Schmid and his deputy, Robert Alcorn, and swore he would kill them because they had the nerve to fire on him and Bonnie, in one of their close getaways, when his and her mother were only ten feet away and might have been killed. He was "unpredictable, irresponsible, and neurotic."

Bonnie Parker was "a highstrung, emotional girl caught in a web from which she could not escape, a mamma's baby all her life." As a child, she was "always up to mischief and as pugnacious as two small boys." When she married Roy Thornton, she set up housekeeping only two blocks away from her mother "but that was too far for Bonnie. She had insisted she couldn't live without Roy, and now she found she couldn't live without her mother. Mother and daughter had always adored each other, and Bonnie had become completely dependent, with a full-grown 'mother fixation.' Practically every night she was either begging Mrs. Parker to come and stay with them, or making Roy take her 'home' in the middle of the night. Finally, in desperation, after a few months the young couple moved back so that Bonnie and her mother could be together again. Mrs. Parker found a larger house, in Dallas itself, and for the next six years they were never separated."

Bonnie, particularly toward the end of her life at the age of twenty-three, was alcoholic. Although she actively participated in many robberies and murders, she angrily considered herself "hounded by the police." She was "a born actress, but she was also a born liar. She was, I am sure, genuinely—neurotically—attached to her mother; and I am also sure that from early youth she lied constantly to her mother, as much to spare Mrs. Parker's feelings as to enable her to go her own way. She was a show-off, a glutton for sensation and excitement, for thrills and the violence they bring.

"In sum," writes Miss DeFord, "Clyde was self-centered, self-pitying, and self-absorbed; Bonnie was self-centered, self-pitying, and self-dramatizing. There was absolutely no Depression-born social protest involved in their stick-ups—made purely for gain—or in their shootings—inspired either by their need to escape or by the cop-hating common to all small-time criminals—as the motion picture based on them seems to imply."

Don Moser and Jerry Cohen have written a book about the murderous deeds of "The Pied Piper of Tucson," Charles Howard Schmid, Jr., one of America's most repulsive multiple slayers. Schmid was convicted of killing fifteen-year-old Aleen Rowe in May, 1964, and of later murdering seventeen-year-old Gretchen Fritz and her thirteen-year-old sister, Wendy. He is described as "an implausible burlesque of American manhood. He had dyed his reddish hair black, bronzed his features with pancake makeup, whitened his lips with cosmetic cream, adorned his face with phony imperfections, and, to appear taller, had stuffed a three-inch layer of tin cans and rags in his knee-high boots."

Schmid fairly obviously had deep-seated feelings of inferiority all his life, for which he often tried to dramatically compensate. After he killed Aleen Rowe, he just couldn't resist bragging about the murder to a friend, Paul Ginn, as well as to another friend, Bruns, and probably several others. Somewhat similarly, earlier in his life, he had pretended to be a fine guitarist, when he actually faked strumming a guitar and played a hidden tape recorder to impress others with his "playing."

He was insanely jealous of his girlfriend, Gretchen, one of the three girls he killed, and actually spread the rumor that she had a venereal disease "to belittle her reputation so that nobody would want her except him." He paranoiacally suspected every fellow in town of running over to take her out; and he sent anonymous letters to her parents accusing her of promiscuous sex relations, so they would keep a closer eye on her.

At Schmid's trial, "he seemed indifferent to what went on." After conceding his guilt, repudiating his guilty plea, and then reinstating it again, he finally sobbed uncontrollably. He was judged technically sane by two court psychiatrists; but his attorney, F. Lee Bailey, told the court: "The defendant is in need of psychiatric help, although under the law as it now stands, he is not legally insane. But I believe such help is needed, and the defendant wishes it."

After the trial was over, Bailey urged that society take the opportunity to "study killers like Charlie to learn what it can about them. Don't execute the Charlies to exact an ounce of retribution. He's sick. What's behind the sickness? I don't know. That's for the psychiatrists to find out, and I'm not a psychiatrist. But there's another Charlie somewhere else, and your daughter might be next."

Dr. Carlos A. Leon, chairman of the department of psychiatry of the Universidad del Valle Medical School, Cali, Colombia, South America, gives brief portraits of several of the multiple murderers who participated in *La Violencia,* a recent period of sustained violence in his country. He writes: "Most of the *bandoleros* show religiosity, in some instances of an intense nature, together with their aggressive and promiscuous trends. When the notorious bandit Efrain Gonzalez, author of 117 murders, was killed in Bogota after a great struggle with the army, it was found that he kept several religious images, a scapulary, and a request to call a priest in case of danger of death.

"*Desquite* kept in his wallet, together with formulas of witchcraft, the prayer *'El Justo Juez'* (the Fair Judge) and a long poem to his dead child, Cielo, in which he expressed his longing to have been a kind and loving father to her, described himself as a very unhappy man, implored with tears her love, and stated his hope to join her soon in the hereafter.

"*El Mosco,* a ferocious bandit of the Caldas region, was said to be a very religious man. He prayed often and forced his men to pray with him. He was convinced that, due to divine protection, bullets would not enter his body. A detective posing as a bandit gained his confidence and was appointed as his bodyguard. After waiting for months for a suitable opportunity, he shot him in the back. Then he went into a panic when after five shots the body did not fall. Just as he was convinced that the bandit was bulletproof the body fell, and even after it lay on the ground the detective kept firing.

"A *bandolero* in Tolima had the skin of his chest opened, then placed a crucifix inside the wound, and had it sewn up. He wanted to carry the crucifix under his skin as a protection against the bullets of his enemies. Some *bandoleros* in the same area used to wrap a scapulary around the muzzle of their rifles in order to secure sharpest aiming and be fortunate in combat. The dreadful bandit *'El Turpial,'* who used to poison his bullets with cyanide, was reputedly a religious fanatic and kept with him a walletful of prayers, among them one to the 'Fair Judge' and another one to 'St. Mark of the Lion.' "

One of the main multiple—or, more accurately, mass—murderers in history was undoubtedly Adolf Hitler, who was directly responsible for the demise of about six million Jews and other "non-Aryans" and who indirectly (as a result of famine and disease spread by his military machine) may well have killed tens of millions of additional victims. On a more personal level, it is also possible that he murdered his niece, Geli Raubal, who was found shot dead in his flat in Munich on September 18, 1931. Although the inquest verdict was suicide, Andrew Ewart reports that "it has been said that Hitler himself pulled the trigger in a passion of jealousy."

Ewart also gives evidence of Hitler's basic state of emotional imbalance. In his youth, before the outbreak of World War I, "he seems to have been lazy and moody, with a marked distaste for regular work but capable of bursts of activity—a strange amalgam of ambition and indolence. . . . Even at this time his few acquaintances noticed his vehemence in airing his pet 'hates'—the greatest of these being the Jews. Indeed his remorseless hatred of the Jews provides a monotonous theme for all his adult life: he never stopped excoriating them from his first soap-box to his last will and testament. . . . Hitler believed that inequality was an absolute law of Nature. He despised the fundamentals of a democratic society—freedom of speech, Press and Parliament. His megalomania was chronic—even as a jobless, half-starved pauper he never wavered in his belief that he was one of nature's superior beings. . . .

"His racial prejudices are, of course, well known, but his megalomania extended in all directions. He believed that he could have been a great artist or architect—his views on art were held with the same opinionated dogmatism as his views on international affairs—and, as usual, he would tolerate no contrary opinion."

Hitler continued his highly emotionalized, monomaniacal way of looking at things into his chancellorship days and may well have lost World War II because of it. Ewart reports: "It was this same insufferable and overweening arrogance in his character that brought him to disaster in Russia. The successful campaigns of 1939 and 1940 convinced him that the German armed forces under his direction were invincible. He would listen to no warning against his plan to invade the east. He was certain that the war in Russia would be over in three months at the outside; accordingly, he refused to take precautions for a winter campaign."

Eliot B. Wheaton, after a most objective study of the rise of the Nazi revolution, holds that "strictly speaking, the fanatical anti-Semitism displayed by Hitler's government was not essential to his grand design. . . . But Hitler was a man born for hatred: He lived by it, reveled in it, constantly arousing it by his tirades and counting on this most diabolic of passions to generate among his followers a seething and irresistible force. Ever since his Vienna days, moreover, the fury of his own personal hatred had been concentrated on the Jews. They were his prime obsession, and he longed to humiliate them, hurt them, crush them, whether or not the realization of his basic program demanded it."

Albert Speer, Hitler's chief architect and one of his closest associates throughout his later political career, gives us even more first-hand observations of his disturbed behavior: "As anxieties mounted, he made himself into a strictly disciplined worker. But such discipline ran counter to his nature and this was inevitably reflected in the quality of his decisions. Overwork and isolation led to a peculiar state of petrification and rigor. He suffered from spells of mental torpor and was permanently caustic and irritable. . . . From month to month Hitler became more taciturn. Lunch with him became an ordeal. In silence, we spooned up our soup. . . .

"The dog was the only creature at headquarters who aroused any flicker of human feeling in Hitler. Hitler's deep estrangement from people proceeded slowly, almost imperceptibly. He used to make one remark all too revealing of his unhappy isolation: 'Speer, one of these days I'll have only two friends left, Fraulein Braun and my dog.' "

Speer continues: "Hitler frequently set schedules that were completely unrealistic. Since he invariably ordered immediate action, the advance detachments came under fire before the task force could bring its full firepower to bear. The men were led piecemeal up to the enemy and annihilated. . . . In the last weeks of his life, Hitler was shriveling up like an old man. His limbs trembled; he walked stooped, with dragging footsteps. Even his voice had become quavering. Its force had given way to a faltering, toneless manner of speaking. When he became excited, as he frequently did in a senile way, his voice would start breaking. He still had his fits of obstinacy, but they no longer reminded one of a child's temper tantrums, but of an old man's. . . . Perhaps that was why no one said a word when he more and more frequently took flight from reality, when he spoke of the clash between East and West which must be on the point of erupting—when he bade us realize that it was inevitable."

Many of Hitler's henchmen, of course, were also individuals with serious disturbances—for example, the egomaniacal Hess and Goebbels, the sexually obsessed Roehm, and the drug-addicted Goring. The same may be said of a whole host of political murderers, only a few of whom we are specifically examining in this book since it is difficult to determine whether many of their crimes were "natural" results of the social climate of their day or "unnatural" results of their own idiosyncratic sadistic tendencies. Thus, Genghis Khan exterminated about 10 percent of the population of the world during his reign, and callously had thousands of his enemies boiled alive in cauldrons, tortured, raped, and massacred. And Richard III of England had several of his own royal relatives butchered, including Henry VI and his son, the Prince of Wales.

But it is not clear how much this murdering had to do with these rulers' personal lust for blood and how much it was caused by their desire to build and maintain their empires. At the same time, Francois Ribadeau Dumas has recorded in his book, *Madness in Power,* some thirty-one instances in history where rulers of nations have suffered from varying degrees of mental derangement and where their crimes (such as those of King Saul and of Mad King Ludwig of Bavaria) had little or nothing to do with their political ambitions.

Adolf Eichmann was captured in Buenos Aires, put on trial in Jerusalem, and ultimately hanged for crimes against the Jewish people, crimes against humanity, and war crimes during the period of the Nazi regime. Although on the surface Eichmann was a psychiatrically "normal" individual, with a good family life, Hannah Arendt provides ample evidence that this was not so: "He left no doubt that he would have killed his own father if he had received an order to that effect." Gideon Hausner reports that he was psychiatrically judged, before his trial, to be "a man obsessed with a dangerous and insatiable urge to kill . . . a perverted, sadistic personality." Miss Arendt finds him to be hardly stupid, but believes that his pathological thoughtlessness "predisposed him to become one of the greatest criminals" of recent history.

T. C. Fest, Simon Wiesenthal, and many other writers provide us with considerable evidence that, like Hitler and Eichmann, most of the well-known Nazi leaders, many of whom were convicted of serious war crimes and murders, were seriously deranged individuals.

When all the facts are in, it may be that Joseph Stalin will turn out to be the greatest murderer in history, since in one way or another perhaps thirty-five million people died as a result of political and economic moves which he directed. As Andrew Ewart conservatively puts it: "So vast and terrible was the extent of the Stalin reign of terror in the decade after 1929 that the full toll of human suffering and death can be measured only statistically. In these years in Russia a minimum of one million were slaughtered, according to Western experts who have examined the large amount of official Soviet information which has since become available. That is only part of the total. In the same period *at least another sixteen million perished.* Half of that total died in the great famine; the other half died by administrative murder in the terrible forced labor camps in the Arctic and Siberia. . . . The statisticians have discovered also that in a single year Stalin's murders exceeded by twenty times the total number of people officially executed by successive Czars in their programmes of repression *in a century.* For political massacres committed against his own people Stalin easily beats even Hitler's record; there is no comparison in the whole of recorded history. In addition, as a result of his deportations, *one Soviet citizen in every fifteen had become a convict.*"

Coincidentally enough, where Hitler was rumored to have murdered his favorite niece, Stalin may have done in his young second wife, Nadia Alliuyeva: "The terror and misery began to prey on her mind. One night in November, 1932, at a gathering in Voroshilov's home attended by other members of the Politburo, she spoke her mind. That was too much for Stalin. In front of their friends he poured out vulgar abuse on his wife. She walked out. Later that night she was found dead. Reports circulated that she had committed suicide. But there have been rumors that Stalin murdered her in a fit of drunken fury."

In a brief biography of Stalin, Ewart gives ample evidence of his emotional instability: When he attended the Orthodox Theological Seminary at Tiflis during his youth, "his fellow students did not find him an easy colleague. Easily incensed when his arguments were challenged successfully, he would nurse a grudge against an opponent and seek to revenge himself by malignant gossip and slander.

"As he advanced into his fifties, two traits which had always been integral parts of his character, prudence and distrust, became more marked. . . . As Stalin overcame one group of opponents after another and battered down all opposition to his forced collectivization and industrialization policies, he became obsessed with a psychopathic fear of enemies, both real or imaginary. He saw danger to his absolute rule in everything and everyone. . . .

"At a dinner for some of his European satellite leaders given in the Kremlin in April, 1945, Stalin became drunk and hysterical. This was to happen often in his later years. . . . After the war, . . . Stalin became ever more capricious, irritable and brutal. His persecution mania reached unbelievable dimensions. He took an almost fiendish delight in humiliating his closest associates in public. . . . By 1949 Stalin's paranoia had reached such an advanced stage that he did begin to murder members of the Politburo itself. . . .

"Stalin's own personal life was even worse than that of his son. In the years after the war Stalin, like his boon companion Beria, developed a 'Lolita' complex. Former members of Stalin's personal guard who deserted to the West have told of how Beria used his police to pick up forcibly pretty under-age girls off the streets for the satisfaction of his own lust and that of Stalin. If the minors refused they were threatened with deportation and the extermination of their families. . . .

"By 1952 Stalin was quite mad. He even believed that his lifelong friend, Marshal Voroshilov, President of the Soviet Union, was a British spy. And he began to make plans to 'physically annihilate' various members of the Praesidium: it is said that he had in mind Molotov, Malenkov, and Khrushchev whom he suspected, possibly correctly, of plotting against him. Probably he also developed a strong anti-Jewish attitude."

Stalin's chief collaborator and ultimate successor, Khrushchev, has written a sizable volume, *Khrushchev Remembers,* in which he frankly gives some details of Stalin's disturbance:

"Our best commanders were exterminated [in the 1937 purge]. The military staff underwent two, three, even four changes of command. Most of the people promoted were honest and loyal, but they needed experience. Their initiation cost our country terrible ruin. . . .

"I had to argue with Stalin many times. Even though he could have blasted me with fire and water, I doggedly tried to persuade him to my point of view. Sometimes I succeeded. However, it was always very difficult to argue with him—and very dangerous. . . . He had also begun to think of himself as a great military strategist, which made it harder than ever to argue with him. But I knew what sort of a hero he was. I'd seen him when he had been paralyzed by his fear of Hitler, like a rabbit in front of a boa constrictor. And my opinion of him hadn't changed.

"During the first part of the war, when things were going badly, I'd noticed that Stalin's signature didn't appear on a single document or order. This practice didn't change even after we repulsed the Germans outside Moscow and Stalin began to regain his confidence. And this was no accident.

"There is another example of Stalin's refusal to accept direct responsibility for what was happening at the front. Many of our generals who were taken prisoner were declared traitors on Stalin's order, and their families were sent to Siberia. The treatment of the rank-and-file troops and junior officers was no better. When a commander reported to Stalin about someone's incompetence or mistake, Stalin used to ask, 'Did you punch him in the snout? If he does something like that again, punch him right in the snout!' . . .

"It was as though the devil himself held a string attached to Stalin's main nerve, and no one knew when the devil would give the string a jerk, sending Stalin into one of his fits of rage."

Khrushchev insists that "there was something unquestionably sick about Stalin." In reviewing his book, Harrison E. Salisbury, once the main Soviet correspondent of the *New York Times,* notes: "From these memoirs you begin to get a deeper conception (already sketched out by Stalin's daughter, Svetlana Alliluyeva) of the emptiness and boredom at the top, of Stalin's loss of touch with life, his total isolation from reality, his inability to break any pattern and, of course, his constant and ever-deepening paranoia."

Evidence on the severe emotional disturbance of a number of other multiple murderers can easily be collected from contemporary news reports. While research on this book was in progress, many more cases occurred. For example, during the month of July, 1968, Angel Angelof, a Bulgarian emigre living in New York City, carried a .45-caliber revolver to Central Park, and suddenly started shooting. He killed a young woman and an elderly man completely unknown to him, and before police fatally wounded him he also shot two policemen. Investigation showed that Angelof had an extreme hatred of Communist rule in his native Bulgaria, which, according to *New York Times* reporter T. Buckley, "was transformed in his loneliness in New York into murderous mental derangement." "He was very secretive, very moody," said his roommate, Kyril Dikov. "In the three months we were together I never learned anything about his past." He had ultra-right sympathies and had pictures of Nazi leaders pinned to his wall. He was a member of a Bulgarian fascist group—legionnaires who sided with Hitler during World War II. He had no real friends; but an acquaintance said that "he was a crazy man, always talking about pistols, pistols, but I never thought he had one." Mr. Dikov said that Angelof had possessed "an old and rusty revolver" earlier in the year. "He would twirl it and look at himself in the mirror. I wasn't worried. I knew that it couldn't shoot." From these reports, Angelof was obviously disturbed.

On a cold day in March, 1967, in Wautoma, Wisconsin, Jim McBrair, who was known to most of the town citizens as a former high school hero and a highly respectable citizen, suddenly took his .22-caliber semi-automatic rifle and within a few minutes shot and killed his twenty-four-year-old wife, Carol; her father, Marv, who ran the Pontiac agency in town; her sister, Barbie; and a fifteen-year-old baby sitter, Cheryl Oleson. Jim had a long history of emotional instability. He had no particular goals in life; he seemed unable to keep a job; and he wasn't able to adjust to the army. Later in life, things got worse. As Bruce Porter reports:

"In the countdown months leading up to the murders, McBrair was going through personal hell. The relationship with his wife, Carol, begun five years earlier as a casual flirtation during a Saint Patrick's Day party, was always in a precarious state near misery for both of them. They were separating constantly; it got to be so often that McBrair can still rattle off the pattern: 'First there would be family fights,' he says, 'started with little or no reason. Then she would begin the anti-Jim campaign with her mother. The third step would be filing papers for divorce and then she'd be seen in public with other men.' McBrair was so afraid of a second divorce that he was incapable of asserting himself. He thought he knew where the blame lay—it was, in his eyes, always his own fault. 'Maybe I was causing the trouble,' he remembers thinking. . . . It was then he experienced the 'tired' feeling. 'It was not sleepy-type, like I wanted to vomit—but not from the stomach, from the brain.' Even wild escape attempts provided no relief. . . . He injured his back on the job at a local sand-and-gravel company and after that, just didn't bother going in to work. He lost 20 pounds within a few months. Along with the tired feeling then came thoughts of suicide, of lying down in the middle of the highway and letting a truck run over him."

Rafael Torres, forty-year-old proprietor of a grocery and candy store in Jersey City, was accused of stabbing and beating his wife and seven of their children to death. Torres was apparently tormented by a family tragedy and the fear of imprisonment on a murder charge under which he was free on bail. He had been "extremely depressed" since the death of a sister, Carmen, from burns suffered in her Hoboken home two years before the homicidal tragedy. Neighbors told of his erratic behavior: One called him "a wild man." Only a week before the killing, Torres had shouted "I shoot people" at an ice cream vendor who had parked his sales truck in front of the Torres store. After being freed on bail in the murder of Jose Ortiz in Hoboken, he agreed to a psychiatric examination and, on the recommendation of a Summit psychiatrist, was committed to Trenton State Hospital; but he was released two days after admission at the request of his wife, who said that her husband was "very unhappy" at the hospital.

Donald Lambright, the son of the famous Negro comedian, Stepin Fetchit, killed himself after wounding fifteen persons on the Pennsylvania Turnpike and killing his wife, Annette, and two motorists. A year previously, he was told by a psychiatrist that he needed help or he would commit suicide; but he refused psychotherapy. His uncle, Howard E. Johnson, said that Lambright had been "very sensitive to infringement on the freedom of all people and almost paranoid about race relations. . . . He also said that his nephew had slept with a rifle in his bed."

Frank H. Woyke, Jr., a minister's son, was charged with beating his mother and grandmother to death in Oak Park, Illinois. Gallagher and Felcher report: "Police said Woyke told them he saw the image of a demon on his mother's face and 'had to beat the devil out of her and beat the evil off her face.' Woyke told them he punched her several times, knocked her to the floor, and then began jumping up and down on her. When Mrs. Jacopian tried to intervene, Woyke said, he saw the image of a demon on his grandmother's face also, and then began to beat her and jump on her. Woyke was naked when arrested in the women's second-floor hotel room and told police he felt clean without clothes. He said it cleansed him to go naked, police said. . . .

"The elder Woyke told police his son had a birth defect and had brain surgery at the age of six months. . . . Woyke, who had no steady job, read the Bible constantly. . . . Woyke also ripped his Bible and threw it into a garbage can on Sunday," just before the murders.

Ernest L. Bishop, Jr., charged with murdering a University of Michigan coed, and probably involved in a series of seven killings that terrorized girls on two Michigan campuses, was found not guilty of murder by reason of insanity. "Bishop was on parole from a rape conviction when he became acquainted with Margaret Phillips, 25, a University of Michigan graduate student in sociology. Bishop's attorney admitted that Bishop shot Miss Phillips last July at her apartment but said he was insane at the time. Miss Phillips had apparently been trying to rehabilitate Bishop as a personal project. In a tape recording taken when Bishop was under the influence of truth serum, he cried: 'I shot her, I shot her. Why her? Why her? I just kept shooting and shooting. Why her? She was always sweet, always an angel' " (*New York Times,* January 25, 1970).

One of the most sensational instances of multiple murder in recent years occurred when Sharon Tate, a beautiful Hollywood actress and wife of the noted film director, Roman Polanski, was savagely killed, along with her house guests, men's hair stylist Jay Sebring, coffee heiress Abigail Folger, Polanski's colleague and friend Voyteck Frykowski, and her caretaker's friend Steven Parent. The following day, August 9, 1969, the killers of Miss Tate and her guests also bloodily slaughtered a prosperous California grocer, Leno LaBianca, and his wife. After months of searching for the killers, the police located and obtained indictments against Charles Manson, thirty-four-year-old leader of what has been called by the *New York Times* "a nomadic band of hippies" and five members of his band: Susan Denise Atkins, twenty-one; Linda Louise Kasabian, twenty; Leslie Van Houten, nineteen; Patricia Krenwinkel, twenty-one; and Charles Watson, twenty-four. According to an article supposedly by Miss Atkins, the Manson "family" may possibly have murdered, in the course of their relatively brief activities as car thieves, burglars, and drug takers and peddlers, a total of eleven victims.

The murder trial of Manson and three of his "family" members (Linda Kasabian turned state's witness, was given immunity, and was not herself tried, and Charles Watson was not tried because he was adjudged legally insane) was one of the most spectacular ever held in the United States. It took six months of almost incredible fracases, with Manson, Patricia Krenwinkel, Susan Atkins, and Leslie Van Houten all acting outrageously in court and fighting with almost everyone else (including their own lawyers). *New York Times* reporter Earl Caldwell reported: "As the trial progressed, it was the unusual that came to be expected. Once Manson angrily lunged across the defense table at Judge Older with a sharpened pencil in his hand."

An incredible mass of testimony was collected, both before and during the trial, which makes it almost certain that Manson's tribe, including himself as its unmistakable head, consisted of exceptionally disturbed individuals. The girls allowed themselves to be almost totally dominated by Manson; and his control of them was said to have been so great that some of his followers called him God and Satan, while others called him Hymie, by which they meant Hitler. The three convicted girls, as well as Linda Kasabian, submitted to Manson's every whim, felt they were under his hypnotic, mystical spell, and blindly obeyed him, even to the extent of the girls' having sex relations with any male he designated.

All the members of Manson's group seem to have been deluded into believing he was a genius (although his tested IQ was merely 114). They were inveterate drug takers, particularly of LSD and methedrine. They unhesitatingly accepted his bizarre edicts (such as the emanation that they were to cleanse their bodies by eating peanut butter and honey when they were in jail). Most of them, in the opinion of a San Francisco psychiatrist who got to know them, were "hysterics, wishful thinkers, seekers after some absolute" who regarded Manson as a high-priest "all-powerful, all-knowing." The girls in the troupe saw serving Manson and his male associates as their sole purpose in life; they allowed themselves to be intimidated by his regular threats of physical violence and death; they unquestioningly accepted his indiscriminately hostile attitudes toward members of the Establishment; and they seemed to go along, almost without exception, with Susan Atkins's admission that, "I never questioned what Charlie said. I just did it."

As for Manson himself, there is considerable evidence that he never was emotionally stable and that, as his life progressed, he became increasingly aberrant. Reared by an alcoholic mother who had been a teen-age prostitute, by an aunt and uncle, and by various foster parents and schools, he managed to spend thirteen of his first twenty-five years of life in reformatories and prisons; subsequently, he added another four years to his prison record. His misdemeanors and felonies seem to have included juvenile delinquency, car-stealing, burglary, pimping, cashing stolen U.S. Treasury checks, forgery, physical assault, possession of illegal weapons, possession and selling of "soft" and "hard" drugs, and various other offenses.

Dr. David Smith, who knew Manson and his "family" well

when they visited the Haight-Ashbury Free Clinic, which he founded, has commented that the violence which Manson inspired and participated in "was not the kind of sociopathic 'escape' violence we see in the Haight but a psychotic, Rasputin-type violence. If you believe God is on your side, anything is justified. The communal thing is very spiritual. Belief in magic, astrology, cosmic consciousness—that explains everything. . . . He would probably be diagnosed as a schizophrenic, but ambulatory schizophrenics were very much looked up to in Haight-Ashbury because they could hallucinate—without drugs." Dr. Roger Smith (quoted by P. O'Neil), who served as Manson's parole officer after his release from prison in 1967, has stated: "Charlie was the most hostile parolee I've ever come across. He was totally up front about it. He told me right off there was no way he could keep the terms of his parole. He was headed back to the joint [prison] and there was no way out of it. . . . Drugs give you something but they also take. In the case of Charlie, he redefined what reality was. He began to drift farther and farther away. He certainly wasn't operating on anything vaguely related to reality. . . . Tenderness toward girls? Not a damn bit. I never sensed he had any real warmth toward the girls. They were his possessions."

Other indications of Manson's emotional instability are easily picked up from those who personally knew him: He read the Bible when he was in prison, somehow merged its teachings with those of the quasi-religion and crackpot "psychotherapy" system of Scientology, decided that the Book of Revelation had predicted the coming of the Beatles and also decided that one of the Beatles's songs, "Revolution 9," really was a reference to the Book of Revelation, Chapter 9, Verse 21: "Neither repented they of their murders, nor of their sorceries, nor of their fornication, nor of their thefts." (This kind of thinking, incidentally, is typical of schizophrenic confabulation.)

Going a step further in his muddled philosophy, Manson seems to have become exceptionally hostile to (1) the rich, who he said in his soft voice, were "pigs" who needed purging and liberation—preferably by death—to atone for their materialism; to (2) whites in general, especially the white Establishment; and to (3) some blacks and black militants, whom he thought would be falsely blamed for some of his group's depredations against whites and would therefore help speed up a racial war which he believed was imminent. According to Susan Atkins, he was specifically hostile to Terry Melcher, who once owned the house which was occupied by Sharon Tate and her guests at the time they were murdered, and whom Manson presumably hated "because Terry had given his word on a few things and never came through with them." In regard to his overweening hostility, P. O'Neil remarks: "He also collected guns and ammunition. The family, he prophesied, was one day going into Los Angeles to set off the apocalypse foreordained for them in Revelation, Chapter 9: 'They were given the power of scorpions . . . the noise of their wings was like the noise of many chariots . . . and they have as king over them the angel of the bottomless pit.' There was no doubt who was king. Charlie Manson talked about it to visitors: 'He was going to shoot all the white people he saw, all the established people; then the black people would get enthralled and destroy everybody while he would retreat into the desert.' Charlie did not just talk. He took incredible pains, with the aid of the family's males, to prepare for the day. They stole Volkswagens, stripped them and turned them into reinforced dune buggies, some with machine gun mounts."

We also learn from O'Neil: "Charlie's word was law: he carried and fondled a Bowie knife, his scepter. 'He really loved knives,' recalls an acquaintance. 'He used to say, "Man, everybody in this world is afraid of getting cut." ' "

O'Neil, with the help of a whole bevy of *Life* reporters, additionally notes: "Charlie billed himself as a 'roving minstrel' come to fulfill their [the Haight-Ashbury hippie girls'] dreams with magic, strike off the chains of male chauvinism and lead them to the promised land—although in fact he regarded them as squaws, treated them like cattle and excommunicated those who complained. 'I was hitchhiking to San Francisco once with Charlie,' says a girl who used to know him, 'and we had these two big packs. He wanted me to carry both of them. I refused. I said I'd share, but I wouldn't carry both. He got more and more angry and finally said I had to carry both bags and walk 10 steps behind him. When I wouldn't do that, he took my guitar from me and smashed it into little pieces against a post.' . . . Charlie preached a confused but vehement philosophy. Everything in the world belonged to all its people—thus there could be redivision of valuables, but no theft; all humans were part of some homogeneous and mystic whole—thus there could be no real death."

E. Malnic gives some more details on Manson's view of racism: "Charles Manson talked of triggering a war between blacks and whites by killing whites—including white police—and making it appear that blacks were responsible. Friends recalled: 'He said he was building a bunch of dune buggies. He said he was going to mount machine guns on them.' 'He said he'd take his army of dune buggies and kill every white mother—every white pig—between here and the desert. Then he was going to make an exodus —take his people to a big hole up in Death Valley and hide there. From there he could just sit back and watch the revolution.'

" 'You see, he hated the Establishment. It wasn't that he felt it owed him anything. He just didn't belong.' 'He had strong anti-black feelings, too. They came from those years he spent in the penitentiary, I think. But he didn't talk about it much. It was just one of those feelings you get.' "

We may well imagine that there is some amount of prejudice in these reports, especially since the narrators all seemed aware of the fact that Manson had presumably ordered and participated in the cold-blooded and unusually cruel murders of close to a dozen people. But too many of the independent reports of Manson's peculiarities overlap for us to believe that they are entirely exaggerated. The objective evidence alone indicates that this alleged multiple slayer has always been an exceptionally disturbed person and that most of his alleged accomplices are also perilously close to psychosis.

The severe emotional disturbance of Manson's co-defendants was demonstrated during the many months they were on trial in a Los Angeles court. Linda Kasabian, who admitted complicity in the murders and who turned state's witness against the other defendants, testified that she had experienced extrasensory perception, could communicate with animals, and perceived that Manson was giving off "vibrations" in the courtroom. She said that she had thought Manson was Jesus Christ; that she now believed he was the devil; and that she also believed that she was an "emissary from God." Also, at the time of the seven killings for which the "family" was on trial, she thought she was a witch. When granted immunity for testifying at the trial, she said she thought that some supernatural source had given her this immunity.

The three girls who stood trial for the murders acted most bizarrely on many occasions in court and in prison and were consistently reported to be severely disturbed by friends, associates, and even their own lawyers. Susan Atkins, scheduled at first to testify against the others, repudiated her early "confessions" (although they almost exactly agreed with independent testimony of others brought out at the trial). She said that she had no interest in saving her body but was only interested in saving her soul, which presumably would "live forever." She often claimed to be deathly sick in court, in spite of physicians' statements to the contrary. She continually fought with Judge Older and said to him at one point: "You are not my judge."

A former prison inmate, Ronni Howard, testified at the trial that Susan had described the stabbing of actress Sharon Tate as a "sexual release" and said that killing people was like a drug habit: "The more you do it, the better you like it." Another witness, Virginia Castroa, testified that she talked freely of the murders and seemed "elated, living it over."

Dianne Lake, a former Manson "family" member, similarly reported at the trial that Leslie Van Houten, one of the defendants, told her about the murders after they occurred and "said that she stabbed someone already dead. . . . She said she didn't want to do it, but the more she did it, the more fun it was." When Judge Older tried to stop Miss Van Houten from impulsive outbursts in court, she said that she was unwilling to abide by the court's rulings. "You are no longer my father," she told the judge. Patricia Krenwinkel acted similarly and told the judge: "I'll judge myself. You don't speak my words. You are taking yourself to destruction. I do not accept this courtroom." The chief defense counsel, at one point in the trial, attempted to change her plea to not guilty by reason of insanity.

Miss Van Houten, testifying at the penalty phase of the trial, which resulted in the three girls and Manson all being sentenced to the death penalty, admitted that she and Miss Krenwinkel stabbed Mrs. Rosemary LaBianca, one of the dead victims. She said: "I had a knife and Patricia had a knife. We just started stabbing and cutting up the lady." When she was asked by her lawyer, Maxwell Keith, whether she felt ashamed of this deed, the following dialogue with him ensued:

"What is ashamed?"

"Do you feel you want to cry?"

"For her death? If I cry it's for death itself. She's not the only person who died."

Patricia Krenwinkel admitted stabbing women at the Tate and the LaBianca homes. When her lawyer, Paul Fitzgerald, asked what she felt after stabbing Abigail Folger, she replied, "Nothing. What is there to describe? We were just there and it was right." She later told the jury: "I am perfectly willing to face anything—my own death. I judge myself. I know that everything that was done is done—has been done is perfect." She also reported that she once saw Manson turn another man into a skeleton and that on another occasion he made an old man young again.

The three girls, despite the seriousness of the charges against them, spent much of each day in court chatting and smiling, showing little reaction to detailed accusations against them. During pretrial hearings, they turned their backs on the judge as a sign of contempt and after much disruptive behavior in court had to be ordered from the courtroom. They continually chanted at the judge; they demanded the right to represent themselves, when they obviously were not able to do so; they insisted on testifying in court, in spite of their lawyers' opposition to their testimony; they engaged in shoving matches with court bailiffs, with Miss Krenwinkel slapping one of the bailiffs; and they were generally disruptive and self-defeating in their courtroom behavior. Maxwell Keith, Miss Van Houten's attorney, endorsed the prosecution's "robot theory" of the girls' engaging in murderous activities; held that they (and Charles Watson) were "robots" who did only what Manson ordered; said that there was something "mystical" about the relationship between Manson and his three co-defendants; and contended that the record showed that the women "really believed that he was God."

Manson's overt indications of severe emotional disturbance at the trial proceedings were, if possible, more pronounced than those of the three girls. He kept interrupting the judge and the prosecution, and had to be continually banned from court. At one point, he leaped at the judge and said, after being subdued, "someone should cut your head off!" When the judge threatened to have him removed, he replied: "I'll have you removed if you don't stop. I have a little system of my own." He punched his own lawyer, Irving A. Kanarek, several times. He repeatedly insisted that he was totally alien to the society around him and to the government, and when Mr. Kanarek asked him to describe what effect this had, he replied: "It makes me stronger." He insisted on defending himself, in place of his lawyers, even when Judge Older stated: "It's my conclusion that you are hopelessly incompetent to defend yourself in a case of this complexity." His attorney, Paul Fitzgerald, reported to the court that several witnesses the defense would have liked to present were not cooperating because Manson refused to ask them to help him.

Many witnesses, in and out of court, have testified to Manson's lifelong history of hositlity, violence, and disturbance. Richard Meltzer, who knew him as a bunkmate at Boy's Town, when Manson was a teenager, observed: "That boy had rocks in his head even then, he was what we called *flakey*." Phil Kaufman, who met Manson when they were both serving a sentence at Terminal Island Federal Prison, told Nat Freedland that Manson might have made it as a singer and composer of popular songs but "the reason Charlie never got out a record was he'd always take off for someplace else after he'd done one of those studio demos. He had a very short attention span, he was too undisciplined to follow a producer's orders or work out an arrangement with a back-up band. But the companies wanted to record him, it was just that he'd disappear on them before anything was finished."

Linda Kasabian testified at the Tate murders trial that Manson had said, "I'm the Devil doing the Devil's work" after the murders had been committed and described to him. She (and several confirming witnesses) reported that Manson's philosophy revolved around his conviction that the black people were ready to stage a revolution against whites and that the family would hide in the desert until the fighting was over and the blacks realized they needed the Manson group to help them run the country.

She noted that Manson believed that the Beatles' recorded song, "Helter Skelter," was a term for the forthcoming revolution between blacks and whites (a conclusion later stoutly denied by ex-Beatle John Lennon); and she linked this belief with the words "Helter Skelter," which were scrawled in blood at the scene of the murder of Mr. and Mrs. Leno LaBianca of Los Angeles, who were stabbed to death the night after the Tate murders. Dianne Lake fully corroborated this by independently testifying at the trial that Manson had told his "family" they were going to have to kill "pigs" to launch blacks into a "helter skelter" revolution.

Brooks Poston also testified that Manson had once urged him to kill a law enforcement officer, and that Manson felt that black people were destined to enter into a race war with whites and that they had to be shown how to start such a race war. Gregg Jakobson, a Hollywood record producer who knew Manson before the murders occurred, testified that Manson became convinced that Armageddon, the violent war predicted in the Bible as the end of civilization, was approaching; and that he found evidence of this in the song, "Helter Skelter," as well as in another Beatles' song, "Blackbird."

According to Martin Waldron, "Manson, playing the Beatles' songs over and over, would argue that 'hidden messages' from the 'four prophets' (the Beatles) included one asserting that it was time for blacks to rule, becoming the 'establishment.'

"Mr. Jakobson said Manson believed that Negroes were created to serve whites and that, after Negroes had been rulers of the earth for a time, they would slowly conclude that it was not in their nature to be rulers. They would then come seeking him and his followers in their 'bottomless pit' in the desert and Manson would reign. In his role as future king of the earth, Mr. Jakobson said, Manson portrayed himself as Jesus Christ and Satan at the same time."

"Tex" Watson, who was first scheduled to be one of the main co-defendants in the Tate and LaBianca murder trials, was psychiatrically examined after his apprehension, and the state conceded that he was psychotic and placed him in a state mental institution. He will presumably never be tried.

On October 20, 1970, a prominent and highly respected Santa Cruz eye surgeon, Dr. Victor M. Ohta, was found shot to death, together with his wife, two of their young sons, and the doctor's secretary, Mrs. Dorothy Cadwallader. Their bodies were dumped into the swimming pool at the doctor's mansion in the rugged hills overlooking Monterey Bay. Dr. Ohta was shot twice in the back of the neck, apparently with a .30-caliber weapon. Lieutenant Kenneth Pittinger of the Sheriff's Department said that "it was like an execution."

The alleged killer of the five victims, John Linley Frazier, is said to have left a note at the scene of the crime indicating that the murder was of a cultist nature. The note read: "Today World War 3 will begin as brought to you by the People of the Free Universe. From this day forward anyone and/or company of persons who misuses the natural environment or destroys same will suffer the penalty of death by the People of the Free Universe. I and my comrades from this day forth will fight until death or freedom, against anything or anyone who does not support natural life on this planet. Materialism must die or mankind will." As *New York Times* reporter Douglas E. Kneeland indicates, "The note was signed with the names of four knights from Tarot, the fortune-telling cards once favored largely by Gypsies but now undergoing a popular vogue." The suspected killer is said to have been extremely devoted to Tarot readings; and is quoted by a witness as saying that people who lived as the doctor's family did were too materialistic and "should be snuffed." Although most of the facts on Frazier are still obscure, he (or whoever actually perpetrated this senseless multiple murder) certainly appears to have been severely deranged.

After the longest war crimes trial in American military history, First Lieutenant William L. Calley, Jr., was found guilty of the premeditated murder of at least 22 South Vietnamese civilians at Mylai in March, 1968. The government had charged Lieutenant Calley with four specifications of premeditated murder involving at least 102 men, women, and children; but, because witnesses at the trial disagreed on the exact number of dead, the military jury convicted him of only 22 killings. Calley conceded some of the killings; but pleaded that he only did so under orders. Many other witnesses insisted that he took a personal, nonmilitary part in the killings of unarmed civilians, including children and babies, whom he gunned down at point-blank range; and the six members of his court-martial jury credited these witnesses more than they did Calley.

An Army sanity board, after extensively examining Calley at Walter Reed Hospital in Washington, found him "normal in every respect." This seems exceptionally questionable, in view of the facts of Calley's life, his own testimony, and that of several psychiatrists who testified at his trial. He originally got into trouble in the seventh grade—"for cheating, basically, sir"—and continued thereafter to get poor marks as he went on through military schools and a junior college. In spite of his education, he had a series of menial jobs, such as busboy, dishwasher, short-order cook, and strikebreaking freight car conductor.

Lieutenant Calley said that, after spending awhile in Vietnam, he had come to regard all Vietnamese, including children, as potential enemies and to regard them all with deepening suspicion and hate. At Mylai, he considered every man, woman, and child "all enemy. They were all to be destroyed." He said that the army never told him that his enemies were human. In spite of the fact that several witnesses reported that Calley shot for an hour at women, children, and old men whom he caused to be shoved into a trench by his soldiers, that when a small child scrabbled out of the ditch and tried to run back to the village, he picked it up by the arm, slung it into a deep part of the ditch and fired one shot at it, and that he poured automatic rifle fire into the ditch and blew the head off a woman who tried to rise from a pile of corpses, Calley showed no remorse over the killings of these civilians. The only remorse he felt, he testified, was for losing some of his own men in a minefield and being helpless to stop them from being killed.

Several psychiatrists insisted that, although Calley was not outrightly insane or psychotic, he had more than his share of emotional problems. Dr. David G. Crane of Indianapolis testified that his psychological make-up made it impossible for him to grasp the enormity of the killings he directed and participated in. Calley did not "consciously understand" what was happening, he held. At the time of the murders, he was suffering from "transient situational disturbance" which led him, unpremeditatedly, to engage in the shootings.

Dr. Albert A. LaVerne, senior psychiatrist at the New York University-Bellevue Medical Center said that at Mylai Lieutenant Calley was suffering a "virtual paralysis of will" so that he "was acting as a robot." He also felt a compulsion to obey his company commander and "father image," Captain Ernest L. Medina. "He was like a person with a compulsion to turn off faucets or avoid walking on cracks. He had a compulsion to obey orders, to do his duty as an officer." While being examined by Dr. LaVerne, a defense psychiatrist, Calley felt that he was being placed in some kind of trap, became hostile, gesticulated with his hands, and exhibited what Dr. LaVerne called a pronounced "paranoid reaction."

Dr. Wilber Hamman, a psychiatrist from Washington, testified that when Calley killed a man in a hut, as he himself admitted he had done, he did not intend to kill him. "He had the intent to waste the man. But waste is not the same to Lieutenant Calley as kill. He had this capacity, to know he wanted a group of people dead, but he did not have the volition to order that." The prosecutor, Captain Aubrey Daniel III, asked Dr. Hamman: "What's the difference between wanting someone to die and wanting to kill them?" Hamman replied: "For Lieutenant Calley there is a difference. Lieutenant Calley perceived the act he was doing not as killing but destroying—destroying an enemy. This is one of the factors limiting his volition. His capacity for appreciation was diminished. . . . In my opinion he did not have the mental capacity to form the mental intent to kill. He was deprived of that choice by his state of mind. He does not have a labeled diagnosable mental illness, but he does have certain things which interfere with exercising free choice."

Although most of the testimony about Lieutenant Calley's emotional problems was, as to be expected, contributed by defense psychiatrists, we believe that they may have not been too far from the mark. Calley's entire history was emotionally shaky; and it is fascinating to note that, even though he would have greatly benefited from being held to be disturbed, he himself (like several of the killers we examine later in our chapter on the psychology of assassination) bridled at the very thought of such a diagnosis. When the court referred him to an army sanity board, whose certifying him as insane would probably have resulted in all the charges against him being dismissed, he said: "I think it's unwarranted and unnecessary. I don't think we're trying to say I was insane. So I don't like it."

Significantly, the most emotion he showed during his lengthy trial was at the very end, when in his final plea for understanding he choked and sobbed while he said to the court: "Yesterday, you stripped me of all my honor. Please, by your actions that you take here today don't strip future soldiers of their honor, I beg you." As the army prosecutor, Captain Daniel, quickly rebutted to the jurors: "You did not strip him of his honor. What he did stripped him of his honor. It is not an honor—it has never been an honor—to kill unarmed men, women, and children." But to the very end, and most typical of the distorted way he tends to see things, Lieutenant William L. Calley, Jr., seemed to be much more interested in his and the army's "honor" than in keeping alive at least a score of unarmed civilians.

The foregoing cases are typical: Whenever a new instance of multiple murder occurs, and whenever psychological information on the killer is available, it is almost always found that he is an exceptionally disturbed individual, often in the psychotic range or at least suffering from a psychotic episode at the time of his crimes. This kind of killer usually has a long history of emotional disturbance prior to committing plural homicide and he frequently has an intense period of mental stress or breakdown immediately before he takes two or more human lives.

Is the same true of single murderers? Not entirely. A minority seem to be moved, at least in part, by extenuating circumstances. A slayer may be drunk at the time he kills; he may have been treated with rank injustice by his victim; he may get into an ordinary kind of brawl and accidentally kill his opponent; he may rightly or wrongly believe that he is protecting his own life by murdering some adversary; he may be ruled by motives of greed; etc. By and large, however, these factors do not seem to be as important as murderers and defense attorneys would like us to believe they are. Usually, some degree of emotional derangement is involved.

Take, for example, the two cases in Reinhardt's book where only a single incident of homicide was involved. In the first case, Carl Austin Hall kidnaped young Bobby Greenlease, and with the help of his female companion, Bonnie Brown Heady, murdered the child and buried him in Bonnie's backyard in St. Joseph, Missouri. Hall then sent out a ransom note and collected six hundred thousand dollars for the safe return of the boy. On the face of it, this looks like a simple murder for profit, with the boy being killed to keep him quiet and to protect the murderer from being identified later.

Carl was forced to wear fastidious clothes by his parents when he was a child, was called a "sissy" by other boys, and never got over the feeling of inferiority which overwhelmed him at that time. When his father died during his eleventh year, he became disobedient and domineering toward his mother, and terrorized her. He rebelled against military school and repeatedly urged his mother to let him return home. He then exhibited behavior which was described by his schoolmates and neighbors as consistently "impulsive," "arrogant," "impatient," "unconscionable," and "unfeeling." Drinking bouts and sexual delinquencies led to recurrent arrests during his senior year in high school. At the age of eighteen, he entered the United States Marines and spent considerable time in the "brig." When his mother died, he squandered his inheritance of two hundred thousand dollars in less than four years, pouring much of it down the drain in a senseless, gorging rage for recognition. When his funds ran out, he tried various get-rich-quick schemes, resorted to armed robberies, and became a drug addict. Reinhardt notes that "his powers of reasoning, and his sensitivities, were dulled by an excessive intake of chemical poisons. Medically, he was an alcoholic and a drug addict. . . . Whatever the frame of reference, Carl Austin Hall at the age of thirty-four was mentally diseased, physically debilitated, and utterly cut free from the motive springs of socialized men."

In the second case of an individual who committed only one homicidal act, Dr. Reinhardt interviewed and investigated the details on G. L. At the time he spoke to him, G. L. had served fourteen years of a life sentence for the murder of an eight-year-old boy. Meeting the boy by accident, he took him to a barn, where he wanted to put on some new clothes he had just gotten from the Salvation Army, and had a sudden impulse to choke the boy. He choked the boy into unconsciousness, took a beer can opener from his coat pocket, stripped off the child's pants, and with the can opener tore open his victim's rectum and slashed his testicles. He then sat down beside the mutilated body and masturbated.

G. L. was a sickly boy who got into trouble with school authorities and juvenile officers at an early age. By the time he was thirteen he had wandered over three states and had been arrested and repeatedly returned home. He had also spent thirty days in a state hospital for psychiatric observation. Several psychiatrists and agencies pronounced him a "psychopathic personality." By the time he was seventeen, he had served sentences in several jails, one state reformatory, and a penitentiary. At his trial for murder, psychiatrists for both the defense and the prosecution reported him to be a psychopathic personality, with ideas of reference, paranoid tendencies, immature emotionality, marked deficiency of judgment, and deficient reasoning ability. As a child, in spite of good intelligence, he was slow to speak and walk, had two attacks of sleeping sickness, and was diagnosed as having encephalitis. He had very peculiar eating habits, started stealing quite early, and was a known liar. The prosecuting attorney at his murder trial described him in this manner: "His ego is the sort that demands cruelty, and he found a great deal of ego satisfaction in an abnormal sex act involving the infliction of cruelty on a relatively helpless creature. It seemed as if he were saying, 'now I am even.' He knew what he was doing, but the ego delights of the moment outweighed any possible inhibitory influence." He showed no ability to love or to really hate. Before he murdered the eight-year-old boy, he admitted, he had previously dwelt upon murderous scenes in his mind; and he had returned to them in imagination in order to create sexual excitement.

From the facts taken from the lives of these two single murderers, it can be seen that they are just about as emotionally disturbed as were the multiple slayers explored. This may be because of Reinhardt's biased selection of cases; but there is a great deal of other evidence which indicates that individuals who murder only one person during their lifetime are usually emotionally aberrated. For example, in Miriam Allen deFord's book, *Murderers, Sane and Mad,* practically all the single murderers on whom sufficient personal evidence is available turn out to be pretty deranged; and in several instances indicate data that their parents or other close relatives are far from emotionally normal.

Other sources which contain histories of individuals who killed only one other person also almost invariably show, where sufficient information is available about the murderers, that they had a lifetime record of severe neurosis, psychopathy, borderline psychosis, or outright psychosis. Thus, G. Bishop tells us that William F. (Billy) Rupp, who violated and killed a fifteen-year-old baby sitter in California on August 8, 1952, and was executed for this crime, "was an admitted schizoid"; and that Timothy Stokes, who drowned Marcella Tyle on the banks of the Thames River in London and then had intercourse with her dead body, was declared to be "legally insane." R. Trainer reports that Amos H., a cabdriver who confessed to the rape-murder of an eight-year-old girl, was continually involved in problems—debts, traffic violations, drinking, and fighting, and always tried to solve matters by running away. "He had married four times. The marriages were always casual, so casual that Amos did not bother getting a divorce before taking a new wife."

Shultz, in her book on sex criminals, finds that just about all the murderers of one victim whom she examined were highly disturbed. Thus, Fred Thompson, killer and rapist of four-year-old Edith Kiecarius, "had been confined in Pilgrim Hospital in Brentwood, New York, after beating one of his daughters in a drunken rage. (At this time, according to the newspaper, he had been diagnosed as having an alcoholic psychosis.)" After his conviction for the Kiecarius murder, Thompson was sent to Bellevue Hospital in New York for examination, where he was found to be insane and therefore sent to the Matteawan State Hospital for the Criminally Insane. Emmett O. Hashfield, a fifty-three-year-old man who had spent most of his adult life in jails or prisons for offenses against children and who was out on parole at the time eleven-year-old Avril Terry's body was found in the Ohio River, cut into seven pieces, was convicted of her murder. He admitted being with Avril "but insisted that he had 'blacked out' after getting the girl into his car and had no recollection of what had happened until he found himself with the body at the riverbank." Less than a month before this crime, Hashfield had apparently lured an eight-year-old girl into his car and had driven her to a deserted place, where he smilingly told her, "Now I am going to kill you." She was saved by the purely accidental arrival of a couple who had lost their way. At his trial, four intimates of Hashfield, two psychiatrists, and one neurologist testified that he was mentally ill and unable to control his antisocial impulses. The neurologist held that he was brain-injured, and was probably a sex offender because of a severe blow on the head he had suffered two years before the first of his many sex offenses.

Franklin finds that the one-victim murderers he writes about in *The World's Worst Murderers* are almost as severely disturbed as mass murderers. Thus, he thinks that Nathan Leopold and Richard Loeb, the notorious killers of fourteen-year-old Bobby Franks, suffered "from that kind of communicated insanity known as folie à deux," as well as being involved with each other homosexually. Leopold and Loeb, following Nietzsche's philosophy of the superman of supreme intelligence who is beyond good and evil and is above the law, felt they were superior to ordinary mortals. "They agreed with tremendous enthusiasm and conviction that they were both supermen who could do no wrong and were a law unto themselves." They first embarked on a series of petty thefts and then decided that only by committing a perfect murder would they really prove themselves.

When captured for their crime, they remained totally unrepentant. Fortunately, the famous lawyer, Clarence Darrow, was able to convince the jury how emotionally deranged they were: "Loeb was a schizophrenic and Leopold a paranoiac. Although they each worshipped each other's stupendous intellect, Leopold was the slave of Loeb, who fancied himself king. This interlocking of their fantasies, the slave-and-king relationship, was the basis of their strange friendship. The opinion was put forward that they were both thoroughly mentally unbalanced, an opinion, one would have thought, with which no one would have disagreed."

Franklin also depicts the case of Pauline Yvonne Parker and Juliet Marion Hulme, who coldly planned and executed the bloody murder of Pauline's mother, Honora Mary Parker, who had threatened to break up their highly intimate, lesbian relationship. Pauline was sixteen and Juliet was fifteen at this time. "They believed they were geniuses, set apart from the ordinary race of human beings. They had their own religion and developed a rather alarming philosophy. Their fantasy world was peopled with bizarre characters like Charles II, Emperor of Borovonia, Deborah, the Emperor's mistress, Lancelot of Trelawney and the Empress of Bolumnia. They wove voluminous fiction around these characters, in which each girl played the characters, and which contained lurid descriptions of bloodshed and violence." According to Juliet's mother, who examined her correspondence with Pauline, "The early part of the correspondence is extravagant and grandiose, but it later becomes full of murder, suicide, and sudden death. Later violence and bloodshed figure to a disproportionate degree."

Dr. Reginald Warren Medlicott, the superintendent of a psychiatric hospital at Dunedin, interviewed the accused girls at Paparua Prison and diagnosed them as "suffering from paranoia of the exalted type in a setting of folie à deux, which he described as a form of systematized delusional insanity. . . . 'There was a gross reversal of the moral sense. They admired those things which are evil and condemned those things the community considers good. . . . They said they had their own paradise, god, and religion.'

" 'They have no appreciation,' Dr. Medlicott said, 'that the natural result of this matter will be their separation for many years at least. They have no idea anyone would be so illogical as to separate them. . . . The whole thing rises to a fantastic crescendo. In my opinion they were insane when they attacked Mrs. Parker.' " Dr. F. O. Bennett, who was the doctor of the Hulme family, "said that these two girls had delusions of grandeur, had turned their backs on society and lived in their own world, 'where every prospect pleases and only man is vile.' . . . Dr. Bennett said that both girls had since steadily maintained that the murder was justified. Neither would admit contrition or regret, and Pauline said she would still feel justified in killing her mother today if she was a threat to their being together."

Elwyn Jones has written an entire book on the last two murderers to hang in Great Britain, Peter Anthony Allen and Gwynne Owen Evans, who brutally beat to death Jack West, a fiftyish homosexual. Allen, according to Jones, seems to have been an inadequate and inept individual who was led by the more vigorous and persuasive Evans. Evans was a pathological liar, who claimed to have German descent when he did not and who insisted that he had married a German girl when he hadn't.

"His mental health had caused someone concern when he was only ten, for between September 1950 and March 1952 he was an out-patient at Dovenby Hall Mental Colony, Cockermouth. When he was sixteen, "he was before the juvenile court as being beyond parental control." He was later discharged from the Royal Air Force ostensibly as "physically unfit for Air Force service," but actually "his mental fitness was also demonstrably in doubt." He committed various larcenies as well as several driving offenses. When charged, with Allen, for ten petty thefts and ordered by the court to pay one hundred pounds in fines, he induced Allen to join him in robbing and killing Jack West in order to get money to pay these fines.

Chapter 3

General and Sociological Theories of Murder

Murder is one of the most dramatic and usually the worst of human crimes. But its very dramatic impact partially obscures the fact that it *is* a crime and is therefore similar to various other crimes of violence. Many murders are, of course, premeditated and therefore differ from other cases of homicide, where the victim is accidentally killed. Innumerable crimes, however, are also premeditated—as, of course, are many kinds of rebellious uprisings.

For every individual who is actually murdered, moreover, perhaps several more come within a hair's breadth of being slain; and some of them literally lie at death's door for a long period of time until they recover. In a bank robbery, in a racial riot, or in a family quarrel, for example, several individuals (sometimes a score or more) are seriously injured, and yet only one may actually die. The survivors may remain alive mainly because their assailant had bad aim, left them for dead when they were still alive, was balked by outside parties in his murderous attempt, or failed to kill for some other accidental reason. The main point we are making here is that premeditated murder is hardly as rare as the actual homicide statistics show. It is attempted much more often than it is achieved; and it is thought about and planned much more often than it is actually attempted. It is, therefore, part and parcel of a general tendency of many human beings to be violent in general and murderous in particular. If we thoroughly understood, therefore, why and how men become physically violent toward each other, we would probably also understand why and how they become murderous.

In this and the next few chapters, we shall examine the human impulse toward homicide, in an attempt to discover its basic causes. We shall look at the general, the sociological, the psychoanalytic, the psychological, and the biological theories of murder and try to see, in the light of some of the material we have already examined, which of these theories seems to make sense. First, in the present chapter, let us look at the general and sociological theories.

One of the most general explanations of murder is the criminosynthesis theory of A. Stevens Giannell, which broadly states that "any crime (deviancy) results from the high need frustration, low internal inhibitors, low external inhibitors, low contact with reality, high situational crime potential, and high potential satisfaction" existing at the time a murder is committed. The synthesis theory is reasonable in the sense that it cites conditions that must exist for a killing to occur; it does not provide insight into motivation, however.

Fredric Wertham, in *A Sign for Cain,* proposed that "the grounds for why men kill are not so different from those for other wrong things they do. They are based on all kinds of negative emotions: greed, jealousy, fear and the persisting memory of fear, distortion and frustration of sexual development, hunger for revenge, petty angers and irritations, hostility, wild ambition, sadistic fixations, resentments, unforgiven humiliations, rivalries in almost any sphere. These emotions are kindled by very different circumstances always in close relation to the mores and customs of the time." Wertham provides us with a bizarre example: "It was to be expected that the frequent irritations and frustrations with the upkeep of household appliances could lead to an extreme case of violence. Recently a thirty-two-year-old TV repairman had a disagreement with a man whose set he had repaired. And soon afterward, the customer walked into the repair shop and shot and killed him."

Both Wertham and Giannell rightly stress the social as well as the individual reasons for homicide. Wertham asserts that "scientifically, it is misleading to emphasize the isolated phenomenon of an impulse. What we see instead is a human being in whom such an impulse works. The decisive point is often not why one does it, but how one justifies it, rationalizes it, to oneself. The impulse is individual, the rationalization is social. This is where the individual and the social meet. If the environment itself is ruthless, it is easy to take a cue from that and find a plausible rationalization for violent behavior. The idea that an impulse to murder may arise momentarily in and by itself is not tenable. Nothing has a longer preparation than an impulsive violent act. . . . The reason why men kill, in short, is always to be found in negative factors in the personality and in society. For a murder to be committed, it takes two people *and* their social environment."

While plausible, the Giannell and the Wertham individual-social theories of the causation of homicide leave some sizable loopholes. For example:

1. The hypotheses do not account for all possible causes or conditions. They do not account for such possibilities as high suggestibility, imitativeness, and ego-bolstering demands. Juvenile delinquents, by way of illustration, have committed murder by suggestibly imitating the behavior of their neighborhood buddies or because of the hope of achieving great prestige by their deeds. All of Giannell's conditions of motivation do not always exist for these circumstances. Such a slaying could take place under very high external inhibitors, high contact with reality and low potential satisfaction—even abhorrence—for the actual act of murder itself. If one of Wertham's motivations fits, it is only vaguely suited.

2. Neither Giannell nor Wertham seems to give much weight to accident or pure impulse. Wertham states that an impulse to murder cannot arise momentarily in and by itself, because a person obviously does not live in just a single moment of time, and has antecedent training and behavior that make him much more likely to act one way than another. Wertham may be correct, technically. Nevertheless, it is likely that a good many murders are committed because some circumstance *did* happen to arise quite by chance (such as an individual's accidentally finding, when he is knocked down in a brawl, that a dangerous weapon is within reach), and that this did largely determine (a) his idea of killing

and (b) the act of killing. If Wertham wishes to contend that this is not the usual cause of murder, he is doubtless correct; but if he denies that it is sometimes a major cause, he is upholding a dubious thesis.

3. Giannell's and Wertham's lists contain reasons for homicide which hardly have equal weight or relevance. Although a great many murderers probably have some degree of low contact with reality—since at the moment they commit their crimes they may delude themselves that they will not be caught, convicted, and penalized—relatively few may be in a situation which has high crime potential. Five psychologists reporting in a symposium on "Murder within the Family" chaired by J. R. Hurley at the American Psychological Association Convention, indicated that murder is usually a family affair or an action among friends and is mostly committed by "nice guys." Most homicides perpetrated in family atmospheres can hardly be said to have taken place in a situation which has high crime potential, unless the fact that the homicide took place is used as evidence—the only evidence—of the potential.

4. Giannell, Wertham, and other theorists who list causes for human killing fail to emphasize that these causes are much more likely to affect one person than another. The individual who murders from high need frustration usually tends to have an unusually low tolerance for frustration, and much of his "high need" is created by his belief that frustration is intolerable and that *therefore* he cannot bear it. Frustration, even when it is consistent and severe, does not *have* to lead to low frustration tolerance and hence to physical aggression. Many individuals who live in conditions of great frustration tolerate these conditions very nicely, while many who are relatively little frustrated can't stand—or at least *think* they can't stand—almost any frustration. It is these latter individuals who seem to turn up on the list of murderers far more than do the former; and the generalized theories of frustration do not exactly indicate how they grew to be intolerant of life's difficulties or how their intolerance interacts specifically with other factors to induce them to resort to bloodshed.

Another generalized theory of murder is that of J. H. Gillin, who studied ninety-two Wisconsin prison inmates and noted some important factors that may contribute to this crime. Gillin found these factors to be loss of status, economic insecurity, culture conflict, marital conflict, and social inadequacy. Gillin also found that murderers, as compared to a control group of nonmurdering criminals, tended to leave school earlier, start work earlier, change jobs more often, live more disharmoniously with their wives, feel that they were someone's "favorite," be less likely to be farmers, and tend not to be professional criminals.

While Gillin's study may have turned up some factors that are fairly consistent in the lives of murderers, it has to be emphasized that these factors are *correlates* not *causes* of homicide. People who tend to lose status, be economically insecure, have culture and marital conflict, feel socially inadequate, and have various other traits mentioned by Gillin may easily be *peculiar individuals* who (1) have these kinds of undesirable traits, and (2) actually commit murder. In fact, if our theory of the importance of philosophic factors in aberrant behavior is true, we would predict that individuals with a poor or self-defeating philosophy of life *would,* appreciably more often than those with a saner, more assertive outlook, have various kinds of conflict and inadequacy in their lives and also the greater potential for committing murders.

Reporting on the "sudden murderer," J. W. Lamberti and his associates investigated common factors in the life patterns and offenses of thirteen individuals who were selected from a larger sample of criminals because they fitted the category of having suddenly murdered their victims. These individuals were seen at the Social Maladjustment Study Unit of the Malcolm Bliss Mental Health Center in St. Louis.

The investigators particularly studied parental attitudes and conditions of rearing of their subjects. They reported: "A striking finding was the overt attitude of the parents toward the patient during the childhood period." No father had a warm or even overprotective relationship to the child; the father's attitude was generally characterized as hostile, rejecting, or overstrict (five cases), or indifferent (two cases). The father was absent during the rearing period in three cases, and his attitude toward the patient was unknown in three cases.

Even more consistent was the mother's overt attitude toward the patient during the childhood period. It could be characterized as overprotective in eleven cases (being unknown or undetermined in the remaining two). In no case was the mother's attitude that of satisfactory warmth or even indifference or overt hostility.

At the same time, the patient considered himself to have been, as a child, attached to his mother in eleven instances and hostile to her in only one. Except for three cases in which the overt emotional ties of the patient to his father were not known, the attitude toward him was generally hostile (eight cases) or indifferent (two cases).

The closeness of the emotional tie to the mother is demonstrated by the fact that only one patient out of thirteen ever made a complete break away from home. These patients were not well educated, only one having been graduated from high school. The majority also had poor job stability as well as marginal economic status.

With respect to their character and personality traits, Lamberti and associates reported that "striking and consistent patterns were noted in several subjects. . . . In general, these patients showed some degree of ambivalence in their attitudes toward authority and some degree of feeling not wanted or loved or recognized or appreciated. Most of them showed as well some degree of fear of failure or defeat and some feelings of resentment. Most patients showed some surface ability to get along with others but all tended to blame other people for their troubles and all expressed definite feelings of isolation. In general, they expressed marked feelings of sexual inadequacy. All showed some small degree of chronic depression, although this was not marked in any case. Most of these patients could be characterized as introverts, only one being definitely extroverted and one being an ambivert."

Regarding the crimes of these individuals, the investigators found that "in twelve cases there appeared to be some later precipitating factor or 'insult' that threatened the patient's stability in his most important relationships." They also noted: "It appears that persons who have committed or attempted to commit sudden 'inexplicable' murders have certain consistencies in their life patterns. Although the families of origin are generally large and of marginal economic status, they tend to be relatively stable geographically, living in the same area throughout the patient's childhood, and there is a definite tendency toward cohesiveness and toward an apparent family attempt to conform to social norms. . . ."

At the same time, there is a strong tendency for the mother to dominate in the family pattern, and the mother and father do not generally get along well. The father is consistently a negative figure (either absent from the family picture or indifferent or overtly rejecting the child). The mother is even more consistently overprotective. Despite reasonably adequate intellectual capacities and good physical constitutions, these murderers generally do not do well in school, at work, or in the armed forces, and tend to drift from place to place, perhaps looking for greater opportunities—which they are not able to handle successfully when they become available.

Because their societies demand a great deal from them and because they sense their inability to meet social standards adequately, murderers are easily triggered by some "insult"—one that may seem trivial to an objective observer. Although Lamberti's data are indicative of a good many important social conditions which may encourage individuals to become sudden murderers, they are perhaps even more indicative of the kind of personality disturbance which we shall discuss in the chapter on psychological theories of murder. For the investigators note that these murderers demonstrated certain schizoid traits (emotional coldness and isolatedness, difficulty in forming close relationships with other persons, and trouble in expressing hostility directly) and that they also exhibited certain qualities of the passive-aggressive personality (feelings of hopelessness, inefficiency, and persistent reaction to frustration with resentment). In four of their cases, an outright diagnosis of schizophrenia was ultimately made; and a follow-up study which was done after most of the murderers had been incarcerated for a period of time indicated that "the behavior patterns of all thirteen offenders were essentially unchanged from the time period of our last observations. . . ." This confirms the impression that psychological rather than sociological factors may have been primarily responsible for the homicidal acts of this intensively studied group of murderers.

Henry and Short have theorized that homicide varies positively and suicide negatively with the strength of external restraint or discipline experiences over behavior: "When external restraints are weak, aggression generated by frustration will be directed against self and when external restraints are strong, aggression generated by frustration will be directed outwardly against another person." They define frustration as "a loss of status position relative to others in the same reference system."

They raise the question of individual differences in expressing aggression—that is, all other things being equal, why does one person choose homicide and another suicide? Their answer seems to be that "the internalization of harsh parental demands and discipline produces a high 'psychological probability' of suicide and a low 'psychological probability of homicide.' "

They also note: "The highly tentative interpretations presented . . . suggest the reasonableness of our hypothesis that suicide and homicide are acts of aggression undifferentiated with respect to their common source in frustration generated by business cycles. . . . Our argument based on the frustration aggression hypothesis and the childish formulation of suicide as a form of aggression has attempted to tie together into a more or less coherent whole the disparate correlations of both suicide and homicide with the business cycle and tentatively explain them as aggressive reaction to frustration generated by differential changes in status position accompanying the ebb and flow of economic forces."

Littenun and Gaier tested the Henry and Short hypothesis by studying the effects of social control in both Finnish and American subcultures. Although they found that the American subculture showed a higher degree of social control, a higher homicide rate, and a lower suicide rate than the Finnish subculture, they point out that the evidence to support the Henry and Short hypothesis is inconclusive.

M. Gold examined the suicide and homicide rates of males and females, enlistees and officers in the army, Negroes and Caucasians, and rural inhabitants and urban dwellers. He felt that the first of each of these pairs has greater experience of physical punishment, and he found that the suicide rate—as compared to the combined suicide and homicide rate—was lower for these groups. This affirms the Henry and Short thesis.

D. Lester did a study on homicide and suicide which casts doubt on the Henry-Short hypothesis. He explored the aggressive behavior of nonliterate societies, as shown in their suicide and homicide rates, to see if they were related to the socialization practices in these societies. He found no significant association.

B. B. Whiting rated societies according to whether murder is settled by retaliation or by referring the case to a delegated authority. She found that the mean importance of psychological punishment in the societies where murder is responded to by retaliation was −5.23, and in societies where it is referred to a delegated authority, −6.36. This difference is not significant and is in a direction opposite to that suggested by Henry and Short.

L. W. Simmons found that, for societies in which sacrifice was common, the mean importance of psychological punishment was −14.33, and for those in which it was rare, −4.50. This difference is significant at the 1 percent level and tends to support the Henry-Short thesis.

Simmons also discovered that, for societies in which infanticide is present to a moderate extent or more, the mean importance of psychological punishment was −7.00, and for those in which it is of little importance, −8.43. This difference is not significant and is in a direction opposite to that predicted by Henry and Short.

S. Palmer found that murderers, when compared with their brothers, had been subjected to greater physical discipline and stress than had these brothers. This supports Henry and Short. Palmer also found that the mean incidence of murder for fifteen societies who subject children aged less than two years old to stress was 9.87, and for those who do this after the age of two (or not at all), 8.57. This difference is not significant but is in the direction indicated by the Henry-Short theory.

Lester, in a study of aggression, used the Simmons ratings on the mean importance of aggression and calculated that, in societies where warfare is common, this was −7.35, and in societies where it is rare, −5.40. This difference is not significant but is in the expected direction. Using the same ratings, he found that the mean importance of psychological punishment in societies that hunt heads and scalps was −4.29, and in those that do not, −7.00. This difference is not significant and is in a direction opposite to the Henry-Short findings.

D. Horton rated the aggression resulting from alcohol for its intensity and found that the mean importance of psychological punishment for societies in which the resulting aggression was moderate was −7.80, and for societies where aggression was violent, −5.67. This difference is not significant and is opposite to the Henry-Short prediction.

Lester sums up the result of many relevant studies, including those just mentioned, as follows: "The results from comparisons of the discipline practices of societies and various indices of aggressive behavior in these societies have on the whole failed to substantiate the proposition derived from empirical studies using individuals. Obviously, the data are open to criticism. The samples of societies have been small and not randomly selected, and historical connections between them have been ignored. However, other studies have faced similar problems and yet have found results that accorded well with predictions based on empirical and theoretical psychological writings. It may be that aggressive behaviors are differently determined at the societal level than the individual level. It may be that the samples used above were biased in some way, or that the indices were poor. It is the case that the 'societal' findings are cross-cultural and largely exclude America. Further investigation is necessary to determine whether societal aggressive behavior follows laws different from those that individuals within a society follow."

One of the most thorough modern investigators of homicide has been Marvin E. Wolfgang, who wrote a book, *Patterns in Criminal Homicide,* which gives a sociological analysis of his and others' researches. Working with material from the city of Philadelphia, Wolfgang made an analysis of 588 murders listed by the police in that city between January 1, 1948, and December 31, 1952. He devoted a major part of his book to such problems as the motivations of murderers; temporal and spatial patterns in the commission of their crimes; the interpersonal relationships between them and their victims; race, sex, and age differences; methods and weapons used to inflict death; the relationship between the presence of alcohol and homicide; homicide while committing another felony; victim-precipitated homicide; unsolved homicide; homicide-suicide; tempo and legal procedure; insanity; and court disposition. He considered these problems in the light of "the most important reports and studies on criminal homicide in this country . . . to provide perspective to the local patterns in Philadelphia."

Most of Wolfgang's findings, though interesting and important, have little to do with the possible causation of murder. Some of his relevant conclusions are as follows:

1. Criminal homicide is largely an unplanned act. It, however, has tangible empirical uniformities of special social phenomena—for example, "a significant association between criminal homicide and the role and sex of both victims and offenders." The proportion of female offenders is reportedly much higher in England than it is in the United States.

2. During the hot summer months, criminal homicide tends to increase, but there is no significant association either by seasons or by months. Other studies report inconsistent conclusions; and Wolfgang's findings cast considerable doubt on the hypothesis that climate plays a significant role in the etiology of murder.

3. Homicide is significantly related to days of the week and hours of the day. The weekend in general, and Saturday night in particular, are significantly associated with murder, as are the hours between 8:00 P.M. and 2:00 A.M. These findings, in general, agree with those discovered in other studies of temporal patterns in criminal homicide.

4. "Criminal homicide usually results from a vaguely defined altercation, domestic quarrel, jealousy, argument over money, and robbery. These five police-recorded motives are involved in eight out of every ten cases."

5. When committed by or against women, homicide seems to be more personalized; that is, acquaintanceships of murderer and victim are usually more intimate and of longer duration.

6. About one-quarter of the murders studied appeared to be largely precipitated by some kind of action or attitude on the part of the victims.

7. "Suicide following homicide is five to six times more frequent in England than in the United States."

Wolfgang, in a sociological analysis of the data he collected, makes this conclusion: "Our analysis implies that there may be a sub-culture of violence which does not define personal assaults as wrong or antisocial; in which quick resort to physical aggression is a socially approved and expected concomitant of certain stimuli; and in which violence has become a familiar but often deadly partner in life's struggles. Attacks against the person are made without compunction, despite the middle-class value-system which views such acts as the most heinous of crimes. A conflict or inconsistency of social norms is most apparent, and the value system of the reference group with which the individual differentially associates and identifies, determines whether assaultive behavior is necessary, expected, or desirable in specific social situations. When an insult or argument is defined as trivial and petty by the prevailing culture norms, but as signals for physical attack by a sub-culture tradition, culture conflict exists. When a blow of the fist is casually accepted as a normal response to certain stimuli, when knives are commonly carried for personal defense, and a homicidal stabbing is as frequent as Saturday night, then social control against violence is weak. Under such circumstances there appears to be a subculture where the collective *id* dominates social consciousness—*i.e.,* where the basic urges, drives, and impulses of the group members are less harmonized with each other or external reality; where basic desires are less inhibited, restricted, or restrained; where reduction of tension and satisfaction of needs are characterized by immediacy and directness; and where the social regulators of conduct are weak and less omnipresent than in the larger culture of which this collectivity is a part. Thus altercations that lead to homicide become symptoms of unconscious destructive impulses laid bare in a subculture where toleration—if not encouragement—of violence is part of the normative structure."

Wolfgang's analysis sounds eminently sensible. However, a few factors may be mentioned which may throw some light on *why* a conflict or inconsistency of social norms is apparent between the general American culture and the subculture—which largely consists of individuals of lower socioeconomic status and of Negroes—that produces a significantly greater percentage of murders:

1. This subculture tends to consist of individuals who are more deprived and frustrated than the members of the general culture; and frustration, as we keep noting, is one of the main sources of encouragement to the rise of aggression.

2. The individuals in this subculture, because of their work and living habits, may be subject to mounting weekday pressures which abet increased anxiety and hostility; and may therefore be more likely to let out their pent-up anxiety and hostility on weekends, because of the lessened work responsibility, the greater alcohol intake, and the increased intimacy conducive to potential frustration, which often occur at that time.

3. A certain percentage of individuals—such as those who are mentally retarded or emotionally disturbed—are members of this subculture partly *because* of their mental and emotional handicaps. For in our society people who are mentally, emotionally, or physically handicapped tend to become members of the lower socioeconomic classes, even though they may have originally been reared in a higher-class group.

4. Members of the deprived and often unjustly treated subculture frequently are resentful of the discrimination they feel is being waged against them by the general culture; and consequently they directly or indirectly become more hostile and violent and may take out their hostility either against members of the general culture or against members of their own subgroup.

5. Members of the subculture may, for a variety of reasons, be reared with more irrational ideas than are members of the general culture. Thus, studies of lower socio-economic groups tend consistently to show that individuals in these groups are more superstitious than are individuals in higher socio-economic groups. It is likely, therefore, that the murder-prone subculture which Wolfgang is describing believes far more strongly in such irrational ideas as (a) if someone calls you a nasty name, you have to be terribly hurt; (b) the only good way to deal with an insult is physically to assault your insulter; (c) the police and the courts are

going to excuse your crimes as long as you follow an eye-for-an-eye and a tooth-for-a-tooth philosophy when you commit them; etc.

The sociological analysis of Wolfgang includes a good many of the important psychological and attitudinal reasons for murder, which we will discuss in more detail in other chapters of this book. John Bartlow Martin has independently noted this inevitable coalescence of the so-called sociological and the so-called psychological causes of criminality:

"As everybody knows, children who grow up in slums, badly treated at home and poorly educated at school, surrounded by teenage delinquency, are likely to end up in prison. Studies have documented it, from such great sociological works of the 1920s and 1930s at the University of Chicago as *The Gold Coast and the Slum, The Gang and Delinquency Areas,* down to the *Haryou* work of the 1960s. They show that certain areas of the city favor criminal behavior—slums in the older parts of the city where housing is bad, schools are crowded, poverty is great, family and community life disorganized, recreational facilities few, and a tradition of delinquent behavior is passed on from one generation to another, as is the tradition of eating with a spoon. Other studies showed, too, that 'white-collar-crime'—embezzlement, tax evasion, and so on—increased as urbanization increased, removing the brake of neighborhood disapproval.

"But the sociologists could not explain everything, as they themselves said. What of the slum boy who grows up straight? What of the suburban boy enjoying all the outward 'advantages' who goes wrong? The sociologists called attention to many important problems of our cities, problems that are today made screamingly acute by the Negro revolution. But in the end, they concluded that of all the factors involved in criminality, the most important was the subtle emotional relationship among members of the family. And this is far closer to psychiatry than to sociology."

In a sociological analysis of murderous assault in Ceylon, A. L. Wood notes that the high incidence of this kind of behavior in that area "is a manifestation of persons strongly alienated and demoralized." Feelings of alienation and demoralization, he further hypothesizes, are "in turn derivative not of all low status persons, but of those who feel their social deprivation."

Somewhat similar conclusions are reached by Pittmán and Handy, who made a survey of a random selection of one-quarter of 965 serious crimes listed by the St. Louis Metropolitan Police Department during 1961. Their purpose was to establish "patterns" of aggravated assault, as Wolfgang did for homicide, and to test his hypotheses in regard to assaults. Their collected data, like his, were analyzed in terms of a set of formulated hypotheses concerned with the variables of time, location, and season of the year, weapon, reporting, injury, police processing, alcohol involvement, victim-offender relationship, and arrest records.

Regarding the relationship of offender and victim, Pittman and Handy state:

1. "Prior to the act of aggravated assault, the offender and victim have generally been in interaction with each other. Verbal arguments usually precede the aggression. These quarrels may range from domestic incidents to tavern disputes over who was to sit on which bar stool. On the surface the quarrels appear to have little rationality. They must be understood in terms of the social and psychological mechanisms which the offenders and victims have developed to handle their aggressive impulses."

2. "A comparison of the findings in this study with those of Wolfgang for criminal homicide reveals more similarities than differences, even though the two studies represent different time periods, cities and police departments."

3. "The ingestion of alcohol was more common in homicide than in assault, as was a drinking episode between offender and victim prior to the crime."

4. "Alcohol was involved in the arguments in homicide situations more often than in aggravated assault cases."

Pittman and Handy conclude: "This comparison of findings concerning acts of homicide and aggravated assault indicates that the pattern for the two crimes is quite similar. Both acts, of course, are reflections of population subgroupings which tend to externalize their aggression when confronted with conflict situations." Like Wolfgang, Pittman and Handy do not clearly indicate *why* members of one population subgrouping tend to externalize their aggression when confronted with a conflict situation more than do members of another population subgrouping. We would hypothesize, in this connection, that members of the more assaultive population subgrouping tend to think more irrationally about conflict situations and their own ego-involvement in such situations, that their crooked thinking tends to lead to more inappropriate and self-defeating emotional reactions, and that their thinking and emoting impels or compels them to assaultive behavior. More details of our hypothesizing are presented later in this book.

Looking at murder in terms of economic factors, R. Quinney investigated suicide and homicide in 48 countries from data obtained from the World Health Organization publications. He calculated the mean annual suicide and homicide rates per 100,000 population for the years 1953 to 1960 and also calculated an urbanization and an industrialization index for these years. He concludes that "the evidence just reviewed indicates that urbanization and industrialization bear a fairly constant relation to the relative frequencies of suicide and homicide. Suicide rates tend to be high and homicide rates tend to be low in highly urbanized and industrialized countries. On the other hand, suicide rates are likely to be low and homicide rates are likely to be high in rural non-industrial countries. Countries at medium levels of urbanization and industrialization tend to have intermediate rates of suicide and homicide."

Quinney also notes that his findings disprove the hypothesis that suicide and homicide are functional alternatives, which was advanced by Henry and Short and Karl Menninger. He claims that they are causally separate phenomena: "Societies vary according to their economic development in the extent to which they produce conditions that are conducive to suicide and homicide. . . . High rates of homicide, on the other hand, seem to be characteristic of rural, non-industrial countries. S. M. Lipset has suggested that populations with a low level of education, lack of sophistication, isolation from heterogeneous values, and a limited frame of reference are predisposed toward concrete and immediate solutions to problems. Homicide, thus, may become institutionalized as the most appropriate solution to a number of interpersonal situations. Studies of homicide in underdeveloped countries or among people in lower socio-economic strata support this hypothesis. Another interpretation, consistent with this hypothesis, is that homicide as a response is learned through socialization in a subculture stressing aggression and violence."

Ball and Butes tested the hypothesis that crime in general is associated with urbanization migrations and residential mobility by studying 925 drug addicts at the public health service in Lexington, Kentucky. In spite of previous studies suggesting such an association, their findings indicated that addicts are not more mobile from birth than are members of the general United States population, and that they do not lead a more transient life after their initial hospitalization. However, variations in mobility patterns were noted among certain ethnic groups. Thus, they suggested that the relationship between crime and mobility has been oversimplified, and that the evidence indicates the bulk of crime to be committed by local residents.

S. Parker, utilizing concepts proposed by Abram Kardiner, studied the Wiitiko psychosis which accompanies violent and homicidal cannibalism of the Ojibwa Indians. He found that the Ojibwa personality and culture are related to the structure fostered by the specific socialization techniques of the group; and this, in turn, results in social factors acting on the individual members of the group and producing anxiety and hypertension in some of them. Parker, along with Kardiner, holds that personality in general, and specific personality distortions leading to homicidal cannibalism in the Ojibwa, are products of man's social environment. This may in part be true. But it is to be wondered whether those Ojibwa Indians who feel so pressured by certain social factors which exist in their environment and who do *not* commit homicidal cannibalism are not also prone, for biological or other reasons, to be less influenceable. It is possible that, if all the facts were known here, a heredenvironmental hypothesis, rather than a purely environmental one, would better fit the facts of the observed cannibalism.

McKnight and associates studied 100 individuals who had

killed 100 others and wounded 28, and found some interesting sociological factors prevalent among them. In particular, they noted that (1) homicide occurred within the murderer's family in about half of the cases; (2) the peak age of the murderer was 30 to 35 years; (3) the main seasons for murder were spring and fall, with an increase during the Christmas period; (4) most homicides occurred in or close to either the offender's or the victim's residence; (5) shooting was the chief method of killing; and (6) the majority of the offenders did not attempt to escape after the homicide. From this kind of sociological evidence alone, it could be surmised that a great many of these murderers were highly disturbed individuals; and actually they were, since they were examined in a psychiatric hospital and more than half of them were found to be schizophrenic.

Before concluding our discussion on the sociological theories of murder, we should consider briefly the sociology of crime in general.[1] Sociologists have on the whole concerned themselves more with explaining crime than with outlining the causes of specific crimes; and the major sociological theories, while sometimes applied to such areas as white-collar crime, forgery, or violence, generally are not directed to narrow but to broad categories. That is, sociologists have asked why people violate the norms of society, why they risk punishment, and in what conditions such violations increase. Much less frequently have they asked why some people murder, rape, or steal.

Edwin Sutherland, the dean of American criminologists, posited a theory of crime—the concept of differential association—which was later revised and updated by his colleague Donald Cressey. The theory has been sharply criticized by many sociologists, particularly by Sheldon Glueck. Sutherland started from the premise that all behavior is learned behavior. If it is learned, it must be taught; and, just as normative and law-abiding activities are learned, so is law-breaking. By a process of communication, largely within intimate personal groups, people presumably learn

[1] The material in this and the next eight paragraphs was written in collaboration with Dr. Edward Sagarin of the Department of Sociology of the City University of New York and Donal E. J. MacNamara of the New York Institute of Criminology.

how to break laws and what motives, values, and attitudes they can bring to their lawbreaking. They define their legal codes, or parts of them, as favorable or unfavorable; and this definition is determined by their associations. Consequently, they become criminals "because of an excess of definitions favorable to violation of law over definitions unfavorable to violation of law. This is the principle of differential association." Again: "When persons become criminal, they do so because of contacts with criminal patterns and also because of isolation from anti-criminal patterns."

While this theory may explain a good deal of antiauthority sentiment in certain areas, as well as the delinquency and criminality that thrive in these areas, it hardly explains the criminality of the social isolate or psychopath, or that of the person who commits murder although he has not followed a criminal path prior to his slaying, or that of the murderer who was reared in a highly law-abiding milieu. So, at best, it only partially applies to crime in general and murder in particular.

Thorsten Sellin used the theory of culture conflict as an explanation for crime. According to his views, conflict between groups of people—often ethnic groups—occurs within a society, either because they are living in contiguous areas or because migration has brought together people who have different interpretations of the norms of their community. Some individuals take with them, upon migration, the norms of their motherland, or they may move to a region in which they find that the norms of one authority group are imposed upon the norms of another group. Because these individuals are unable to have a single view of right and wrong, they clash with the members of other groups in their community; and out of this culture-clash a rise in criminality occurs.

Sellin's view may throw some light on the occurrence of murder, even though this act is not condoned as a mode of behavior in the sanctioned mores of any known society. For some individuals are probably more prone to violence as a way of "problem-solving" than are others; and in certain cultures these individuals may be less likely to have their violent outbursts condemned, particularly if these outbursts are directed against authority groups in their culture who are seen as oppressors. Nonetheless, Sellin's theory of crime appears to cover, at best, only a small part of its social causation, and many other factors have to be accounted for until a comprehensive theory is formulated.

Social disorganization, or normative conflict, has also been suggested as a cause of crime, and this theory is somewhat related to that of culture conflict. Not only in the United States but all over the world people tend to live in pluralistic, complex societies. They therefore can identify with a number of different groups within their community, but not with their society as a whole—or with what has been termed the "community." In urban areas, particularly, there is often a strain on the individual, as he notes various kinds of behavior going on around him and as he finds that he does not have to swear allegiance to one taken-for-granted way of righteousness. There is so much heterogeneity in his society that there comes into being, simultaneously, both a criminal and an anticriminal subculture. Because he is pulled in both or many directions, the individual can be tempted to commit acts which in a more homogeneous group would not be attractive to him; and his resistance to some criminal activities therefore becomes weak.

Similarly, mobility, both geographic and social, sometimes makes for crime. Geographic mobility makes it easy for an individual to commit depredations against those with whom he does not have roots; and social mobility makes it easy for him to commit crimes in order to further his ambitions. If it were impossible for the individual to raise himself from one socio-economic class to another, he would have little incentive to engage in crime. Where it is possible for him to rise by criminal means, he can elect to plot and scheme, or at least to go along with such means.

Starting from the theory of anomie originally proposed by Emile Durkheim and later developed by Robert Merton, Cloward and Ohlin proposed that crime largely arises out of a mode of behavior in persons who have been inculcated with goals of society—success, money, social climbing—but not with the necessity of following normative courses of arriving at such goals. Where the conventional pathways of achievement are blocked, or where people wrongly believe that they are blocked, some individuals have such strong drives to reach the socially approved ends that they willingly take the forbidden roads of arriving at those ends.

Sykes and Matza have presented a sociological theory of understanding the states of mind of people who decide to become criminal. They contend that people who violate the law—and particularly youthful offenders—create defenses, justifications, and rationalizations in their minds in order to neutralize the internalized norms of their society that they would otherwise use to restrain themselves. Among these "techniques of neutralization," they list denial of responsibility, denial of injury, denial that they really meant to victimize anyone, condemnation of their own condemners, and insistence that they acted out of loyalty to some higher cause. Although Sykes and Matza's theory may not account for all or most of the crime that occurs in any society, it is clear that the kinds of defenses and denials that they list are important in murder and assassination. In fact, the insistence that the assassin acted out of loyalty to some higher cause or authority frequently plays an important part in killings such as those of Senator Robert Kennedy and Dr. Martin Luther King.

E. M. Schur identifies criminal behavior with the same kind of values as those normally expressed in conforming behavior; and he believes that the individual's decision to commit a crime is a product of socially structured pressures on him and opportunities open to him. In addition, his propensity to commit crimes is often exacerbated by the irrationality of certain laws under which he lives and by the injustices perpetrated against him (and his fellows) by law enforcement agencies.

R. B. Textor did a cross-cultural summary of the Human Resources Area Files at Yale University and found that a comparison of a sample of thirty cultures taken from these files showed a correlation between incidence of personal crime and emphasis on military glory. In cultures where military glory is emphasized, personal crime has a high incidence, and in cultures with low emphasis on military glory personal crime has a low incidence. An emphasis on military glory, therefore, would presumably encourage the commission of homicide.

Wolfgang and Ferracuti, in their important book *The Sub-*

culture of Violence, show that subcultures where physical assault is lauded and encouraged—such as the black ghetto, the *machismo* aspect of the Mexican peasants, and frontier and vigilante "justice" in the United States—accept violent behavior as part of their values, take a permissive view toward it, and rear their children to conform to it. Consequently, the norms of one's reference group in these subcultures of violence actually promote violent "solutions" to personal and group conflict. Thus, Wolfgang and Ferracuti point out that lower-class males in our culture tend to be much more oriented toward direct expression of violence than are middle-class boys—who are more likely to turn their violent impulses inward and castigate and harm themselves.

Some evidence supporting this thesis is presented by C. A. Leon, who reports on the period known as *La Violencia* in Colombia. This period lasted from about 1949 to 1962 and was characterized by an enormous amount of assaultive crime, including arson, atrocious sex crimes, and sadistic murders. According to Leon's summary, "*La Violencia* affected characteristically the Andean region of the country. It did not occur in Nariño, and the Atlantic coast was virtually free with the exception of isolated actions in a small area in Bolivar and toward the south of Córdoba." Leon holds that "the contamination caused by violent attitudes is quite real. The witnessing of violence and constant exposure to messages of violence may finally succeed in creating a violent atmosphere and leading people to criminal acts. . . . Once the seed of violence is sown, it may continue growing if there is no effective way of preventing its development."

Evidence such as that presented by Wolfgang and Ferracuti and by Leon is fairly convincing, in that it tends to show the real effects of attitudinal factors on overt violence by members of a given subculture. We feel constrained to repeat, however, that certain groups of individuals may well be more predisposed, by both biological and early environmental factors, to respond to proviolence suggestions than are other groups.

Leon found, for example, that the two main nonviolent groups in Colombia during *La Violencia* were (1) the Atlantic Coast inhabitants who "are on the average outgoing, fun-loving, friendly people who display a truly hedonic sense of enjoying life in a rather carefree environment where social inhibitions and religious pressures are relatively low. Racially, they are predominantly mulatto and Negro" and (2) the inhabitants of the Andean plateau in Narino, who "are predominantly Indian and mestizo; they are generally introverted, retiring, and shy; they lead rather austere lives, behave in a socially submissive manner, and pay great respect to religion and traditional forms of authority." Both these somewhat extreme groups may have been significantly different, temperamentally, from the groups in central Colombia who were—or, shall we say, who easily allowed themselves to be—seriously affected by proviolence attitudes.

Wolfgang, in an article, "Who Kills Whom?" reviews various studies, including his own and those of several other sociological investigators, and notes that "it is in the network of neighbors, friends and relatives that homicide has its highest chance of occurrence. That we kill the ones we love may not be entirely accurate but it is a phrase that indicates the ambience of amiability within which most murders take place. Every homicide detective knows that the circle of investigation around the victim of a homicide is generally smaller than for the victim of any other crime against the person or against property. Determining the perpetrator is usually the least difficult in homicide cases, mainly because the offender is one with whom the victim had an intimate relationship prior to the slaying. . . ."

Using data on victim-offender relationships among 456 murders in England and Wales from 1957 to 1960, Terence Morris and Louis Blom-Cooper (quoted by Wolfgang) report that in 53 percent of the cases the duo in the homicide drama were related, and another 28 percent were friends and acquaintances, making a total of 81 percent with relatively close relationships. . . . In a 1956 Danish study of 172 murderers, Kaare Svaslastoga found that of every 10 murderers, six selected victims among members of their own family, three selected victims among acquaintances, and only one selected a stranger as a victim. . . . Murder of kinsmen or sex partners was very high among the Soya (63%), Gisu (41%) and Tiu (54%) tribes of Africa, reported Paul Bohannan."

Voss and Hepburn evaluated 395 cases of homicide occurring in Chicago in 1965 and found (1) that males and nonwhites were overrepresented both as victims and offenders; (2) "the home was the most common location"; (3) intoxicants were present in slightly more than half" of the cases; and (4) "almost half were killed by a family member or close friend."

Lalli and Turner analyzed United States statistical data on about forty million people in regard to annual homicide and suicide rates by white, Negro, and six occupational groups. They found that the white homicide rate was less than half the aggregate and that the Negro homicide rate was more than six times the aggregate. They hypothesize that the higher rate of murder among blacks results from the blacks constituting a "closed society" in a larger "open society." They believe that the "open society" causes depersonalization which reduces the homicide rate, while the "closed society" emphasizes close interpersonal relations, which facilitate murder.

Ted Robert Gurr, after reviewing considerable data on collective violence, comes up with the thesis that its overt expression varies strongly with the intensity and scope of relative deprivation experienced by members of a group. By relative deprivation he means a perceived discrepancy between what people believe they are entitled to and what they actually attain. When they see a sharp discrepancy between the "ought" and the "is," they tend to violently rebel. Though Gurr's theory does not explain all the important aspects of collective assault and killing, it appears to be much better supported by the evidence than are most other theories and in all probability has a good degree of credibility.

Surely one of the most important and relevant theories of crime in recent years has been the statement issued by the National Commission on the Causes and Prevention of Violence on "Violent Crime: Homicide, Assault, Rape and Robbery." The Commission pointed out that between 1960 and 1968 "the national rate of criminal homicide per 100,000 population increased 36 per cent, the rate of forcible rape 65 per cent, of aggravated assault 67 per cent, and of robbery 119 per cent." It made the following observations:

"1. Violent crime in the United States is primarily a phenomenon of large cities. This is a fact of central importance. . . .

"2. Violent crime in the city is overwhelmingly committed by males. . . .

"3. Violent crime in the city is concentrated especially among youths between the ages of 15 and 20. . . .

"4. Violent crime in the city is committed primarily by individuals at the lower end of the socioeconomic scale. . . .

"5. Violent crime in the cities stems disproportionately from the ghetto slum where most Negroes live. . . .

"6. The victims of assaultive violence in the cities generally have the same characteristics as the offenders; victimization rates are generally highest for males, youths, poor persons and blacks. Robbery victims, however, are very often older whites. . . .

"7. Unlike robbery, the other violent crimes of homicide, assault and rape tend to be acts of passion among intimates and acquaintances. . . .

"8. By far the greatest proportion of all serious violence is committed by repeaters."

On the basis of its findings, the Commission made some grim predictions: "Lacking a sharp change in Federal and state policies, ownership of guns will be almost universal in the suburbs; homes will be fortified by an array of devices, from window grills to electronic surveillance equipment; armed citizens in cars will supplement inadequate police patrols in neighborhoods closer to the central city, and extreme left-wing and right-wing groups will have tremendous armories of weapons which could be brought into play with or without any provocation.

"High speed, patrolled expressways will be sanitized corridors connecting safe areas, and private automobiles, taxicabs, and commercial vehicles will be routinely equipped with unbreakable glass, light armor and other security features. Inside garages or valet parking will be available at safe buildings in or near the central city. Armed guards will 'ride shotgun' on all forms of public transportation.

"Streets and residential neighborhoods in the central city will be unsafe in differing degrees and the ghetto slum neighborhoods will be places of terror with widespread crime, perhaps entirely out of police control during nighttime hours. Armed guards will protect all public facilities such as schools, libraries and playgrounds in these areas.

"Between the unsafe, deteriorating central city on the one hand and the network of safe, prosperous areas and sanitized corridors on the other, there will be, not unnaturally, intensifying hatred and deepening division. Violence will increase further, and the defensive response of the affluent will become still more elaborate.

"Individually and to a considerable extent unintentionally, we are closing ourselves into fortresses when collectively we should be building the great, open, humane city-societies of which we are capable."

The gist of this report seems to be quite clear: that when a large group of individuals becomes economically deprived and is forced to live in close quarters in certain sections of a big city, violent crime becomes almost inevitable. A subculture of violence then springs up; and, self-defensively, people living in the surrounding subculture of lesser violence feel that they have to resort to armoring and counterviolence. These tactics, in turn, encourage the individuals in the violent subculture (1) to arm themselves to an even greater degree and (2) to fight more viciously among themselves when it becomes too difficult or dangerous for them to combat the members of the surrounding subculture.

On the surface, if the predictions of the National Commission on the Causes and Prevention of Violence are actually borne out, two major interconnected theories about violence would seem to be substantiated: (1) Rage and violence largely stem from economic causes, particularly from poverty, crowded living conditions, and other forms of economic deprivation. (2) They appreciably stem from feelings of frustration and injustice.

Although there is probably a great deal of truth in both these theses, they are still oversimplified "explanations" of a much more complicated state of human affairs than a first-blush examination of the facts of violence and crime would reveal. Several important biological and psychological factors also lie behind the evidence and predictions presented by the Commission and may fairly easily be connected with its findings. For example:

1. Something besides poverty obviously attracts people, and

particularly members of minority groups, to large cities. Not all blacks and Puerto Ricans in the United States by any means run to and stay in highly populated ghetto areas in urban areas.

2. Most of the members of a poor minority group in a large city do not resort to much violence; and certainly only a minority of this minority engage in forcible rape, aggravated assault, homicide, and robbery. Some ghetto dwellers—such as the Jews—seem to have a greater participation in violence when they live in crowded conditions than when they live in suburban or urban areas; but they have a considerably lower proneness toward violent crimes than do other minority groups who live in ghettos.

3. Ghetto residents (as well as nonghetto residents) who habitually use alcohol or hard drugs are much more prone to crime and violence than those who do not. Most such residents are not, of course, alcoholics or drug addicts; and those who are usually are psychologically different from those who abstain or imbibe occasionally or moderately.

4. The National Commission on the Causes and Prevention of Violence found that crime in the cities is overwhelmingly committed by males—especially by youths between the ages of fifteen and twenty. Males in general and young males in particular are no more economically deprived or otherwise frustrated than are females or older males who reside in ghettos. Indeed, the latter are frequently more deprived. Deprivation, crowding, and frustration themselves, therefore, can hardly be the only factors in causing crime. Obviously, biological and psychological conditions, such as low frustration tolerance and ego-bolstering drives, also contribute to city violence.

5. We would be highly unsophisticated to assume that people live in ghettos today only because they are poor or that they are poor only because they are members of a minority group that is discriminated against in their society. Some of them are poor and live in ghettos because (a) they to some degree prefer that kind of existence; (b) they refuse to work very hard; (c) they have close ties to other ghetto dwellers; (d) they could move but are too inert to do so; (e) they are not well educated and/or intelligent; (f) they are addicted to drugs or alcohol; (g) they are physically ill; (h) they are severely emotionally disturbed; (i) they have other defi-

nite, and sometimes unique, reasons for being poor or living in crowded conditions. There may be a significant correlation between some of these individual reasons for ghetto living and the reasons that certain city dwellers habitually commit crimes. This hypothesis is perhaps partially supported by the Commission's finding that "by far the greatest proportion of all serious violence is committed by repeaters."

In summarizing the general and sociological theories regarding murder, we would say that these theories indicate that crimes of violence, and homicide in particular, tend to occur with significantly greater frequency among individuals who have relatively low socioeconomic status and who live in ghetto areas of large cities. However, a good proportion of murders also occur among individuals living in rural, nonindustrialized areas. Consequently, certain populations or subpopulations in our society do seem to be more prone to murder than are other groups. But before we jump to hasty conclusions and theorize that violence and murder are largely dependent on socioeconomic factors, we would better look more closely at some of the psychological and biological influences which are correlated and interact importantly with sociological conditions.

Chapter 4

Psychoanalytic Theories of Murder

When we think of psychological theories of murder today, we almost inevitably think in psychoanalytic terms. Unfortunately, psychoanalysis is often used as a virtual synonym for psychological analysis or psychotherapy. The Freudians and the neo-Freudians (many of the latter actually being neo-Adlerians but still identified by the public with psychoanalysis rather than with what Adler called "Individual psychology") have had, until very recently, the best public relations of any group of social theorists. They have influenced academic thinkers and reached a vast public through psychoanalytically influenced novels, plays, films, television productions, paintings, dance productions, and other forms of art and entertainment.

The general psychoanalytic theory of aggression, sadism, and murder has perhaps best been outlined by one of the analytic pioneers, Ernest Jones in *Hamlet and Oedipus*: "The main discoveries here may be summed up in the statement that, side by side with loving attitudes and peaceful contentment, there are always to be found mental processes reminiscent of the most primitive aspects of savage life of an intensity that is only faintly mirrored later on by the distressing aspects of our international relations, including even the tortures and other atrocities. Violent and ruthless impulses of destruction (*i.e.,* murder in adult language) follow on the inevitable minor privations of this [early childhood] period. The jealousies, hatreds, and murderous impulses of which signs may be detected in childhood are, in fact, the weakened derivatives of a very sinister inheritance we bring to the world and which somehow has to be worked through and chastened in the painful conflicts and emotions of infancy. To say that a later reaction to a situation is excessive is simply to say that contributions have been made to it by the unconscious, *i.e.,* the still living infantile mind. Before humor and other aids to mental digestion make their appearance, these aspects of the infant's mind are entirely tragic, and all the tragedies of poets are ultimately derived from them."

Jones goes on to say that the main jealousy is that which a boy experiences toward his father, especially when the latter disturbs, as he necessarily must, his enjoyment of his mother's exclusive affection. "This feeling is the deepest source of the world-old conflict between father and son, between the younger and the older generation, the favorite theme of so many poets and writers, the central *motif* of most mythologies and religions." He continues: "It was Freud who first demonstrated, when dealing with the subject of the earliest manifestations of the sexual instinct in children, that the conflict in question rests in the last resort on sexual grounds."

The Freudian theory, then, is based on the assumption that hostility is largely rooted in sexual jealousy. Males in particular first hate their fathers for depriving them of their mothers' sexual and loving responses; then, by extension, they later hate others because of sex-love rivalry. Their sexual, jealous, and murderous impulses are a product of their *id.*

As Hinsie and Campbell note: "The id, as a psychoanalytic formulation, is part of the energy system of the psyche. It is regarded as the reservoir of psychic energy or libido; it contains all phylogenetic acquisitions and is the source of instinctive energy. The pleasure-principle reigns supreme in it and has control over the erotic and thanatotic (death) instincts. The id resides in the unconscious, far removed from reality, to which the id pays no attention. The id recognizes only its own needs and does not itself undertake to modify its needs in any way. Modification of id impulses are brought about through other agencies, the superego and ego."

The superego "is the representative of society within the psyche (*i.e.,* conscience or morality) and also includes the ideal aspirations (ego-ideal). The superego is mainly unconscious; its functions include: (1) approval or disapproval of the ego's actions, *i.e.*, judgment that an act is 'right' or 'wrong'; (2) critical self-observation; (3) self-punishment; (4) demands that the ego repent or make reparation for wrong-doing; and (5) self-love or self-esteem as the ego reward for having done right."

The ego "is that part of the psychic apparatus which is the mediator between the individual and reality. Its prime function is the perception of reality and adaptation to it. The ego is the executive organ of the reality principle and is ruled by the secondary process. The various tasks of the ego include: perception; motor control (action); adaptation to reality; use of the reality principle and the mechanism of anxiety to ensure safety and self-preservation; replacement of the primary process of the id by the secondary process; memory; affects; thinking; and a general synthetic function manifested in assimilation of external and internal elements, in reconciling conflicting ideas, in uniting contrasts, and in activating mental creativity."

According to Freudian theory, every individual has an aggressive impulse, stemming from his id, which achieves its highest degree of expression in the form of a death impulse. The self-destructive tendency is innate in every individual, but the individual may direct it away from himself, and against others, in order to defend his own ego. Freud in *New Introductory Lectures on Psychoanalysis* states: "We maintain the hypothesis of a special instinct of aggression and destructiveness in man." More specifically, the male child is innately driven toward being jealous of his father and, wanting to murder him, becomes fearful that his father will castrate or slay him instead, develops thereby a full-blown Oedipus complex with considerable consequent guilt, and may be driven to actual murderous acts because of this complex.

Our main criticisms of this general Freudian theory of murder are as follows:

1. Children may well be born with a strong tendency to become enraged and violent when they are thwarted and when they are deprived specifically of attention and love. But the tendency seems to be, much more concretely, that they easily and "naturally" believe that they *should* be omnipotent, they *must* get what they immediately want, and that it is horrible and catastrophic when they are not and do not. They are therefore born with the

predisposition to (a) strongly desire certain things and goals, (b) feel thwarted when they do not get them, and (c) conclude falsely that it is awful when they are thwarted. Their final belief, that it is awful for them to be frustrated, is what mainly causes their rage and violence.

2. There is little evidence, as Jones contends and as Melanie Klein states in more specific detail, that normal children are preoccupied with jealousies, hatreds, and murderous impulses much of the time and that they are entirely tragic. Some children—especially autistic or schizophrenic children—may continually think and feel this way; but most children most of the time probably do not.

3. There is no reason to believe that boys invariably demand the *exclusive* attention of their mothers and that they therefore inevitably hate their fathers. Many boys obviously care more for their fathers than their mothers and resent the mothers for taking away paternal affection from them; and other boys are easily able to get along with both parents and to resent neither out of jealousy. It is very likely that many *non*sexual frustrations, probably even more than sex-love deprivations, help boys (and girls) to resent their parents.

4. When there are love or jealousy problems encouraging children to resent one or both parents, there is no clearcut evidence, as Freud states, "that the conflict in question rests in the last resort on sexual grounds." Many male children do not in the least lust after their mothers, or have sex problems regarding them. They may be very jealous of losing the mother's *attention* or *affection* on entirely nonsexual grounds. The Freudians unfortunately *read* sexuality into all kinds of sensual and amative desires and responses; but this hardly proves that it is truly extant.

5. The id-ego-superego system is largely fictional and consists of an unscientific reification of "parts" of the personality which really have no independent existence, are not laden with "instinctual energy," and do not "drive" the individual to do anything. Many biologically based *desires* (of which the individual is often quite conscious) prejudice or motivate human behavior; but it is inaccurate and vague to lump them together as the "id." Similarly, the individual has many guilt- and shame-producing attitudes,

thoughts, beliefs, values, and philosophies which prejudice him in various ways and cause him to "feel" guilty or conscience-stricken; but it is inaccurate to combine these views, call them his "superego," and then insist that this collective entity makes him do or not do various things. Again, the person perceives, acts, organizes, thinks, feels, etc.; but saying that his "ego" does these things or makes him do these things is to invent an intervening variable that explains nothing and sets up problems in its own right. *He* perceives, acts, organizes, thinks, feels, etc.; and if he does have an "ego" (or self-preserving attitude), *he* possesses it and to some degree can change and control it.

6. Although "normal" human beings almost always seem to have strong self-defeating tendencies, in that they go for short-range instead of long-range gains and thereby defeat their own best ends, there is no evidence that they have true self-destructive or death instincts. Aggressive drives, moreover, though they may actually to some degree be biologically based, as we show in our first chapter, hardly seem to merely be defenses against the individual's self-destructive tendencies. There is reason to believe that they exist in their own right, whether or not the person is unusually self-destroying.

For many reasons such as these, we hardly subscribe to the general psychoanalytic theory of aggression, violence, and murder. We shall now examine, in the rest of this chapter, some of the more specific views on murder which originate in psychoanalytic formulations.

Psychoanalytic views of the causation of murder are fairly common. Walter Bromberg, in his book *The World of Murder: A Psychiatric Study of Homicide,* offers one such view. He proposes that "violent crime occurs, with or without provocations, when inhibitory, defensive or sublimating mechanisms of the ego are insufficient to curb direct expression of aggressive impulses."

This hypothesis may have some validity, but it is again—as in the Giannell synthesis theory—too generally stated and does not account for the specific reasons that the individual should lack control over his destructive impulses. If he is inhibited, defensive, or sublimating, there is reason to believe that he uses these ego mechanisms in order to avoid, or at least to attempt to avoid, anxiety. It is his anxiety, therefore, rather than his defenses against this anxiety, which is the real issue; and the Freudian theory does not provide a clear explanation of what anxiety is or how it arises. It vaguely assumes that the individual's superego is in conflict with his ego or his id; and that because he cannot tolerate this conflict, he becomes anxious.

Actually, the individual becomes anxious because he has some strong, irrational ideas—the idea that he should achieve outstandingly, for example, or that he should be approved by all the significant people in his life, or that he should be in control of the forces in the universe—and he finds that these demands are impossible to achieve. His anxiety largely flows from unrealistic goals and expectations. If he tells himself, "I should do outstandingly well in my profession," and there is a likelihood (as there almost invariably is) that he may not, he is forced to the inevitable conclusion, "—or else I am no damned good." This idea, that he is worthless and hence incapable of controlling his own destiny, is what makes him feel insecure or anxious.

If, therefore, the individual is making himself needlessly anxious by not merely wanting but by unrealistically demanding that he do well in his profession, and if he is shown what he is doing and works hard at not creating anxiety in this manner—as provided in the process of rational-emotive therapy—he would have no need to become defensive or sublimating. He could then directly look at his aggressive impulses, determine whether or not they are worth giving in to, and sanely stop himself—because he would merely acknowledge that he was wrong for being so undisciplined and that he'd better make greater efforts to discipline himself next time—and he would thereby prevent himself from becoming compulsively or repetitively aggressive.

The Freudian theory of homicide propounded by Bromberg assumes that the individual has innate aggressive impulses which presumably stem from his id and that he would normally give in to these powerful impulses if his ego did not develop inhibitory, defensive, or sublimating mechanisms to deal with them. He seems to have one set of irrational ideas, which convince him that it is absolutely intolerable if someone thwarts him and that he simply must kill this thwarting individual; and then he has another set of defensive, but still irrational, ideas, which convince him that he would be an utter louse if he killed the individual who is intolerably thwarting him. Normally, his irrational defenses win out over his irrational impulses to kill; but sometimes the former are not strong enough and his murderous id drives break through and he is literally driven to annihilate one or more of his thwarters. According to this theory, the individual has the choice of two evils: Either remaining continually defensive and repressed and sitting on the cauldron of his id impulses in an uncomfortable manner; or becoming sporadically unrepressed and giving vent to his killer impulses.

According to our way of seeing things in rational-emotive terms, the individual may well have underlying tendencies to condemn and perhaps kill others when they thwart him, but he is able to look consciously at these tendencies, see that being thwarted is not really so horrible (though it is often unpleasant), and train himself to abide the limitations of living in a social order, accepting some considerable degree of being thwarted. Once he accepts this reality, and practices calmly letting other people thwart him (when this seems to be an inevitable part of life), or dispassionately showing them that they need not thwart him that much, or objectively moving away from them when they become too thwarting, he then becomes truly inured to being thwarted at times, and does not build up any great underlying hostility toward his thwarters. He also learns that he does not *need* the approval of others and that he does not *have* to denigrate himself if at times he acts childishly and intolerantly toward these others when they do thwart him. With this sensible philosophy of life, he is able to live successfully with (1) his tendency to feel thwarted and (2) others' propensities to frustrate him. He then becomes realistically accepting rather than squelchingly defensive, and he has as good a life as it is possible for him to have in the somewhat difficult social milieu in which he exists. His murderous impulses, though not fading away to zero, become less easily arousable and more easily held in consciously suppressive and nondefensive rather than unconsciously repressive and defensive check.

Another psychoanalytic explanation of murder is given by McKnight and his collaborators, who studied cases of matricide where shooting was the method of killing. They concluded that the constructs of the "Orestes complex" and the "catathymic crisis" warrant further attention as causative agents in murder. The "Orestes complex" they derive (like Freud derived the Oedipus complex) from Greek legends. Orestes was the son of Agamemnon and Clytemnestra and the brother of Electra. After Clytemnestra (with the help of her lover, Agisthus) slew her husband, Orestes (with the aid of his sister) became irate and murdered Agisthus and Clytemnestra. According to McKnight and his associates—following the legend—men who kill their mothers are frequently aping Orestes and are defending their cuckolded fathers' honor.

We frankly take little stock in the Orestes complex as a prime cause of matricide (just as we take little stock in the more famous Oedipus complex of Freud). Although the full facts of such murders are not easy to ascertain, there is no reason to believe that more than a small percentage of mother-killers wreak vengeance on their female progenitors because they know or suspect that these women are (1) cuckolding their father and (2) have actually plotted with a lover to kill him. Matricidal males are much more likely to do their mothers in because they paranoiacally think that they are against them; because they resent their mothers bitterly for frustrations they think they have suffered at their hands for many years; because they stand to gain financially by their mothers' demise; because they are too drunk or demented to know what they are doing at the time they murder; or for other prosaic reasons which have little to do with Greek mythology. Rather than being particularly interested in their fathers' honor, they are much more likely, if irrationally, to believe that they themselves have been unduly persecuted, endangered, or frustrated by their mothers and that they cannot tolerate this kind of treatment a moment longer, and therefore for all time they must remove the horrible source of their danger or frustration.

Another psychoanalytically oriented theory regarding murder is presented by G. J. Rose. He reports that "from the story of the murderer of a three-year-old girl, a hypothesis was formulated that the crime represented the reenactment of consciously remembered, severely traumatic events in the man's childhood. An amytal interview conducted by an independent observer confirmed this hypothesis. From the data, the probability that the primal scene was also reenacted is reconstructed, and psychic functions involved are discussed."

There are several serious objections to this kind of conclusion:

1. It is very easy to connect contemporary behavior with almost *any* kind of childhood traumatic event. All human beings tend to have a good many early traumas, and it is not difficult to interpretively link them with practically anything that later occurs in their lives.

2. Assuming that a given murderer has a specific childhood experience and that this is closely correlated with his subsequently slaying someone, the questions would still have to be asked: (a) Why was the original experience taken to be so traumatic? and (b) Why did this early traumatic event *continue* to influence the individual many years after it occurred? Renaud and Estess did an important study of the life history of a hundred normal American males and found that during their childhood these individuals experienced as many traumatic events and other tensions and hazards as did a control group of psychotic individuals. They found no significant differences between the normals and the psychotics in regard to family tension, excessively rigid or indulgent patterns of discipline, oedipal anxieties, unresolved sibling rivalries, or repressed sexuality. From this study and from other clinical and experimental evidence, there is reason to believe that murderers may be the type of individuals who in many instances *make* the usual traumas of childhood exceptionally severe and influential in their lives and that they later *keep ruminating* about these experiences, instead of letting them go.

3. In regard to psychoanalytic views about the importance of a child's witnessing the primal scene—that is, seeing or hearing the sounds of sexual intercourse between his parents—there is reason to believe that innumerable individuals who later grow up to be emotionally sound witness such scenes and that they *make* much less of them than do children who are traumatized by the

same kind of experiences. It seems much more plausible to hypothesize that a man who later murders his father (or who kills someone who resembles his father) was a somewhat odd kind of individual from childhood on, who easily misunderstood the significance of any primal scene that he may have witnessed, than to hypothesize that simply because he saw his father copulating with his mother he was seriously affected for the rest of his life, became exceptionally hostile toward his father and similar men, and finally killed his male progenitor or some symbolic substitute for him.

4. It is of course possible that in the single case examined by Rose, the murderer actually did kill a three-year-old girl partly or largely because he related her existence to some traumatizing events in his childhood. If so, he seems to have been a most unusual individual and there is no good reason that any important generalizations about murder should be made from this single instance. Moreover, even in such a rare case, it would not truly be the killer's witnessing of any primal scene during his childhood that would cause him to slay a child many years later, but his own interpretations or cognitions about such a scene. Thus, he might tell himself, "It is terrible to witness my parents having intercourse; it is only from this kind of a vile scene that children are born; this presumably innocent three-year-old child was actually conceived in this horrible fashion; therefore she is living a hypocritical, lying existence and does not deserve to live." Underlying this killer's childhood "observations" and "trauma," and motivating him in his adulthood crime, would be his highly irrational *philosophies* that (a) sex is a nasty business; (b) intercourse between his parents is particularly vicious; (c) any "innocent" child born of such a horrible event is actually tainted and deserves to die; and (d) he would be a noble morality-restoring person if he killed such a child. It would be these highly prejudiced value systems (which the Freudians and many other psychotherapists often tend to ignore) that he brought to the primal scene he witnessed that would really make it highly traumatic for him. And it would be his senselessly continuing to believe in these philosophies for the rest of his life, and thereby undergoing a continuing increase

in his anxieties, that would finally move him to commit murder.

Similarly, practically every Freudian view of homicide that has ever been purported reads motives into the killing that are dubiously there in the first place, and then importantly ignores the basic values behind these motives if the latter actually existed.

The Freudians have no hesitation in applying their questionable theories of murder to fictional as well as real killings. Here, as a good case in point, is J. C. Flugel's "explanation" of Hamlet's murder of Claudius, his uncle and his stepfather. In the following passage Flugel closely follows the reasoning of the two masters of psychoanalysis, Sigmund Freud and Ernest Jones.

Hamlet's "mother only marries the stepfather after a period of widowhood during which the boy may have appeared to possess the sole, or at any rate the chief, claim upon her interest and affection. By her re-marriage she will probably seem to the boy's unconscious mind to have been, in a very real and poignant sense, unfaithful to himself, and to have rejected his own love for that of an outsider; an idea which may appear in consciousness in the rationalized form of an imputation of unfaithfulness towards the mother's previous husband—the boy's own father. It is a complex of feelings of this kind which, as Ernest Jones has so convincingly shown, underlies and forms the principal psychological motive in Shakespeare's tragedy of *Hamlet.* It is this which is the cause of Hamlet's vacillation in regard to the contemplated murder of his stepfather; the latter had only done what Hamlet himself would fain have done before him, but was inhibited from doing. The contemplation of Claudius's ill deeds serves dimly to call up the buried tendencies which at one time prompted Hamlet himself to commit a similar atrocity—the murder of the king (his father) for a similar end—the possession of the queen (his mother), and the paralyzing effect of the arousal of such feelings makes itself felt as an inability to carry out the punishment of one with whom he thus has much in common, and whom he feels to be in a sense no worse than himself, the would-be punisher. Moreover, in virtue of his marriage with the queen, Claudius now really stands in the old king's place; in killing him, therefore, Hamlet is to his own unconscious mind becoming guilty of the very crime of Oedipus which had tempted him before his father's death; hence the resistance to the consummation of the act which hatred of the interloper prompts him to perform."

In the foregoing passage a good many fairly wild presumptions are made—and then developed as being indubitable truths, on the basis of which further highly dubious assumptions are constructed. Moreover, the basic philosophic ideologies behind these assumptions (assuming that they contained some measure of truth) are never explicated; and therefore the profound understanding which presumably would arise from truly making man's unconscious thoughts and feelings conscious is never actually achieved. Here are some of the main premises which are cavalierly adopted in the Freud-Jones-Flugel version of Hamlet's murderous deed, together with the basic human ideologies which underlie these premises but are never made clear by any of these three masters of psychoanalysis:

1. It is assumed that Hamlet, as a child, was mainly interested in the sole possession of his mother after his father's death; and that therefore he unconsciously took her marriage to Claudius as (a) infidelity to himself and (b) rejection of his love for her. Although it is possible that Hamlet did want to possess his mother completely, it is also possible that he was really very happy about her "neglect" of him after her marriage to Claudius; since perhaps she was literally and figuratively a royal pain in the neck and he was delighted to have greater freedom to do what he wanted to do in life after she became preoccupied with Claudius and married him. It is also possible—as many lines in the play suggest—that he was much more concerned about the loss of his dear father than he ever was about the lack of attention from his widowed mother. Lots of other possibilities exist here (as they always do); and it is typical of the Freudians that, because we find that *some* children are upset about losing the sole attention of the mother when she remarries, they dogmatically insist that *all* children, including Hamlet, must be similarly distraught. This is a typical psychoanalytic overgeneralization.

Assuming, again, that Hamlet was displeased by his mother's marrying Claudius and thereby taking some attention away from him (a dubious hypothesis because she was obsessed with Claudius *before* she collaborated with him to get her husband out of the way, and therefore could hardly have given the half-orphaned Hamlet much attention immediately after her husband's murder), he would have been terribly disappointed not because of the mere *fact* of his mother's neglect but because he foolishly believed that he *should* have her undivided attention, that he *must* be totally adored by her, and that he *couldn't stand* any neglect on her part. These ideas, which are fairly common to children but which are certainly not held by *all* of them, are the core of Hamlet's original upsetness, if the Freud-Jones-Flugel assumptions are correct. But, typically, these Freudians sadly neglect clarifying such ideas, vaguely talk about Hamlet's "complex of feelings," and miss the main point of why he was disturbed. Moreover, if they ever tried to treat the young Hamlet for his severe "feelings" of deprivation, they would probably let him express his feelings, perhaps in the form of some kind of expressive play therapy if he were young enough when they first saw him, and they would never get to the ideas behind these feelings, would not show him exactly what are these ideas, how asinine they are, and how to challenge and question them in order to give them up and replace them with more sensible notions, such as, "It's too bad that my mother is neglecting me for my stepfather; but that's the way things often are in life, and it won't kill me, since I really do not *need* her complete attention, even though it would be nice to have it."

Moreover, if an orthodox psychoanalyst saw Hamlet in his young adulthood, when he was severely troubled about his mother and Claudius, and was thinking of murdering the latter, he would not be able to understand fully what Hamlet was telling himself at the time to *make,* or *keep,* himself troubled: for example, "I still can't stand the fact that my mother deserted me when I was a child and focused most of her attention on Claudius. How could she have done such a thing! I think I'll kill him or both of them to avenge myself for that horrible wrong. I *must* be totally loved by my mother—even at this time in my life!" Because he would not get to this philosophic source of Hamlet's murderous intentions, the analyst would hardly be able to show him how to forego them; and another of the many failures of psychoanalytic therapy would be in the cards.

2. Flugel assumes that Hamlet unconsciously felt, when he was neglected by his mother, that she was "in a very real and poignant sense, unfaithful to himself, and to have rejected his own love for that of an outsider." This seems to us to be the imposing of a highly sophisticated, adult-oriented attitude onto Hamlet as a child. Granted that he may have been displeased by not having his mother's full love, there is no reason that he *had* to demand that love as he would have possibly demanded it if he were an adolescent or adult suitor for her hand. This is a typical Freudian position looking at the young child as if he were truly a little adult. The evidence, however, as gathered by Jean Piaget and a host of his students, tends to show that children think quite differently from adults and that it is unscientific if we project into them the kind of thoughts and feelings that we would have if we engaged in circumstances similar to those in which they are engaging.

If Hamlet really did feel that his mother was unfaithful to him and if he really were upset about her rejecting his love for that of an outsider, then he would be believing something along the following lines: "Because I want my mother's full attention and she does not give it to me, she is being unfaithful to me and is rejecting me completely. Whenever I want someone's love, like I want hers, I *should* be able to get it fully; and it is catastrophic when I don't. How can she possibly act that way to one who is so needful of her affection as I am? I'll fix her and Claudius's wagon for being so cruel!" It is, again, these crazy, totally unrealistic *views* of Hamlet, and not the mere *circumstances* of his mother's neglect of him, which made him terribly upset. This is what the psychoanalytic interpreters ignore.

3. Freud, Jones, and Flugel make a third assumption—and quite a lulu!—when they contend that Hamlet's conscious imputation that his mother was unfaithful to her first husband, his father, is really a projection of his own unconscious feeling that she has been unfaithful to him. First of all, we really do not know that he does think that his mother was reprehensibly unfaithful to him and that he is afraid to face this thought and therefore only allows himself to hold it unconsciously rather than consciously. There seems to be no definitive reason that he could not quite consciously believe that his mother, when he was a child, owed him

primary love and that it was horrible that she did not give it to him. Lots of children in our day, and quite probably in Hamlet's, consciously and without guilt confess that they are in love with their mothers and that they want to marry them when they grow up; and it is not clear why Hamlet could not have been in this category.

Assuming that Hamlet was ashamed of his sex-love feelings toward his mother (which we shall discuss further below), he still could have *also* felt that she was unfaithful to his father. In fact, the events of the play seem to indicate that she was. So there is no reason to believe that he *only* accused her of infidelity to her first husband because he was really concerned about her infidelity to himself, and that he could not consciously face this concern.

If the Freudian hypothesis about Hamlet's repressing his love interest for his mother is true, and he really did fantasize her being unfaithful to his father, then the philosophic ideas behind his acting in this aberrant way would have been something like these: "I want to have a full sex-love relationship with my mother; but this would be incestuous and wicked, and I cannot bear to admit that I would have such desires. Any male child who lusts after his mother *should not* act in that manner, and is a worthless individual if he does so. I therefore better not admit, even to myself, such fiendish desires; and I'll assume, instead, that it was not me to whom my mother was unfaithful (since if that were true I'd have to admit my own culpability in demanding that she be sexuo-amatively faithful to me), but that she must have been faithless to someone else—that is, my father." If Hamlet's ideas are stated in this form, it quickly becomes apparent how irrational they are and what he might do to change them. When they are obscured with psychoanalytic verbiage, it would falsely appear that their source is in the events of Hamlet's life rather than in his own cognitive-emotional interpretations of these events and that the only thing that is likely to help him is an endless recounting of these events and his feelings about them—rather than his incisively examining his own value system and his working hard to change some of his contradictory and self-defeating values.

4. Freud, Jones, and Flugel all assume (as do innumerable psychoanalysts after them) that Hamlet's real problem is not so

much his relationship with his mother and his uncle, Claudius, but with his father. Having, according to classical psychoanalytic theory, a full-blown Oedipus complex, he lusted after his mother in early childhood, he wanted to murder the king (his father) because his father had the full sexual possession of the queen (his mother), and he thought that his incestuous and patricidal wishes were so horrible that he deeply repressed them. When Hamlet sees that Claudius has actually done what he wanted to do himself, and unconsciously senses that he has much in common with Claudius, he vacillates about the contemplated murder of his stepfather. He feels Claudius "to be in a sense no worse than himself, the would-be punisher," and he is therefore guilty about (a) his original Oedipal feelings and (b) the idea of killing Claudius.

Again, some very fancy hypothesizing! The facts of the play, and of human nature in general, give us no real cause to believe that Hamlet lusted after his mother and consequently wanted to kill his father, that he deeply repressed both these ideas, and that he vacillated about killing Claudius because he guiltily identified with him. On the contrary, it would appear that his *conscious* horror over his mother's conspiring with his uncle to kill his father was pretty much the same as his *unconscious* feelings. For us to insist that he could not possibly have really had the feelings that he did consciously have, and that they must have been a mask for his real or unconscious feelings, is to play a typical Freudian game of never taking *anything* at its face value and of presuming that there has to be some other and often contradictory reason for it.

But if the Freudian theory of Hamlet is true, it still misses the main philosophic point of what was going on in Hamlet's head. For this theory really states that Hamlet (like most males) had several irrational ideas and that these ideas caused his downfall. Freud himself, incidentally, used the word *ideogenic* in the first book on psychoanalysis which he wrote with Breuer to describe how and why individuals become "emotionally" disturbed; but, unfortunately, he and his followers almost completely forgot this very useful term thereafter.

Anyway, the basic self-defeating ideas which Hamlet almost certainly had, if Freud, Jones, and Flugel are correct about his murderous feelings, are something like these: (a) "It is terribly wrong for me to lust after my mother. (b) If I do lust after her and she would rather sleep with my father than with me, I can't stand to be thwarted in such a horrible manner, so I'd better get rid of the old man and then have her completely to myself. (c) If I have any wishes to kill my father, I am really an awful person and cannot even tolerate the fact of having such wishes. I must never admit such wishes to myself, but have to repress them. (d) If my Uncle Claudius conspires with my mother to kill my father, the only thing I can honorably do is to kill him in turn and thereby avenge his murder. (e) But since my Uncle Claudius has done the kind of dastardly deed that I would have liked to do, how can I possibly act as an agent of justice against him? I would be an utter louse if I condemned and killed him for committing a crime that I came close to committing, at least in my mind's eye, myself. So I'd better dilly-dally about doing him in."

These ideas are all irrational because they insist that certain acts, such as lusting after one's mother, are wrong, when they could easily be viewed as being right or harmless; because they demand that the individual *ought* not act in this "wrong" manner, instead of advising him that it is undesirable if he does act that way; and because they postulate that if a person does act in a "wrong" way he is not merely mistaken but is a worthless lout and that he deserves to be punished severely. If all or some men do have—as the Freudians insist they have—an Oedipus complex, they do not have this complex because they lust after their mothers, but because of the irrational ideas they have in regard to such lusting. If we wanted, psychotherapeutically, to ameliorate or eliminate this complex, we would not be so sidetracking as to spend years, as psychoanalysts do, trying to get them to see that they have it, but would quickly and directly show them the irrational attitudes that *created* this complex during their childhood and that now maintain it, and we would also uproot these attitudes.

Still another Freudian-oriented view of homicide is propounded by M. N. Walsh: "The increasing power of weapons for mass annihilation is . . . related to the desire for power surpassing that of the father, with increasing danger of self-annihilation due to the unconscious guilt related to the Oedipal conflict."

We have already given our view, relative to the Hamlet theme, of the implausibility of the Oedipus complex theory regarding murder (or virtually any other human disturbance). We can only repeat that there is no conclusive evidence that the vast majority of males in our society have a full-blown Oedipus complex, though there is evidence that most of them have some kind of sexual feeling at some time during their lives toward their mothers, and some kind of jealousy of their fathers (mainly because the latter are occupying the time and attention of their mother, rather than having sex relations with her). What is more, where an Oedipus complex does exist, there is no reason to believe that it lasts forever and that it is a prime factor in driving the individual to commit a murder many years after his childhood has passed. Certainly, few adults appear to murder because of an unconscious guilt about their Oedipal feelings for their mother and about their drive for power surpassing their father (as Walsh alleges), or contemplate suicide, or kill someone else instead, or invite the wrath of the police to punish themselves for this guilt.

It is much more likely that, when males in our society develop homicidal impulses because of their power drives, they are striving to overcome feelings of inadequacy and worthlessness. They think that by "pulling someone down to their size" (thereby winning the game of one-upmanship) they are proving how "strong" and "manly" they are; and they may go to murderous extremes to prove their "strength." Walsh's proposition that the increasing power of weapons for mass annihilation is related to the desire for power surpassing the father is probably unadulterated psychoanalytic hogwash. Modern technology practically demands more powerful weapons, just as it demands more efficient factory machines. Once one national group hits upon a new weapon, this group's main rivals are virtually forced to put its inventors to work to come up with an equal or more deadly set of mechanical killers. Only a psychoanalyst would think of relating this kind of power struggle to the desire for power surpassing the father!

Not that the psychological power struggle—which has largely

been exposited by the Adlerians—is unimportant in human affairs. It has an enormous import. In order to prove their greatness and impress others with their achievements, men have often resorted to violence—including individual murder and group warfare. But there is reason to believe that the human drives for mastery and power are in part biologically motivated, that they have autonomy in their own right and are not derived from any struggle between fathers and sons. There is also reason to think that, when man does not achieve what he would like to achieve, he makes inordinate demands on himself, perfectionistically believing that he *should* do better than he is doing, and berates himself for being such a nonachiever. At this point, he frequently tries to compensate for his "inadequacy" by "manfully" resorting to violence—even murder.

Many other authors have attempted to give psychoanalytic explanations of crime in general and murder in particular. Melitta Schmideberg, in "The Treatment of Criminals," states that "the only way to really study criminals is to psychoanalyze them." Ben Karpman agrees and deplores the fact that not a single well-authenticated psychoanalysis of a murderer exists in the entire literature. Karpman believes that the choice between right and wrong is determined by emotional motivations that are not consciously controlled by the individual's intelligence. Accordingly, he maintains that a study of murder is and must be a study of the instinctive life of the murderer rather than a study of the "nature, development, and type of conscience of the murderer."

Reviewing the case of a murderer analyzed by him many years earlier, Karpman explores the data he obtained from thirty-five analytic sessions with this individual and he finds "outstanding unconscious factors," particularly a deep-seated Oedipus complex and a strong incestuous attachment to the patient's younger sister. Unfortunately, it is all too easy for Karpman, by using psychoanalytic interpretations that are not convincing to an objective observer, to find the unconscious factors and the Oedipus complex that he is looking for. And, even assuming that these actually existed in the case he presents, a convincing *causal* connection between them and the analysand's motives for homicide is not demonstrated.

M. El-Rawy strenuously objects to this Freudian construct of mother lust being all-important in criminal and other destructive behavior. He points out that "the notion of the Oedipus complex has been originated after a simple and naïve idea. Whatever is forbidden is desired." Instead, he contends, the desire of a child to be with his mother is not essentially sexual and does not require that he hate his father in consequence. He goes on to deny, as have many other psychologists, that the Oedipus complex "should then be responsible for the criminal tendencies which would be shown later in adolescence."

Another proponent of the idea that the Oedipus complex is all-important in homicide is H. A. Bunker. He contends that "the theme of the myth of the Birth of the Hero has as its principal motif, the vanquishing of the father and the winning of the mother. . . . Although frankly expressed in the Oedipus legend, the second part of the principal motif, the winning of the mother, is ordinarily repressed or disguised or it is distorted into what appears its exact opposite, the clearest example of which is found in the drama of Orestes. Thus there is actually a common latent significance in both the Oedipus and Orestes myths, and this is relatively clearly demonstrated in Hamlet."

Bunker here uses the clever psychoanalytic ploy of reaction formation which Ernest Jones also used in his analysis of Hamlet. If the Oedipus complex were really an all-powerful, universal fact of human existence, both Orestes and Hamlet would have been much more interested in killing their father than their mother, since he was clearly depriving them of their mother's bed, thereby "castrating" them. The fact that each of them backed up his father and killed his mother, who was being unfaithful to him, is evidence *against* the Oedipus theory. But, rather than admit this evidence, the psychoanalysts say, "Oh, no! Orestes and Hamlet *really* wanted to kill their father, but could not admit this to themselves, else they would have had to admit that they lusted after their mother. Consequently, they leaned over backward, went in the opposite direction by the process of reaction formation (that is, the process of unconsciously forcing yourself to love what you hate or hate what you love), and deliberately killed their mother. This *proves* that they really wanted to kill their father." The hell it does!

It suggests, rather, that psychoanalytic thinking is distorted and unscientific, and that it is the easiest thing in the world, by its use, to "prove" that black is white.

Fredric Wertham, in an article on the matricidal impulse, also asserted the validity of the Orestes complex as an important factor in homicide: "Overattachment toward the mother can be transferred into a violent hostility against her. This phenomenon, called the Orestes complex, is clearly evident in Hamlet and some cases of matricide." While it is true that overattachment to the mother *can* be transferred into violent hostility against her, the question arises: "In what percentage of the cases of overattachment is positive feeling for the mother actually transferred into violent hostility?" There is no evidence that this usually or always happens; and much doubt that it does. But even when a devoted son becomes violently hostile to his mother, matricide normally would be the last thing he would plan and execute. That he might sometimes *wish* his mother dead is hardly evidence that he would kill her. Moreover, in instances where he did violently hate and physically attack his mother, we would suspect that nonsexual factors far more than sexual factors would be an important influence on him.

G. Bychowski holds that crime is the result of uncontrolled unconscious tendencies or of a conscious intention. The moral order, which arises out of the repression of aggressive tendencies by man, is violated by the criminal. Therefore he "must suffer the penalty which the collective consciousness demands as compensation for the satisfaction he has permitted himself."

To back up his psychoanalytic theorizing, Bychowski appeals to evidence from mythology, history, philosophy, and clinical analytic experience. For the most part, he attempts to support analytic explanations with historical quotations; but in an almost diametrically opposed direction he remarks: "In these speculations we can base ourselves on the psychoanalytic knowledge of the development of the child and on our clinical experience." The psychoanalytic knowledge of the development of the child, however, is itself almost sheer speculation; and analytic clinical experience is normally seen in the light of heavy interpretative biases.

Bychowski finds the origin of man's homicidal impulses in his basic instincts; but he notes that these have to be limited by the realities of nature and of the social structure. As his id drives conflict with reality, man finds a solution to the problem of murder in the growth of a more rational ego and superego. He then sanctions these solutions by religious beliefs and legal institutions. Although much of Bychowski's thinking seems sensible enough, it is consistently couched in vague psychoanalytic terminology which resists operational definition and which makes any truly scientific validation of his hypotheses next to impossible.

This is one of the main troubles with the entire psychoanalytic approach to murder. It is so loosely stated and its theoretical constructs are so inexactly tied to observable evidence that, however plausible it sounds, it resists verification. To say that one's murderous id drives are in conflict with one's ego and superego may not be entirely false. But it would be much more useful to say that man has both conscious and unconscious desires to obtain immediate gratification of his biologically prejudiced and socially learned impulses; that he wishes to give in to these impulses without restriction; but that he soon discovers that he has other desires—particularly, self-protective urges and the desire to win the approval of others—that conflict with his immediate demands. Consequently he must control his impulses (whether they be murderous or sexual) in order to gain some of the longer-range satisfactions that he also desires. What is called his "conscience" or "superego," however, has both a rational and an irrational side. On the one hand, it wisely informs him that certain acts are wrong or self-defeating, and that he'd better not perform them. On the other hand, it foolishly tells him that he is a monster and deserves to be punished on earth or in hell for (a) performing such wrong acts or (b) even *desiring* to perform them.

It is not, therefore (in psychoanalytic terminology), the clash between man's id and ego or between his id and superego that gets him into neurotic and almost insoluble difficulties. Such clashes could be resolved by the normal processes of socialization that Bychowski and other analytic writers keep referring to. Rather, it is man's intra-superego conflicts which really tend to do him in; and these are often ignored or unclearly seen by analysts—with the exception of a few like Melanie Klein, who stressed man's self-castigation tendencies, but then confused her explanations with a great deal of typical psychoanalytic verbiage.

A well-known analyst who presented her interpretation of a man who murdered his pregnant daughter-in-law was Marie Bonaparte. She concluded that the cause of this murder was the "Oedipus complex and the resentment felt in childhood at the birth of a younger sister." Here again the psychoanalytic "explanation" falls far short of plausibility. For, even assuming that this murderer did have an Oedipus complex, how would his lusting after his mother and fearing castration by his father lead him to kill his pregnant daughter-in-law? And, assuming that he did resent the birth of a younger sister when he was a child, why would he (a) still resent this event many years later, (b) identify his daughter-in-law with his resented sister, and (c) go to such great lengths about his transferred resentment as to kill his victim? Rather than our assuming that his early resentment caused his later murderous impulses, would it not be more logical to assume that he was prone, from early childhood onward, to extreme low frustration tolerance and to crooked, overgeneralized thinking which induced him to (a) resent his younger sister without any great provocation on her part, (b) resent other females because they reminded him of his sister, (c) carry a grudge practically forever, and (d) resent his daughter-in-law not only because she, too, was a woman and was about to bear a child, but also because she displeased him in other ways?

P. M. Lehrman discussed the case of a schizophrenic murderer and held that the cause of his act was a series of unsuccessful attempts to resolve problems originating in unconscious conflicts. The murder, he held, represented a fore-stage to the swallowing of the victim, which was the slayer's unconscious goal. He found that constant oral frustration due to the murderer's excessive oral drives ruled his psyche. The victim was therefore symbolically seen as the earliest undifferentiated object of the murderer's oral desires. Going still further, Lehrman claimed that the murder really took on the quality of suicide, "because in the earliest ego-object relationships the victim is also a representation of the murderer."

This kind of totally unprovable gobbledegook reigns almost supreme in the orthodox psychoanalytic literature. First of all, the murderer's so-called excessive oral drives seem to be largely a figment of Lehrman's vivid imagination: The murderer could just as well have been found, by other serious psychoanalytic interpreters, to have pronounced anal, tactile, genital, or other drives. Psychoanalysts usually link orality with dependency, because a dependent child presumably sucks at his mother's breast. An individual, however, even during his childhood can be just as dependent on anal, tactile, genital, or other stimulation as he can be on sucking; and the vast majority of dependents are not desperately seeking any kind of sensual or sexual stimulation, but are generally seeking approval and love. This does not quite fit into the Freudian scheme of pregenital oral or anal desires.

Secondly, even if Lehrman's analysand were orally deprived, in a truly definable sense of that term, there is no evidence that his oral drives would necessarily have to rule his psyche. Lots of individuals have strong desires—such as the urge for food—but manage to live successfully with these desires and not become obsessed with constantly satisfying them. If an individual actually does have strong oral drives and is somehow frustrated in getting them satisfied, to become disturbed he would still have to convince himself of two important points: (1) "I want to be orally satisfied and it is damned inconvenient if I am not," and (2) "I absolutely *need* to be orally gratified and *can't stand* it if I am not." Lehrman and other psychoanalysts usually assume that it is only the first of these things, the strong desire for oral pleasure and the inconvenience of this desire's being blocked, which causes emotional disturbance. Actually, such frustrated desire would be a problem, but hardly a serious one, if the second did not exist: the individual's puerile insistence that he *must* have his oral desires satisfied and that *it is awful* if he doesn't. So it is not, as the analysts insist, the unsatisfied oral longings that lead to the person's obsession and drive, but his unrealistic, self-defeating demands that he *should not* be unsatisfied.

Thirdly, even if Lehrman's analysand was ruled by his excessive oral drives—or, rather, by his childish demand that these drives be fully satisfied—it is quite a magical jump, by himself as well as his analyst, to see his victim symbolically as the earliest undifferentiated object of his orality. If Lehrman is correct, then this murderer was telling himself something along the following lines: "When I was a young child I had great oral longings and needed almost any undifferentiated object, such as my own fingers or my mother's breast, to gratify these longings. Since these desires were never fully gratified, I have been continually obsessed, to this day, with fulfilling them. This individual with whom I now have contact seems to represent symbolically the same kind of undifferentiated object that I once needed for my oral expression; therefore, if I can kill and swallow him I will, for perhaps the first time in my life, be really orally satisfied."

Now it is certainly possible—though unlikely—that Lehrman's patient did think along these lines. If so, it was not his orality that led him into this series of foolish assumptions and non sequiturs but his crooked thinking *about* his oral longings and about the "logical" ways to satisfy them. Any reasonably straight-thinking individual with exactly the same kind of orality would have come up with much different conclusions. Either he would have managed to gratify his unfulfilled oral desires more directly—for example, by finding women who delighted in having their breasts or genitals sucked—or he would have failed to gratify these desires and still managed to lead a tolerable existence. Only in rare circumstances would he be likely to resort to murder (to symbolically swallowing his victim) to become orally fulfilled!

Lehrman and other analysts, therefore, in finding the so-called orality of a murderer central to his homicidal tendencies, are incredibly naïve and superficial. This is like saying that, if a man has the desire for more money (which most of us do) and, if he kills someone to obtain a couple of hundred dollars (which most of us don't!), he was driven to murder because of his cupidity. Obviously, in giving in to his desire for money in this antisocial manner, the man is obsessed with many other magical, unrealistic, and foolish ideas *in addition* to his belief that having more money would be desirable. Obviously, too, the "orally driven" patients whom the Freudians continually find behaving self-defeatingly "because" of their desires for mouth-object satisfactions have many other magical, unrealistic, and foolish ideas in addition to their belief that putting things into their mouth would be fulfilling. Concepts such as "oral fixation" and "severe oral frustration," therefore, at best describe the *results* of an individual's slippery, unrealistic thinking about himself and the world. The concepts by no means *cause* his "oral-driven" behavior. Psychoanalysis uses these descriptive concepts as assumed causes of disruptive activities when there is no evidence of a cause-and-effect relationship. The real causes that are almost invariably involved in such aberrated behavior—the inborn and acquired tendencies of the human individual to philosophize falsely about his desires and satisfactions—are almost completely missed by the superficial "explanations" which are so consistently used by analysts. It is amazing, in these circumstances, that Freudianism is almost universally considered to be "depth psychology" when actually, because it ignores the philosophic underpinnings of human motivation and behavior, it is usually superficial!

Lehrman finally claims that his murdering patient actually was suicidal "because in the earliest ego-object relationships the victim is also a representation of the murderer." This seems to mean that young children confuse themselves with others and are hostile to their parents or peers because they are also angry at themselves. Perhaps so; but hardly always! If Lehrman's patient really was in this category and repeated during his adult life the same kind of ego-object relationships which he experienced during his early days, we'd better clearly note that this repetition did not occur *because* children have confused ego-object relationships but because some children (including this murderer) simply never grow up, and pigheadedly *maintain* their confused early notions of themselves and others.

Why this particular murderer maintained his infantile ideas Lehrman does not make clear. The answer probably is: Because he was schizophrenic, because schizophrenics have strong innate tendencies to remain on an immature level of thinking, and because no one in his environment taught him how to deal successfully with and perhaps to overcome these tendencies toward cognitive slippage, he retained as an adult many of his confused childish thought processes. But Lehrman and most other analysts do not acknowledge that an individual may be biologically predisposed to think schizophrenically. Rather, they insist that his "unconscious conflicts," his "excessive oral tendencies," his "Oedipus complex" or something of that sort *made* him schizophrenic and hence murderous. If anything, the reverse is probably true: His innately predisposed and environmentally unchallenged tendencies to think schizophrenically caused his "unconscious conflicts," "excessive oral tendencies," and "Oedipus complex."

Another psychoanalytic linking of murder with suicide is hypothesized by R. S. Banay. In his careful study and analysis of a murderer, Banay found that this offender had not reached a normal stage of heterosexuality. His victim was for several years viewed by the killer as a mother surrogate; and the wish to murder her, and presumably thereby symbolically to commit suicide, arose when he discovered that she had engaged in a sexual affair.

Banay makes some gratuitous and highly speculative psychoanalytic assumptions here. It is very easy for an analyst to see a murderer's female victim as his mother surrogate, whether or not the murderer really felt that she was. Assuming, however, that Banay's interpretation is correct, then the simplest hypothesis would seem to be that the murderer (1) was horrified at the thought of losing his mother surrogate when she began to have an affair and (2) was scandalized by her having a sex affair when she was supposed to remain something of a madonna image. Out of his jealousy and out of his thinking that she had betrayed him by giving up the mother role, he might possibly have made himself very angry at her and consequently killed her. Why he would want symbolically to commit suicide, however, is not clear. If he really was terribly depressed because he felt he was losing his mother surrogate and could not survive without her, he would probably want *actually* rather than *symbolically* to kill himself. And if he really was extremely angry at her for betraying the madonnalike image that he had created, then he would tend to want to kill her *rather than* himself. His symbolically committing suicide would largely seem to be a highly imaginative surmise on Banay's part; and if this surmise proved to be true, then we would again have to ask: *Why* would this murderer be so upset and suicidal merely because he was losing the mother surrogate that he wanted? And the answer would probably be: Because he foolishly convinced himself that he *couldn't stand* living without her help. This crazy idea, rather than the mere fact that he wanted a mother surrogate and would have been inconvenienced by her loss, is what would truly be upsetting him; and it is exactly this kind of idea that psychoanalysts almost invariably ignore or fail to seek.

Wolfgang and Ferracuti discuss a favorite psychoanalytic interpretation: that homicide is equal to suicide because the murderer unconsciously equates his victim with himself in his unconscious mind. They note that no factual evidence exists to back up this interpretation. In discussing psychoanalytic theory in general, they conclude that the analytic views of murder are based on unproven assumptions and that these assumptions are rooted in vague and obscure interpretations. They also note that psychoanalytic reports are rampant with unconfirmable statements, with tautologies, and with an almost total disregard for observable sociological factors.

M. Rivera Silva gives a general Freudian explanation of crime, including such acts as homicide. He maintains that criminality is not primarily a violation of the social system or even a symbolic act but that it originates in the pleasure principle. Because the id is continually inhibited by society in its attempts to gain satisfaction, it finally reaches a point where it rebels with violence. Thus, crime "is the vengeance of the id against the superego, to which it has sacrificed itself without profit."

The first serious objection to this kind of Freudian thinking is that it invents psychical entities, such as the id, and then reifies them and assumes that they really exist in their own right and that they have the intrinsic power to move their possessors to action. It may well be that human beings have conscious and unconscious drives for pleasure-thinking and that these drives tend to prejudice their thinking and behavior; but it is not the individual's id that truly compels him to act: There is no actual separate part of him —whether it be id, ego, or superego—which makes him do anything. He, as a total organism, has many different aspects; and when he finally behaves in any definite manner, he somehow considers, compromises, and coordinates these aspects—on the basis of various types of evidence about himself and the world which he has, or thinks he has, available.

Even if we more operationally define an individual's id as a combination of many different pleasure-seeking (or, perhaps more accurately, stimulation-seeking) impulses, the fact remains that he basically controls these impulses rather than that they control him. For the most hardened and antisocial criminal rarely urinates in the street, no matter how painful it is to control himself and how pleasurable it would be for him to empty his bladder. So, although the individual's primary pleasure-seeking and pain-avoiding impulses importantly bias and influence his thinking and his behavior, they are largely kept in line by his other values and goals—which, even though they are secondary pleasure-seeking and pain-avoiding processes, are also very important to him. In fact, as a great deal of experimental psychological evidence has shown, man's secondary reinforcers, or his value systems, are usually more influential in his conditioning than are his primary processes.

Therefore, it is not the id which rebels with violence after it has been continually inhibited by society in its attempt to gain satisfaction; but it is sometimes the individual himself who finally decides that inhibiting himself is not worth it and that therefore he'd better resort to crime. He may come to this conclusion vaguely and unconsciously rather than explicitly and consciously; but it is still he, and not his id, which does the deciding for him. In the usual Freudian terms, it would be his ego that decides that his id has been too squelched and that therefore its demands should be more heeded.

As for the id gaining vengeance against the superego, to which it has sacrificed itself without profit, this is more Freudian mumbo-jumbo. For even if the individual's primary drives—for example, his sex drive—suffer because his superego supposedly tells him to curtail them, *he* as a whole person, has *not* sacrificed himself without profit. He thereby saves sexual energy, keeps himself from being disappointed, has more time to devote to other pursuits, refrains from getting into social difficulties, saves money that he probably would have spent on his sexual pleasures, frees himself from some amount of guilt, and otherwise derives a number of specific satisfactions or avoidances of pain.

What Rivera Silva could have far more trenchantly pointed

out, without the Freudian concepts, is that the individual, when he lives in any social group, obviously has to sacrifice some of his primary pleasures in order to get along satisfactorily in that group. If he is a mature person—meaning, if he thinks clearly and has a rational philosophy of life—he calmly (though perhaps reluctantly) accepts this sacrifice for the social gains that he obtains thereby: He gives some concerted thought and action to minimizing the sacrifice and maximizing the gains. If he is an immature person, and runs his life by a philosophy of short-range rather than long-range hedonism, then he angrily rebels against the limitations of his society and childishly insists on getting something for nothing. He thus drives himself into crime in general and sometimes into homicide in particular. Again, it is not his id which drives him to seek vengeance against his superego. It is his foolish, demanding, and whining values, which refuse to keep effectuating a reasonable compromise between his primary urges for pleasure and his secondary desires for sensible group living. It is these values which psychoanalysis keeps unscientifically ignoring or de-emphasizing, because of its obsession with semimythical entities called the id, ego, and superego.

Joseph Belberg constructs a general theory of crime in which he employs several psychoanalytic hypotheses. He emphasizes that, instead of crime leading to guilt, the latter may really cause the former. Because of his castration complex and his consequent consciousness of guilt, and because he acquires passive attitudes with respect to his erotic life and the sexual object, the individual develops the ambivalent situation of sadomasochism. If his masochism prevails, he may become suicidal; if his sadism prevails, homicidal. He may also become homicidal out of love or out of love converted to hate. In any event, his guilty self-accusations cause him to seek punishment—and this search may lead him to further crimes. "Antisocial types result according to the degree of prolongation of oral or anal stages of development."

As usual, Belberg seems to mix psychological sense with psychoanalytic nonsense in his theorizing. He assumes that human guilt is largely attributable to the child's castration complex. Actually the reverse seems to be true. For, when a youngster thinks his parents are going to castrate him, he usually does so because he is already guilty about something that he has done—such as masturbating, lusting after his mother, resenting his father, or some other "bad" activity—and he believes that he is going to be severely punished, perhaps castrated, for such an activity.

But once the individual does make himself severely guilty, for any reason whatever, it is quite possible, as Belberg points out, that his guilt will drive him to crime. For if he is excessively guilty, he may (1) seek out criminal activities for which he will be blamed and punished; (2) become so absorbed in condemning himself that he fails at normal tasks and is consequently encouraged to "succeed" at abnormal ones, such as criminal activities; (3) believe he is not worthy of friendship with respectable members of his peer group and hence gravitate to associating with delinquents or criminals; and (4) become convinced that he is only capable of performing "bad" deeds and hence compulsively continue to perform them.

Belberg accurately perceives that guilt or self-condemnation is the crux of much antisocial activity and that it often (though hardly always) causes rather than results from such behavior. Sticking orthodoxly to Freudian positions, he then muddies his theory with irrelevant ideas about castration complexes and prolongation of oral or anal stages of development. Because Freudians tend, without empirical confirmation, to *define* orality as passivity or masochism and anality as sadism, Belberg drags in these obfuscating concepts to "explain" adult behavior and thereby leads himself and his readers up the garden path.

D. Levinson also emphasizes the theory of "criminality from a sense of guilt." He takes off from Freud's essay, "Some Character Types Met in Psychoanalysis," in which Freud describes a variety of guilt-laden personalities. One of these types is the "criminal from a sense of guilt"—that is, the individual who commits a criminal act in order to be caught and punished. According to Freud, this punishment is sought as a means of alleviating intense guilt feelings relating to Oedipal wishes which exist prior to the criminal episode.

Levinson tests Freud's hypothesis with case material and Thematic Apperception Test interpretations obtained from Will, a young thief who committed his robberies in such a way as to insure his capture and who felt a sense of relief when he was incarcerated. According to Levinson's analysis, the primary theme of Will's Thematic Apperception Test tells of his yearning for a good woman (supposedly his mother) who turns instead to a respectable and powerful but essentially immoral rival (presumably his father).

This kind of research into the validity of Freudian theory is shaky because it relies on the very kind of psychoanalytic interpretation which the research is ostensibly trying to validate. Thus, Will's making up a story, in his Thematic Apperception Test responses, about his yearning for a good woman who turns instead to a respectable and powerful but essentially immoral rival may, and probably does, have little to do with his mother and father. Our stories and movies are constantly full of exactly this kind of theme; and there is hardly a single young male who reasonably often does not wish that he could win an attractive woman but who is afraid that some other male, who is more powerful and ruthless than he, will come along to take this woman away from him. Would Levinson, if he were not highly prejudiced in favor of psychoanalytic interpretations in the first place, ever seriously think of translating the woman Will desired into his mother and the man he lost her to into his father?

Assuming that Will did hate his father, lust after his mother, and feel guilty for his Oedipal feelings, we still would have to ask: *Why* did he make such a big issue of such a common occurrence? According to Freudian theory, virtually every young male has a similar Oedipus complex; yet, obviously, very few of these males feel so guilty as to keep punishing themselves, for virtually the rest of their lives, for the guilt consequent to this complex.

Levinson's reply would probably be that in Will's case his father actually did commit suicide when he was sixteen years old—and he somehow blamed himself for this suicide and felt guilty about it. Possibly so. But several other hypotheses come to mind: (1) Will was ashamed to have come from a family where his father committed the socially disapproved act of suicide and consequently felt like a worthless individual, who deserved to be punished subsequently for having such a father. (2) Will, without ever having seriously lusted after his mother, and without having hated his father, blamed himself for not treating his father well enough when he was alive or not seeing that he was disturbed before his suicide and doing something to help him. (3) Will, as a highly sexed adolescent, lusted after his mother *after* his father's death, when he was living alone with her, and condemned himself for *this* desire. (4) Because his father was seriously disturbed and took his own life, Will inherited a tendency to be depressed, anxious, and guilty; and because his father and probably his mother as well were so preoccupied with their own problems, they had no time or energy to devote to helping Will mature and overcome his self-deprecating tendency. (5) Will's guilt, which possibly drove him to commit crimes for which he would be punished, had little to do with either his father or his mother, or his relations with them, but was a result of his nonfamilial unrealistic demands on himself, which he could not possibly fulfill, and for which he berated himself.

As Levinson notes in the conclusion of his paper, the extent to which his hypotheses about Will and his crime-creating guilt feelings are valid "can be determined only by large-scale research." True! Let us hope that this kind of research, when it is finally done, will test a good many nonpsychoanalytic as well as analytic theories about the interrelationship between guilt and crime.

William Easson and Richard Steinhilber (quoted by Bruce Porter) see murderers as the offspring of a pair of Freudian Fagins who unconsciously use their children to vent their own aggression. Consequently, the child's act of murder becomes largely the carrying out of his parents' inner-felt hostility. This is certainly a far-fetched hypothesis! Several counter-arguments easily come to mind: (1) Obviously, the parents of many murderers are not terribly hostile, though they are frequently disturbed in other ways. (2) When they are exceptionally aggressive, their violence may be quite consciously communicated to their children rather than (a) unconsciously felt by the parents and then (b) unconsciously communicated to the children. (3) If parents have unusual disturbances, as they sometimes do, these disturbances may be transmitted to their children through inherited predisposition as well as an environmental basis, and hypotheses about unconscious Faginism are then inaccurate. (4) Of the millions (or billions!) of parents who communicate both conscious and unconscious hostility to their children, obviously only an infinitesimal number help these offspring to commit murder. Why don't the vast majority of such parents have murdering children? (5) Both the conscious and unconscious hostility feelings of parents may indeed importantly contribute, in some instances, to their children's feeling that they have a right to kill when they desire to do so. But instead of talking, in a direct and honest manner, about these fairly clearcut possibilities, Easson and Steinhilber would much rather do the usual psychoanalytic thing of finding fiendishly clever, much more indirect hypotheses to "explain" children's murdering—and they thereby posit assumptions for which the collection of validating evidence is virtually impossible to achieve.

One of the latest psychoanalytic theories of criminal violence is propounded by David Abrahamsen in *Our Violent Society,* who in a typical dogmatic manner states: "When a man commits a violent crime, it is invariably founded on his unconscious feeling that he must show his mother that he is not insignificant and is able to take revenge upon her for rejecting him." This theory, like practically all psychoanalytic theories before it, is not likely to find any empirical backing, since it exaggeratedly posits (1) that all committers of violent crimes have been seriously rejected by their mothers; (2) that every one of them bitterly resents this rejection; (3) that they are invariably unconscious of their resentful feelings; (4) that they are always intent on proving to their hated mothers how significant they are; and (5) that they all assume that violently attacking or killing other individuals will conclusively prove their significance.

If a single criminal assaulter or murderer fails to fall into these five hypothesized behaviors, Abrahamsen's theory falls apart at the seams. Similarly, virtually all psychoanalytic theories of violent criminality make impossible demands on our credulity and are stated in a manner that almost renders certain their ultimate discrediting.

Chapter 5

Psychological Theories of Murder

A good many psychological, as opposed to psychoanalytical, theories of murder have been set forth in the professional literature. One of the main hypotheses is that murderers frequently have strong feelings of inadequacy or weakness, and that their killings to some degree are compensatory actions to cover these inadequacy feelings and to prove to themselves and the world how worthwhile and strong they truly are.

Tumlirz examined a murderess and felt that her main reason for killing her younger brother and his friend was her feelings of inferiority, to which the younger brother had contributed.

Hellwig found similarly that personality weakness was the principal cause of a thirty-year-old factory worker strangling his wife while she slept. According to the murderer and other reliable witnesses, the wife was a termagant who, by her continual nagging, reproaches, and argumentativeness, made her husband's life miserable. The real cause of the murder, Hellwig insists, was not merely this husband's frustration and annoyance in regard to his wife, but the fact that he himself weakly failed to end the marriage. Goaded by his feelings of inadequacy for allowing this poor relationship to continue, he guiltily and angrily overreacted by killing his spouse.

The other side of this coin of deep-seated feelings of inadequacy is frequently childish grandiosity. Human beings tend to feel inadequate in the first place because they demand that they perform very well in many or most of their life performances; and, once they begin to hate themselves for not being superachieving, they inanely require of themselves even more outstanding performances to "prove" that they are not the worthless individuals they think they are. Many murderers, MacDonald contends, are motivated by the Superman complex, which is related to the philosophy of Friedrich Nietzsche.

Nietzsche, MacDonald notes, "substituted violence for love, evil for good. The masses should be subordinated to Siegfried, the biologically superior man, who tramples under foot the servile herd of the weak, degenerate, and poor in spirit. Milk is for babes, the strong man should be soaked in *blood* and alcohol. 'Evil is man's best strength. Man should be trained for war and women for the recreation of the warrior. All else is folly.' "

A considerable number of murderers, MacDonald holds, uphold these Nietzschean ethical concepts and grandiosely strive for self-inflation at the expense of others. Not only do individual slayers swear by this kind of credo, but on the larger, political scene several mass ideologies—such as those of the Nazis and the nationalistic Communists—promulgate the doctrine that human beings should strive for a superhuman ideal and should consider humanitarianism and democracy execrable. Nazis and fascists in particular stand for violence, racial purity, and world domination; and such ideals not only permit but often encourage the murder of their opponents.

MacDonald's theory that murderers are influenced by the superman ideal is probably not entirely invalid, but it begs the important question: Why do so many individuals take this ideal so seriously? The Nazis, let us remember, were born and reared in a country that for a generation and a half before their rise had been one of the most democratic and socialistic nations the world has ever known; and the Italian fascists before them were brought up largely under the influence of social democracy and working-class syndicalism. Most murderers, moreover, who consciously follow the superman philosophy, have been raised—as was Nietzsche himself—in good Christian homes and were not taught this creed at home or in school.

The answer would seem to be that man is a dualistic rather than a monolithic animal and that he can be a group-centered, rather nauseating conformist on the one hand, and a rebellious anti-Christlike character on the other. Just because he is meek and partially masochistic, he has Walter Mitty-like tendencies to envision himself as superstrong and sadistic. He has difficulty maintaining a moderate, middle-of-the-road policy in many of his affairs, and tends to go from one extreme to another (as we noted earlier). Consequently, when he acts weakly and ingratiatingly and notes that this is undesirable behavior, he tends to jump, at least temporarily, to the other side of the continuum, and become hostile. He wrongly interprets his hostility as strength—when it is really another form of intolerance, hence weakness.

The main point is that the superman or superhostile ideal which MacDonald claims is so influential on many murderers is a philosophy to which many or most human beings naturally and easily subscribe. It is not merely a fiendish idea promulgated by a few Nietzsches, whose powerful writings drill it into the heads of a handful of susceptible followers. It is one of the most common notions humans are prone to believe; and it fairly consistently influences individual and group behavior. It not only is one of the main sources of murderous ideation, but it is an easily available rationalization which is used by many individuals who are hostile and violent for other conscious or unconscious reasons. Thus, a man can be insanely jealous of his wife, because he feels others would think him a fool if she were unfaithful to him; and he may actually kill her to avoid being cuckolded. He may then emphasize in his mind her "low" traits, and those of her potential or actual lover, and feel justified and "strong" about his murderous act.

This illustration may be used as a logical introduction to another theory of murder—that of Mowat, who wrote a book entitled *Morbid Jealousy and Murder.* He studied 110 murderers and attempted murderers who were considered insane and were in an English mental hospital; found that 12 percent of these individuals killed their victims out of morbid jealousy; and concluded that probably no other single delusion is associated with so many deaths from suicide and homicide.

Mowat found a fairly consistent pattern in the jealous reactions of the murderers whom he studied. At the time of his marriage, the average slayer of this type is fairly free of jealousy; but after he has been married for about six years, he begins to feel that his wife no longer cares for him. He becomes convinced, although there may be no evidence to sustain his conviction, that she is being unfaithful to him; and, once he "sees" this, he "finds" confirmatory data. He becomes so deluded that he misinterprets much of the trivia of everyday life and sees in it unmistakable "signs" of her infidelity. He accuses her of adultery and often attempts to extract confessions from her to the accompaniment of high-pitched altercations and sometimes blows. He takes to spying on his wife, to make sure that what he "knows" is true. In the course of an angry scene, he may attack his wife and threaten to kill her; consequently, she often leaves him, but returns home after a short time.

"His false ideas spread," Mowat reports. "He may think he must have caught venereal disease from his promiscuous partner, he may believe he is not the father of his children, or feel that his wife is trying to poison him. He may become hallucinated. The jealous man may contemplate suicide.

"At the age of 47, having suffered his delusions for four and a half years, he kills his wife in anger, suddenly, crudely, and violently with his bare hands or by clubbing her to death. He decides to kill himself but, failing in his resolution or attempt, finds himself confessing to the murder of his wife."

Mowat's fairly typical murderer is probably suffering from severe underlying or overt feelings of inadequacy. He becomes insanely jealous because he cannot bear to lose the full attention of his wife—who, after several years of marriage, may be too preoccupied with family affairs or may have other reasons for not being completely devoted to him. Falsely thinking he not only has failed to keep her love for him alive but that he is a bad person for having failed, he desperately looks around for "proof" of his rottenness—and about the worst thing he can think of is that his wife is having affairs with other men and that everyone in his community knows and despises him because of it.

This murderer, in other words, does what so many paranoid individuals do: lowers himself in his own eyes and then projects his poor image of himself onto others. He is certain they see him as he does. Since he is self-persecutory, his paranoid projection convinces him that others, notably his wife and her lovers, are persecuting him too. The main quick, dramatic "solutions" that he can think of are (1) commit suicide and (2) kill his wife. Sometimes he chooses one of these actions and sometimes he chooses both.

This kind of individual, certainly at the time that he commits murder, is psychotic; and an intensive study of his life history will almost always show psychotic tendencies during childhood and adolescence, although he may then have been able to keep them in check and to refrain from doing anything of a spectacularly self-destructive nature. There are some authorities, however, who insist that, even when a murderer is in the throes of a psychotic episode at the time he commits his crime, he may be basically a healthy individual who has no prior history of severe disturbance.

Fredric Wertham, in *Dark Legend* and *The Show of Violence,* has offered a theory of catathymic crisis as the cause for murder. By catathymic crisis he means that an individual undergoes extremely difficult experiences and under the impact of emotional complexes connected with these experiences he suffers an aberration of reasoning which leads him to an outbreak of violence. He takes care to differentiate individuals in this category from schizophrenics and psychopaths, both of whom he considers to be largely incurable. Where such individuals almost continually get into trouble, including the commission of crimes, the person who undergoes a catathymic crisis only expresses a pattern of violence when this appears to him, at the height of his crisis, as the only way out. Otherwise, he may be symptom-free. Where schizophrenic patients frequently deteriorate, catathymics, according to Wertham, do not.

In Wertham's words, a catathymic crisis is "a circumscribed mental disorder, psychologically determined, nonhereditary, without physical manifestations, and not necessarily occurring in a psychopathic constitution. Its central manifestation consists in the development of the idea that a violent act—against another person or against oneself—is the only solution to a profound emotional conflict whose real nature remains below the threshold of consciousness of the patient."

Wertham postulates five distinct stages of the catathymic crisis:

"1. The stage of initial thinking disorders which follows the original precipitating circumstances.

"2. The stage of the crystallization of a plan, when the idea of a violent act emerges into consciousness.

"3. The stage of extreme tension culminating in the violent crisis in which a violent act against oneself or others is attempted or carried out.

"4. The stage of superficial normality beginning with a period of lifting of tension and calmness immediately after the violent act.

"5. The stage of insight and recovery with the re-establishment of an inner equilibrium."

The weakest parts of his hypothesis are (1) that he defines the catathymic crisis as a completely nonhereditary disorder and (2) that he lays the inception of stage one, the initial thinking disorder, solely at the door of the original precipitating circumstances. These notions of Wertham are probably exaggerated, for two reasons:

First, it is unlikely that any serious personality disorder has no hereditary elements. Man is born the kind of animal who easily becomes emotionally aberrated during his lifetime; and if he were some other kind of creature—say, a Venusian or a Neptuneian—it is probable that he would not as easily pick up the deep-seated anxieties and hostilities that almost all of us are prone to feel. Specific men, moreover, seem to differ widely in their hereditary predispositions. Just as they range enormously in their tendencies to be short or tall, blue- or brown-eyed, rapid reactors or slow movers, there is a high likelihood that they range just as widely in their tendencies to become angry at their fellowmen and to "solve" crisis situations by resorting to murder. Although many or even most of us might commit homicide if the circumstances of our lives were sufficiently crisis-laden, there is no evidence that all of us would do so and there is some evidence that some of us are much more biologically prone to do so than are others.

Second, some of the cases of catathymic crisis that Wertham presents in his writings are not quite convincing. The main example he cites, Robert Irwin, who murdered three people whom he had nothing against while he was waiting to kill another woman (again, for no really good reason), was so *generally* aberrated for practically all his life that it is unrealistic to think of his murderous deeds as merely being the result of a specific *crisis.* Irwin had been seen by Wertham for a good many psychoanalytic sessions because he had literally tried to cut off his own penis several years before his murders.

As a result of information garnered from his analytic sessions and various other investigations of Irwin's life, Wertham reported the following facts:

1. Irwin's mother was a woman with a deep-seated "narrow-minded emotional religiosity" who, in spite of the fact that she was a "well-educated college-trained woman of a very good Southern Family," only managed to work at irregular jobs after she was deserted by her husband, and frequently was a washerwoman, a scrubwoman, or an operator in a shirtwaist factory.

2. His older brothers had a long history of institutionalization for many delinquencies and crimes of increasing severity and finally "landed in jails and penitentiaries for sentences running to many years."

3. Irwin was very sensitive as a child, was mortally afraid of being called a "sissy," and reported, "I could never do anything unless I had some repressed emotions, and as soon as I had a repressed emotion I could knock out anybody."

4. He had a history of several attachments to women older than himself who were often married; several of them were landladies; and he tended to feel quite ashamed of his relations with them.

5. He was frequently obsessed with making "a journey into his own mind in the hope that it would eventually lead him to the 'universal mind,' the central radio station that would permit him to tune in with everything."

6. He became convinced that human energies are commonly sacrificed to the task of reproduction; and he therefore devised "the idea which came to his mind as a definite plan: to cut off his penis in order to 'bottle up his sexual energy' for higher purposes." He consequently broke off his relations with his fiancée, and tried

to cut off his penis with a razor blade, landing in a mental hospital for the first of several times.

7. He was frequently seriously depressed and often thought of committing suicide. At one time, after he had broken with his fiancée, he stated, "I was living with a nice old lady in Brooklyn and she was just like a mother to me. I was only there two weeks and I was so miserable and so sick that I thought I would commit suicide. But I wasn't going to kill myself. I thought I would kill her and go to the electric chair."

8. About his relations with his mother, he reported: "My mother is a wonderful woman. I realize for the first time in my life not only that I don't love my mother, but that I've hated her all my life. I think there was a very, very deep dislike of her. But I never knew anything about it."

9. When first committed to a mental hospital because of his self-emasculating attempt, he absconded after six months. "In a way he had no objection to being there, but he felt too restricted."

10. Says Wertham: "I kept in touch with him and his case through contacts with one of the doctors in the hospital where he was, through letters from him, and through a letter from the superintendent informing me that there was little change in his condition and that their diagnosis was dementia praecox, hebephrenic type. This is about the most serious diagnosis that can be made of a young mental patient."

11. After being in the mental hospital a little over a year, Irwin was discharged; but seven months later he was not doing well and on Wertham's advice he returned to the hospital and stayed there for another two years. He attended theological school for a while, but got into a violent fight with a student and was dismissed from the university.

12. The night he murdered three people against whom he had no grudge, he had the delusion that accusing eyes, like the ghost of Hamlet's father in the closet scene, were on him.

13. When Wertham interviewed him, awaiting trial for murder in the Tombs prison in New York, Irwin said, with tears running down his cheeks: "They say I am a menace. I'm no menace to them. They are a menace to me. I could get along. I proved that

in Cleveland. You know, I'm an unfortunate young fellow who tried to get on in the world and couldn't."

14. Although the lunacy commission of the State of New York found Irwin technically sane and able to stand trial for his crimes, the Committee on the Legal Aspects of Psychiatry later reported: "An interesting sequel of the [Irwin] case is that the district attorney, apparently convinced that the lunacy commission's report would not be sustained as a result of a trial, accepted a plea of guilty in the second degree, and that within about ten days of the prisoner's reception at Sing Sing he was found by the prison physician to be psychotic and was transferred to the state hospital for the criminal insane." Today, some thirty years later, he apparently is still incarcerated there.

15. Wertham reports: "Irwin also wanted acclaim. It was much more than the artist's desire for communication with a public. He wanted omniscience—and that, of course, means knowing more than all the others. He was willing to pay for that the largest price. Like the Nordic super-God Wotan who sacrificed one eye to get omniscience, he was willing to sacrifice his sex organ. After the murders he first thought of giving himself up to Walter Winchell, then gave himself up to a big newspaper chain and evidently enjoyed the proceedings. The price was life, either the electric chair or life imprisonment. He did not have to give himself up, for his chances of escape for a long time were excellent."

16. Dr. Wertham also tells us that Irwin had "a consuming drive for self-perfection. From the age of seventeen, Irwin was possessed by the idea that by mentally visualizing images of pictures he would acquire a degree of mastery over knowledge, art, and himself. To the technique of visualization he added later the practicing of concentration to the ticking of a metronome or clock. This technique of visualization, not entirely absurd in a very limited sphere of application but associated by him with impossible goals, had within it the germ of serious complications. It was closely related to his infantile attitude about his mother, shown by his fantasy of not returning home to her until he had attained this superior power and knowledge. . . . The whole idea of visualization as he conceived and practiced it crossed the line from normal to morbid thought, from belief to delusion."

Almost any professional person—and many intelligent laymen—would conclude that Irwin was schizophrenic and that even in his periods of remission he was acting in the borderline psychotic range. Quite stubbornly, however, Wertham sticks to his diagnosis of catathymic crisis—mainly for two reasons: (1) individuals like Irwin, he notes, do not deteriorate over the years as many schizophrenics do; and (2) they are amenable to psychotherapy, as many schizophrenics are not.

Actually, as Wertham himself implies, although many schizophrenics do deteriorate, *some* do not. And assuming that Irwin has not deteriorated over the years, he could easily be one of those in the latter rather than in the former category. Moreover, while Wertham's views on catathymic crisis were originally propounded in the late 1930's, when few schizophrenics were considered to be treatable or were actually treated by psychotherapy (partly because orthodox analytic methods, which were in vogue at that time, *are* contra-indicated in the treatment of most psychotics) later developments have led to much different theories and practices. John N. Rosen, Whitaker and Malone, Ronald Laing, and a host of other psychotherapists have begun to treat schizophrenics and other psychotics in recent years; and the case of a psychotic murderess who was treated with rational-emotive psychotherapy is included in a later chapter in this book.

Wertham's reasons for not classifying Robert Irwin and other murderers he has seen as psychotic are not valid; and his diagnosis of catathymic crisis is not definitive. It must be admitted, however, that even though the individuals whom he puts in this diagnostic category would seem to be more accurately labeled as borderline or outright psychotics, his diagnosis may not always be inaccurate. There may be a few murderers *not* generally or basically psychotic, who temporarily break down in conditions of extreme pressure and feel that homicide is the only way out of their state of tension. The fact that Wertham's examples, especially Irwin, are not very good ones does not conclusively prove that his concept of catathymic crisis is entirely invalid and that no one justifiably fits it.

Manfred Guttmacher presents a theory of murder that somewhat resembles Wertham's, in that he endorses Dr. Isaac Ray's distinction, first made in his *Treatise on the Medical Jurisprudence of Insanity,* between the behavior of the criminal murderer and the insane criminal, whom Ray designates as "the homicidal monomaniac." Guttmacher, on the basis of his many interviews with murderers, finds that what he calls the "normal murderer" or the "criminal murderer" is much more likely than the "psychotic murderer" to be drunk at the time of his crime, to be nonsuicidal following his slaying, and to take as his victim a person who is not a close relative.

Guttmacher's case for this distinction between "normal" and "psychotic" murderers is not very convincing: As one of his prime examples of the "normal" kind, he presents the case of Robert T., a twenty-one-year-old Negro who shot and killed in a fight a male Negro twice his age. Robert "was a very active truant" when he was a child. Later on, "He had a spotty work record, losing jobs because of absenteeism. The Navy kept him only eight weeks before discharging him. He gambled heavily and used both alcohol and marijuana. His temper was easily aroused, all arguments automatically ended in fights. When he was eighteen he was fined twenty-five dollars for fighting. . . . At nineteen he was sentenced to thirty days in jail because of a street fight in which many youths armed with knives participated. Two months later he robbed a white boy on the street of a small sum of money and was given a penal sentence of two years.

"Two weeks before the murder he and the victim had jointly purchased a bottle of liquor. The other man asserted that he was drinking more than his share and jerked the bottle from his mouth; a fight ensued. . . . Robert learned of a youth in his neighborhood who had paid a group of little children fifty cents for a pistol which they had found. He went to this youth and lied, insisting that the pistol was his, but magnanimously gave him fifty cents to reimburse him for what he had paid the children.

"For two weeks he carried the loaded pistol in his belt. Then one night he saw the other man on the street, walking with a man and a woman. He shifted the pistol from his belt to his pocket as they approached. He claims that the victim made a menacing gesture. He instantly fired one fatal shot and fled to his girlfriend's house, where he had been living.

"Robert was given a life sentence in the penitentiary. A recent inquiry revealed that in the nine years he has been there he has had eighteen disciplinary infractions, including an attempt to choke another inmate, striking an inmate on the head with a brick, and seven fist fights."

Perhaps Guttmacher is right in not considering Robert T. psychotic; but he is hardly an undisturbed individual. He appears to be a classic "psychopath," and most probably has all of his life been in the borderline psychotic range of behavior. If the full facts are determined in regard to Guttmacher's other "normal" murderers and Isaac Ray's "criminal" murderers, we think that it will almost always be found that they, too, may not be fully psychotic but that they are highly disturbed individuals.

E. Tanny, in an article on the "Psychiatric Study of Homicide," bases his conclusions on the observation of fifty-three murderers whom he saw during a period of ten years. He finds that most of these murderers (1) suffered parental violence as children, (2) were afflicted with a severe superego or conscience, and (3) experienced an altered state of consciousness just prior to their murderous acts. He also finds that almost all the murderers in his study were, just before they committed their crimes, dissociating or psychotic. He believes that some murderers are ego-syntonic—that is, they kill without disruption or distortion of their egos—but his data do not give much support for this theory.

Tanny concludes that "perpetrators of homicide seem to be afflicted with an 'overdeveloped superego.' . . . The observation is presented that they are overidentified with the expectations of the behavior appropriate to the middle-class status. Traditional middle-class values prohibit aggressive gratifications on a physical and verbal level. It appears that when these values are reinforced with violent child-rearing practices, the superego becomes a cruel and punitive master, intolerant of any overt expressions of aggression. . . . The function of the superego is to enforce behavior which is acceptable to society, but this very structure can contribute to unacceptable behavior like homicide. The function assigned to a system should not obscure the causal contribution of this system to paradoxical results. Freud pointed out this type of paradoxical phenomenon in the paper, 'Criminals from a Sense of Guilt.' "

Tanny relies on psychoanalytic thinking a little too much for our tastes; but his views contain a good element of validity and may be unanalytically restated as follows: It is probable that murderers frequently come from homes where they are treated violently and cruelly—partially because their parents, being themselves near-psychotic, easily make themselves angry, have low frustration tolerance for their children's wrongdoings, and consequently are overly quick to condemn and punish their offspring. Partly as a result of their innate tendencies to be highly blaming and violent, and partly because of their negative reactions to their harsh early environments, perpetrators of homicide are highly moralistic and tend to condemn themselves and others. Because of their self-castigation, they become highly disturbed and prone to states of panic. Because of their intolerance of others' wrongdoings, they build mild slights into enormous insults and take too seriously any actions directed at them that seem unjust. When a crisis occurs in their lives, and especially when they are in an altercation, they are more prone to resort to extreme violence than are other members of their community.

Thus, what Tanny (and many other Freudian-oriented writers) labels the "superego" is really the individual's propensity to condemn *both* himself and others when some important thing goes wrong in his life; and he acquires this double-edged tendency from his parents both biologically and sociologically. Having this self- and other-flagellating tendency, the individual can kill for a variety of "superego"-related reasons: for example, (1) because he underlyingly thinks of himself as a louse, and would rather project his "lousehood" onto another, and kill this other, than bear the onus of it himself; (2) because he thinks he's pretty worthless and desires, compensatorily, to show how "great" he is by committing some outstanding murderous deed or deeds; (3) because he thinks he is so low and incompetent that he cannot escape from a major life dilemma except by murdering; (4) because he directly and energetically condemns others for their "sins" and honestly thinks they should suffer death for them; (5) because he wants to become a "noble" and self-righteous avenger, and perhaps a suicide as well, and thereby to make up for his previously "sinful" life.

Another theory of murder that has some evidence to support it is that individuals who kill are afflicted with unusually low frustration tolerance; that they take the usual inconveniences of life much too seriously and convince themselves that they cannot stand them; and that once in a while they blow off steam so mightily that they actually kill the persons whom they believe are needlessly frustrating them. Ancona and Fontanes tested this theory by giving a projective test to a group of criminals, most of whom had committed murder. By stimulating their subjects' aggressive tendencies by having them view a stressful film, *Mondo Cane,* they found that the projected hostility, as measured by the test, increased when their subjects did not show external manifestations of hatred and did not subjectively feel hostile, and that they decreased when the subjects did openly display or feel hostility. They also found that the average index of projected hostility, measured on the group of inmates before the experiment, was lower than that found on a group of normal subjects. Their interpretation of these results was that, when an individual's ego is depleted of resources as a consequence of his having a symptomatic or character neurosis, and when he is subject to a good deal of frustration in the environment in which he resides, he tends to resort to violent behavior. In these conditions, he not only fails to learn by frustration and to fight against it in order to get what he wants out of life, he reacts primitively to this frustration by discharging his held-in feelings in an overt, muscular manner.

To some extent, this hypothesis that murderers have lower frustration tolerance than individuals less prone to violence is borne out by other evidence. J. R. Hurley and four fellow psychologists participating in a symposium on murder at the 1967 convention of the American Psychological Association tended to agree that murder is usually a family affair. Various other researchers have come to similar conclusions over the past decade. If this is true, then it may be guessed that people who live closely together in families frequently frustrate each other in many ways; and that individuals with low frustration tolerance cannot take—

or *think* they cannot take—this kind of steady intrafamilial frustration, that they make themselves terribly angry at their family members, and that they sometimes resort to murder, in order to express their extreme anger.

Somewhat similar confirmatory evidence comes from Marvin E. Wolfgang, who finds that the recent sharp rise in murders throughout the United States may be caused in part by the growing number of young adults and by the crowding of more poor people into the cities. It is a known fact that more young people are arrested for crimes of violence than any other age group. It is another fact that young adults make up a larger part of the population of our cities today than they did a few years ago. As to his theory relating to the poor, Wolfgang points out that from 1960 to 1966 there was a 24 percent increase in the number of nonwhite families living in the nation's crowded central cities; that fewer than 4 percent of these families have incomes of more than $10,000 annually; and that there was a 23 percent increase in murders in the first half of 1967 over the first half of 1966.

If Wolfgang is correct, and the correlation between the growing number of young adults and the sharp rise in murders is actually of a causal nature, this might also indicate a causal connection between murder and low frustration tolerance: since youths of eighteen to twenty—the age which he finds the peak years for crimes of violence—are likely to be less tolerant of frustration than are older individuals. If Dr. Wolfgang is correct about the relationship of crowding of the poor in our cities and murder, this again would tend to highlight the importance of low frustration tolerance; since crowding normally tends to increase the frustration of human beings, and a certain small percentage of people who feel that they can't stand such annoyance will erupt into dangerous physical violence, including murder.

The usual mistake made by proponents of the theory that frustration leads to aggression, and that aggression results in homicide, is their stressing of the near-inevitability of these connections. Certainly, most frustrated people sooner or later become angry; and surely some angry individuals display their hostility in the form of physical assaults on others. A lower animal or a young child has little choice about whether it is going to be enraged and whether it is going to resort to some form of violence when rage occurs. An adult has much more "free will" in this regard. Sensible adults can fairly easily choose *not* to be provoked to extreme anger—as millions prove almost every day as they work for nasty bosses or are subjected to the whims of dictatorial professors. And the great majority of individuals who have reached voting age can manage, even when they *feel* frustrated and angry about some injustice in their lives, to refrain from *displaying* their anger in the form of physical violence.

The theory, therefore, that prolonged or intense frustration itself leads to homicide has to be realistically modified. Although it may be statistically true, it really seems to mean that a certain small proportion of people who live under highly frustrating conditions are prone, probably for biological as well as environmental reasons, to take the inconveniences and injustices of their lives over-seriously, to convince themselves that they cannot stand what they don't like, and to agitate themselves into murderous rages. Even these highly susceptible individuals never kill *all* the people they would like to annihilate. Their everyday rages soon pass, and they decide that putting their opponents literally out of the way would not be wise or proper. But when such individuals are in continual contact with the people at whom they tend to be angry, they eventually may slay one or more of these people. That is probably why so many murders are family affairs or are committed against persons who are well known to the murderer. In these instances his hated objects are continually around and keep reminding him, by their undesired behavior toward him, that he *can't* stand them and that they *shouldn't* do the things he thinks it is not right for them to do.

We may therefore conceive of a certain kind of fairly common murder as being a function of frustrating circumstances *plus* repetitive contact by the murderer with people whom he considers to be unusually frustrating *plus* the murderer's inborn and acquired predisposition to define frustration as intolerable and to believe that he cannot stand it for any length of time. Given these three factors (and sometimes additional accidental or repetitive conditions) frustration may be said to lead to homicide in a significantly large number of instances. By itself, however, frustration clearly does not often result in murder. If it did, few of us would be very long for this world!

The theory that murderers in particular and criminals in general tend to be overly emotional and to be relatively free of normal restraints is promulgated by H. J. Eysenck in *Crime and Personality*—who, although he believes in hereditary tendencies toward criminality, presents a detailed learning-theory approach to psychopathy and violence. He theorizes that criminals basically have extroverted personalities and that their consciences are not properly conditioned. Says Eysenck: "We have now propounded our theory, and it is conscience which is, in the main, instrumental in making us behave in a normal and socially acceptable manner. That this conscience is the combination and culmination of a long process of conditioning and that failure on the part of the person to become conditioned is likely to be a prominent cause in his running afoul of the law and of the social mores generally."

Eysenck incorporates two types of learning in his theory: first, the theory of reinforcement, which "says simply that, in general those activities which are pleasurable and which are rewarded will be learned, whereas activities which are not pleasurable and which are not rewarded will not be learned"; and, second, conditioning that works by contiguity rather than by reinforcement: "Two stimuli are associated because they occur close together in time and space, not because they are rewarded in any sense of the term."

Eysenck feels that "it is the person who fails to develop conditioned moral and social responses, due to his low conditionability and his extroversion, who tends to become the psychopath and the criminal. . . . Extroverted people, because they condition poorly, will on the whole tend to have weaker consciences than introverts, who condition extremely well."

Although murderers are commonly seen by members of the public to be uncontrolled, overimpulsive individuals who cannot restrain themselves and who frequently resort to physical violence, a good many of them seem to fall into almost exactly the opposite category. Consequently some authorities theorize that murder is often causally connected with excessive inhibition. George Bach pointed out to a large audience at the American Psychological Association convention that murderers are often "very nice guys" who suppress their hostility toward others and who use "the punishment of death to take out their frustrations in trying to love or be loved." Dr. Bach found that inhibited or "supercovert" murderers outnumbered overtly aggressive murderers by three to one. Edwin I. McGargee, speaking at the same symposium on murder, reported that his studies indicated that many murders, especially those that take place within families, are committed by "chronically overcontrolled" persons.

For a certain type of murderer, the theory of overinhibitedness seems to have some validity. This kind of individual is usually shy and retiring, largely because he is afraid that, if he asserts himself, others will not approve of him. He harbors grudges underneath and may literally seethe with covert resentment. A good case in point is Leo Held, a thirty-nine-year-old chunky, baldish laboratory technician in a paper mill in Sugar Valley, Pennsylvania. Held seemed to be a quiet, peaceful citizen, devoted to his wife and four children, a member of the Sugar Valley School Board, a director of the Loganton Boy Scout troop, and an ardent deer hunter and woodsman. H. Bigart reports that "he was not a good mixer; he was retiring almost to the point of being shy. But on the school board he'd take a firm stand and be obstinate and inflexible."

In October, 1967, with no ostensible provocation, Held walked into the Hammermill Paper Company, a .45-caliber automatic pistol in one hand and a .38-caliber Magnum revolver in the other. Coldly and methodically he wiped out four of his fellow employees. He then sped toward his home town of Loganton, strode into the bedroom of his neighbors, the Floyd D. Quiggles, and opened fire, killing Mr. Quiggle instantly and critically wounding Mrs. Quiggle in the face and neck. Before Held was taken into custody on his own lawn, with his wrists and right thigh shattered by police bullets, he had killed six persons and wounded six others.

It is significant in Held's case—as in so many other instances where without any visible provocation an individual suddenly kills several other people—that he was clearly suffering some of the classic symptoms of paranoia, or a persecution complex. His neighbors reported that he was gnawed by suspicion that someone was out to get his job (though there was no foundation for this belief), and that he felt he had been passed over for promotion. He thought his telephone was being tapped, and he feuded with a neighbor over an inconsequential strip of boundary land. He thought neighbors burned leaves just to spite him, knowing he hated smoke, and that some of them, including those in his car pool, unfairly criticized his driving.

In a case like this, we have to suspect that it was not simply the murderer's shyness or inhibition that caused him to pen up his anger against others, and eventually to feel impelled to blow off steam in a bullet-filled tragedy. Rather, he seems to have been a generally disturbed—and quite likely schizoid—individual who (1) demanded that he be outstandingly accepted by others and that they be unusually considerate of him; (2) condemned himself severely when he did not measure up to his own or to other people's standards; (3) made himself so disturbed at the mere thought of his own inadequacies that he was unable to face his failings calmly and try to do something to correct them; (4) felt more comfortable in finding severe fault with others than finding it with himself; (5) projected his negative views of himself onto other people and believed that they saw him in the same dreadful light that he saw himself; and (6) finally felt that others were completely against him and were persecuting him, and that therefore he had to self-protectively kill them.

Something like this probably often happens when a shy, inhibited individual suddenly becomes a violent killer. He is inhibited because he feels, underneath, that he must have people's approval and is afraid that he is not going to get it if he acts outgoingly toward them. And when he does not get their approval and even gets their opposition or hostility, he thinks he can't stand this, that he is being destroyed, and that he must fight back in a deadly manner. He may also feel so weak and cowardly, because of his lifetime habit of suppressing his feelings and actions, that an act of violence, such as gun-shooting, gives him the illusion that he is strong and powerful and that he no longer will permit himself to be taken advantage of.

A lifetime pattern of inhibition is a symptom of emotional

disturbance. An individual who is sufficiently disturbed to act in this manner may easily think crookedly in other respects, may find "evidence" for others persecuting him when there is no evidence, and may convince himself that the only way out of his difficulties in relating to others is to kill some of these others, and sometimes himself as well. Therefore, it is not the inhibitedness itself which leads some people to break out into uninhibited acts of murder—although a long period of suppressing their feelings may contribute to their suddenly letting them out in aberrated ways. Rather, it is their generally irrational ideas which lie at the root of both their overinhibitions and their paranoid thinking or other misperceptions which impel them to murder. Usually a murderer is driven by complex motives to commit his homicidal deed; and in more ways than one he is likely to have irrational philosophies that underlie these motives and encourage him to kill.

This brings us to perhaps the most important psychological reasons for murder: psychosis in general and paranoid thinking in particular. In some primitive societies a man may murder his neighbor, family member, or enemy for fairly trivial reasons. In committing this deed he may not be particularly emotionally disturbed or aberrated. But among civilized peoples, where the taboo against murdering one's fellowman is strong and the penalty for doing so is great, it requires an enormous impetus for one deliberately and violently to kill another; and in a large proportion of actual murders, this impetus is provided by the slayer's being psychotically pushed, sometimes against his own will and sometimes when he is in a state of confusion and near-amnesia, to commit his deed.

It should be remembered in this connection that, even though most lower animals have pronounced aggressive drives and readily protect themselves in a combative manner, they rarely fight to kill. Compared to the rest of the animal kingdom, man may perform more senseless and needless murders than any other species. Consequently, it cannot unequivocally be said that homicide is an urge that has deep-seated biological underpinnings—though this *is* true of violence in general.

Murder, then, usually is accompanied by some *special* motivation; and that motivation is quite frequently psychotic. Even

Wertham, who so stoutly insists that murderers like Robert Irwin are not schizophrenic but that they suffer from some kind of "catathymic crisis," means by this term that they are at least temporarily insane at the time they commit their deeds and that they may, with sufficient stress, revert to insanity and commit similar homicidal or suicidal deeds. In Irwin's case, Wertham specifically testified to the New York State lunacy commission that he was psychotic at the time he murdered, that he had a fairly long history of similar psychotic episodes, and that therefore he should not be tried as an ordinary criminal. Although Wertham's testimony was not endorsed by the commission, there is little doubt that he was correct.

When murderers, such as Irwin, are not labeled psychotic by professionals or commissions who examine them, they are most frequently called "psychopaths" or "sociopaths." But even though the "psychopath" technically knows what he is doing, and is not entirely deranged, he is hardly sane. As John Bartlow Martin aptly describes him, "His emotions are out of kilter; his moral development, his 'character,' is deficient. He 'knows' the consequences of criminal acts, but is unable to 'feel' them. He never learns by experience. He never feels remorse or shame. He is never sorry he killed. He is the stranger among us. He rejects society and any obligation to it. He has never learned to wait. He lacks brakes. He is unpredictable. He is cold, remote; he cannot be reached by the chaplain's exhortations or the jailer's blows or the psychiatrist's ministrations. He is a wanderer. . . . He is impulsive, immature and unstable. He commits the daring, dangerous crimes—bank robbery, assault, rape, cop killing. He is the mob's hired killer. He commits the 'senseless' crimes. One man called him a 'rebel without a cause.' " H. Cleckley, noting these same traits twenty years before Martin incisively described them, pointed out that the "psychopath" is very close, in many ways, to the schizophrenic individual with dulled or flat affect, and that he is basically psychotic.

Our experience leads us to concur strongly with Cleckley. One of us (Albert Ellis) was Chief Psychologist of the New Jersey State Diagnostic Center and then Chief Psychologist of the New

Jersey Department of Institutions and Agencies for several years, and in these capacities interviewed, tested, and treated scores of "psychopaths" who had engaged in a wide variety of sexual and nonsexual crimes, and also interviewed several murderers who were in the death house at Trenton State Prison and several women who had killed their own children, who were incarcerated in the New Jersey State Prison for Women. The other of us (John M. Gullo) was Senior Psychologist at the Jacksonville (Illinois) State Hospital for several years and also interviewed, tested, and treated a good many "psychopaths," including murderers, who were incarcerated as a result of their criminal behavior. We find that practically all these individuals whom we examined intensively were at least borderline psychotics and that a high proportion of them were outright psychotic. Although they were not completely insane, in the sense that they could not get along in society or take care of themselves effectively, they almost always were seriously out of contact with reality in some ways, had a good deal of the kind of "cognitive slippage" which Paul Meehl finds so typical of schizophrenics, and kept getting into one social scrape after another, even though apprehended for some crime and incarcerated for it.

Our reading of the case histories of murderers whom we have not personally encountered almost invariably leads us to the same conclusion. Whenever sufficient material is given on the murderer's background, it is consistently found that (1) his upbringing, particularly in relation to his being treated kindly by his parents and his being emotionally close to them and to his other family members, left much to be desired; and (2) from an early age, he acted peculiarly, especially in his interpersonal relations with others, and began to get into some kind of school, social, or vocational difficulties.

This is particularly true of those who become multiple or mass murderers. Although multiple murder is rare compared to single homicide, the tendency to commit it is more common than is apparent from published statistics. In many instances of simple murder, the slayer tries to kill two or more victims but only partially succeeds. In bank robberies, the robbers time and again shoot two or three bank employees or customers, but only one of them dies. A great many killers, once they have committed one murder, shoot it out with the police officers who are trying to capture them; and only because of their bad aim or other fortunate circumstances are they captured or slain before they become multiple murderers. Still other individuals go out with the strong intent of killing two or more of their relatives, friends, or associates but get into so much difficulty after the first attempt (which itself may not succeed) that they never get around to becoming the mass murderer that they intended. A good many other persons (such as those who murder their mates) seem really to have killed more people during their lives; but, after they are apprehended for one slaying, clearcut evidence cannot be found linking them with previous ones. Still other mass murderers may never be caught at all, so that we have no real knowledge of their deeds (as in the case of paid gangland killers, most of whom seem never to be caught or convicted).

Thus, actual and would-be multiple murderers are probably much more common than the newspaper reports and court convictions indicate. When such murderers are caught and examined, they almost always seem to be near-psychotic or outright psychotic. Many of them, such as Howard Unruh, who in 1949 went out on the streets of Camden, New Jersey, and slaughtered thirteen strangers, are quickly judged to be paranoid schizophrenics and are either not tried for their crimes or are tried and placed in mental hospitals instead of prisons. But most of them, because of the peculiarities of our law, are judged sane enough to be tried and, when convicted, are given long prison sentences or executed.

Chapter 6

Biological and Physical Theories of Murder

Many psychological, sociological, and anthropological authorities have claimed that criminal behavior in general and homicidal behavior in particular have distinct biological roots, and that violent criminals are born rather than made. Cesare Lombroso, for example, who was a professor of psychiatry at Pavia and who later became professor of criminal anthropology at Turin, held that a criminal represents a distinct anthropological type, that he has definite physical and mental stigmata, and that his criminal behavior is a product of heredity, atavism, and degeneracy.

Ernest Hooten studied fifteen thousand criminals and found them to be biologically inferior to noncriminals. William Sheldon and his associates discerned the quality of "primary criminality" in some of the boys they studied psychologically and somatically and suggested that additional biological researches may indicate that "delinquency may reside in the cellular morphogenotype." Eleanor and Sheldon Glueck used Sheldon's body-typing techniques in their study of five hundred delinquent and five hundred nondelinquent boys and found that these groups differed significantly in both body type and personality structure.

Hans J. Eysenck, one of the best-known British psychologists, has done a long series of studies which present some evidence that human personality traits are biologically based and that criminals tend to be extroverted and, therefore, relatively difficult to condition in usual ways. Consequently, he contends, they do not learn the ordinary socializing processes.

Professor Steven G. Vandenberg presented evidence to the Twelfth International Congress of Genetics at Tokyo that hostility may be inherited. He gave cartoons depicting frustrating situations to identical and nonidentical twins and asked them to select one of several possible reactions to describe their feelings. He found that identical twins were far more like each other in aggressive tendencies than the nonidentical pairs. This suggested that heredity was a significant factor in hostility.

Ashley Montagu reviews some of the most important recent evidence in regard to the theory that criminals have "bad genes." He first disposes of the old notions of Hooten, Sheldon, and Dugdale that criminality is inherited, and calls their ideas "quite unsound." He then summarizes the more scientific evidence that a man's genetic make-up may be responsible for his committing acts of violence, and points out the following findings in this regard:

1. In December, 1965, Patricia A. Jacobs and her colleagues at Western General Hospital in Edinburgh published a report on 197 mentally abnormal inmates undergoing treatment in a special security institution in Scotland, all of whom had dangerous, violent, or criminal propensities. They found that 3.5 percent of these individuals had XYY chromosomal constitutions—an incidence significantly higher than that found in a sample of normal individuals.

2. About a dozen reports since that time have confirmed the findings of Jacobs and her co-workers.

3. In France, during 1968, Daniel Hugon, who confessed to the murder of a prostitute and who attempted suicide, was found to be of XYY chromosomal constitution. Richard Speck, the convicted murderer of eight nurses in Chicago in 1966, also is reported to be an XYY.

Montagu comments on these findings: "It appears probable that the ordinary quantum of aggressiveness of a normal XY male is derived from his Y chromosome, and that the addition of another Y chromosome facilitates the development of aggressive behavior. . . . Most violent crimes are committed by chromosomally normal individuals. However, the high frequency with which individuals with XYY chromosomes commit crimes of violence leaves little doubt that in some cases the additional Y chromosome exerts a preponderantly powerful influence in the genesis of aggressive behavior."

Dr. Montagu is careful to point out that chromosomal deficiencies, when they exist, only endow the individual with a genetic *tendency* to be overaggressive, and that environmental factors are generally necessary to bring out these tendencies. He also notes that the XYY aberration may not be directly inherited but may arise primarily from nondisjunction of the sex chromosomes in completely normal parents. He concludes:

"Although we are in no position to control the genetic inheritance of an individual, we can do a great deal to change certain environmental conditions that may encourage the XYY individual to commit criminal acts. A society does not properly acquit itself of its responsibilities if it places the entire burden of caring for abnormal individuals upon the parents. What we are talking about here is not a program of eugenic control, but a program of social therapy. There is every reason to believe that if we can successfully develop effective methods of help for the aggressive XYY individual, then we will be moving in the right direction to control those social conditions that drive men to crime—regardless of their genotype."

J. E. Brody reports: "Recent studies indicate that a genetic abnormality that has been linked with criminality may occur in as many as one in 300 men. The abnormality, which has been found in nearly 4 percent of inmates in a Scottish maximum-security prison, is the presence of an extra Y chromosome in the men's genetic make-up. . . . If this incidence of one in 300 men holds for the United States at large, there could be as many as one-third of a million American males who are XYY's, according to Dr. Park S. Gerald, pediatrician at Harvard University, who presented a summary of the new findings. Adult XYY men who have been studied to date show a tendency toward tallness, acne, mental dullness and aggressive—sometimes violent—behavior. Several are convicted murderers."

Bartholomew also reviewed recent studies on the extra Y chromosome and criminal behavior, and noted the following:

1. Chromosomal-positive males are about five times more

frequently found in institutions for the mentally deficient than in the normal population, and about one-third of them are committed as a result of antisocial acts.

2. Casey and his associates found a high incidence of chromosomal-positive males in special institutions for male criminals. Casey and his associates also found an incidence of XYY in 24 percent of men who were mentally subnormal and who were detained because of antisocial acts, as compared to no examples of such a chromosome in "normal prisoners" and a "normal" population.

In evaluating these and other results, Bartholomew concludes: "The present position with regard to the incidence of the XYY constitution would appear to be that the highest figure so far found has been 24 percent in a highly selected population. . . . At this time one may say only that the present researches are interesting and exciting but there is need to guard against making unduly extravagant claims and resisting the tendency to confuse established fact with speculation. . . . Although L. S. Penrose commented that 'a human being is a physical entity with a chemical constitution ultimately determined genetically' it must be remembered that individuals with any type of chromosome constitution are born into a society, are educated and mature in a society where they experience stress and learn to cope or suffer as a result of these stresses."

Subsequent to writing his review, Bartholomew testified in the trial of Laurence E. Hannell, a twenty-one-year-old laborer who apparently stabbed a seventy-seven-year-old widow to death in her apartment in a Melbourne suburb. Partly because of Bartholomew's testimony, Hannell was acquitted on the ground that he was legally insane. In spite of Hannell's acquittal in Australia, a French jury convicted thirty-two-year-old Daniel Hugon of a self-confessed murder and sentenced him to seven years in prison. Distinguished geneticists, doctors, and psychiatrists testified to the jury that Hugon is an XYY individual who has an extra male, or Y, chromosome; but their testimony largely went unheeded.

Nonetheless, the facts of Hugon's trial showed that he was an abnormal individual and that his abnormality was in all probability related to his chromosome imbalance. L. Garrison tells us that, at the age of sixteen, "He made his first of several suicide attempts. By twenty-five he was judged to be an alcoholic. A drifter, he held a long string of menial jobs. Employers generally found him polite, shy and a good worker, but prone to nervous breakdowns. . . . He has twice attempted suicide in prison and his attorney argued that a long term would prove fatal. . . .

"The main burden of medical testimony was shared by Dr. Leo Derobert, professor of legal medicine and former president of the French National Association, and Prof. Jerome Lejuene, an authority on chromosome disorders. Professor Lejuene contended that 'the born criminal does not exist' but that those born with chromosome abnormalities have a thirty percent greater chance of becoming criminals than others. Everything about Hugon's life history, he said, indicated that he was doomed to be a 'sick man' from the moment of birth and that this hereditary affliction prevented him from exercising normal responsibility. Professor Lejuene suggested putting the defendant in a 'protected milieu.' Dr. Derobert added that, while there is no known cure for a chromosome imbalance, Hugon could be successfully restrained by tranquilizing drugs and could lead a normal productive life while in the custody of a guardian."

A very conservative *Report on the XYY Chromosomal Abnormality* from the National Institute of Mental Health points out that research has not yet established a definite causal link between chromosomal abnormality and deviant, criminal, or violent behavior, but that "the individual with an XYY chromosomal anomaly appears to incur some increased risk of developing behavioral problems, in comparison to XY [normal] males."

There have been various other studies and theories which attempt to link the commission of crime in general and homicide in particular to different kinds of biological or other physical influences. Thus, a somewhat novel theory of why men—or at least some men—kill is presented by H. Von Hentig, who makes a case for redheads in America being significantly more prone to gangsterism than nonredheads. Behind this seemingly physically based theory obviously lie important psychosociological considerations. For, if it were ever conclusively proved that red-headed individuals were more prone to become mobsters than those with differently colored hair, it would probably mean that in our society redheads are looked upon somewhat differently than are their fellows and that they consequently take a unique attitude toward themselves. It would be these socially promulgated and individually accepted attitudes that would tend to be at the source of the propensity of redheads to kill; and the color of their hair per se would probably have little to do with the case.

One theory of the physiology of murder that has not proven valid is the hypothesis tested by Pokarny and Mefford that violently disturbed people are pushed into homicidal or suicidal actions by geomagnetic storms caused by solar activity. Pokarny and Mefford correlated data obtained on 2,479 suicides, 2,017 homicides, and 4,953 psychiatric admissions to a Veterans Administration hospital with the occurrence of geomagnetic storms. They found: "The majority of comparisons showed no evidence of any relationship between the geomagnetic fluctations and suicide, homicide, and hospital admissions. Use of sets of random numbers yielded correlations with the human behavior variables as high as did any of the geomagnetic variables. It is concluded . . . that fluctuations do not influence psychiatrical hospital admissions, suicides, or homicides."

C. A. Mills claims that the number of suicides and homicides from 1924–28 shows definite time relationships to changes in weather as low-and-high-pressure centers approach and pass over. He believes it is probable that the wide shifts in pressure and temperature in North America play a significant role in emotional instability and the rising rate of psychosis. To our knowledge, his findings and conclusions have not been confirmed by other observers.

Clark M. Garber discussed Eskimo infanticide and concluded, after examining all the significant and valid reports that he could find on this practice, that it is a "blind biological response to the rigid economic factors" with which Eskimos are faced. Recently, however, the practice has been dying out or is clandestinely performed. This, Garber thinks, is due to the influence of the white man's civilization. It is doubtful whether Garber's hypothesis fully fits the facts of infanticide, since many cultures with rigid economic factors and low subsistence standards existed where infanticide was not practiced, and there is no reason to believe that the Eskimos alone (or members of other civilizations where infanticide has been frequently practiced) would have a unique "blind biological response" to economic stress.

The linkage of criminal and homicidal activity with specific brain injury or disease has been suggested by several investigators. G. H. Maria claimed that, in the commission of major crimes where the criminal had been diagnosed as having a psychiatric disorder, a high percentage of the criminals not only were schizophrenic and manic-depressive but also had cerebral deterioration. E. Podolsky studied two homicidal individuals in whom defective physiology of the hypothalamus and the surrounding regions of the brain was demonstrated. He concluded that it is "reasonable to assume that certain cases of homicide are due to anoxia of the cerebral area." A. E. Walker studied murders done by epileptics and felt that sometimes their acts resulted from an epileptic furor.

Vernon H. Mark and Frank R. Ervin raise the question of how many law violators guilty of murder, rape, and assault are afflicted with focal brain dysfunction. John N. Wilford cites Dr. Ervin's continuing studies of people who have recurring, obsessive urges to commit violent acts, and reports: "Dr. Ervin said that 28 percent of the 134 sociopaths he studied in detail had 'clear, unambiguous evidence of classic temporal lobe brain disease.' In addition, 25 percent, he said, had clinical histories similar to brain disease. The same pattern was observed in additional surveys at several prisons and other hospitals. . . . Of the 134 persons studied, 60 percent had been arrested for violent acts, and four had been arrested for homicide. Several said they were afraid to drive a car because of tendencies to use it as a weapon. But most of them directed their rages at members of their own family."

Temporary brain malfunctioning may be involved in murder, as indicated by the high correlation between drunkenness and homicide. Although alcohol is not a direct cause of criminal behavior, it seems to be frequently associated with crime—especially crimes of violence. This may be because certain centers of cerebral cortex, which normally inhibit anger and overimpulsive behavior, are relaxed or rendered inoperative by sufficient quantities of alcohol, thus making it easier for the individual to become enraged or to act out his underlying desires.

Wolfgang and Strohn studied the files of 588 cases of the Philadelphia Homicide squad to ascertain the relationship between alcohol and murder. They found that in 67 percent of the cases where a Negro was the offender, the individual was under the influence of alcohol at the time of committing his crime, and in 58 percent of the cases where the offender was white, overimbibing of alcohol had occurred. A. L. Porterfield obtained different results and found that chronic alcoholism is not highly correlated with the homicide rate. But J. C. Baker, studying American Indians living on a government reservation, found that all 36 Indians whose cases he investigated were under the influence of alcohol when they committed murder. Baker also discovered that most of the Indians he studied had a simple schizoid adjustment, with a previous alcoholic history and patterns of antisocial difficulties that were related to intoxication. Moreover, most of them continued a simple, isolated, withdrawn mode of living while they were imprisoned.

Baker's study points up the difficulty of looking for the causative factors in murder in either brain disease in general or alcoholic addiction in particular. There is good reason to believe that many brain-injured individuals, as well as a good percentage of those who are seriously under the influence of alcohol, commit more crimes, including more murders, than do non-brain-injured and nonintoxicated individuals. However, brain damage is often a concomitant of severe emotional disturbance; and alcoholism is also heavily associated with schizophrenia and other psychological disorders. The individual who is psychotic or in the borderline psychotic range of behavior frequently finds, by accident or by trial and error, that alcohol is one of the best and most available tranquilizers; and he may resort to it habitually. When, after he becomes alcoholic, he commits murder, it is difficult to say whether his basic tendency toward severe disturbance or his concomitant alcoholism is the "real" inciting force. Often, the two "causes" are inextricably combined and tend to reinforce each other.

Alcohol, like many other drugs and substances, acts differently on various individuals: Many persons become happy and peaceful when inebriated, others become depressed, and still others violent. M. Nash points out that among the Cantelense Indians, who are generally aroused easily into aggressive or hostile behavior, "I know of only one man in the hundreds of inebriated Cantelenses I have seen who does not normally become aggressive when his control mechanisms dissolve in alcohol. When drunk, men seek someone to brawl with, some object to pit themselves against, some wrong to redress, or commonly a domestic infraction which necessitates the beating of the wife."

Fredric Wertham, although a vigorous opponent of the thesis that human beings are strongly influenced by biological or hereditary factors to become violent and to commit homicidal acts, emphasizes the role of alcohol in criminal violence: "In contrast to our knowledge about accidents, the contribution of alcohol to acts of violence is still underestimated. It is often repeated that a man under the influence of alcohol will not do anything he would not do when sober. Clinical psychological studies tell a different story. Some people under the influence of alcohol will commit an act—especially a brutal act—which they would otherwise never do. . . . Often there is nothing seriously wrong with these individuals' superego, or conscience. The trouble is that conscience is soluble in alcohol. . . .

"In the now so frequent brutal juvenile violence, committed by individuals or gangs, alcohol is a very important though much over-looked factor. When Michael Farmer, a fifteen-year-old boy handicapped by infantile paralysis, was beaten, kicked, and stabbed to death in a Manhattan park by a group of boys, one of the boys said later, 'I didn't wanna hit him at first. Then I kicked him twice. He was laying on the ground looking up at us. I kicked him on the jaw or someplace. Then I kicked him in the stomach. . . . I stabbed him with the bread knife. You know, I was drunk, so I just stabbed him (giggling). He was screaming like a dog. He was screaming there. And then I took the knife out, and I told the other boys to run.' 'Drunk' and 'giggling' are the important words here."

Wertham also believes that alcohol plays an important part in many cases of the "battered child syndrome." In these cases, of which there are about ten thousand each year in the United States, children are found to have been abused by their parents and to have burns, wounds, ruptured internal organs, broken ribs, arms, and legs. More than half of the children so abused are under four years of age; and more than a quarter of them die of their injuries—although in few of these cases are the parents actually charged with homicide. Frequently, the child makes some kind of fuss when the mother or father is under the influence of alcohol, the parent reacts with rage, and a battering of the child ensues which leads to its serious injury or death.

Jordan Scher, a well-known American psychiatrist, has this to say about violent crime and alcohol: "If there is a drug of violence par excellence, it is alcohol. Alcohol is involved in 67 percent of all crimes of violence, 87 percent of stabbings, and apparently 40 to 50 percent of shootings, and at least 50 to 70 percent of these victims are friends or family, particularly spouses. Alcohol is also involved in 50 percent of automobile and plane accidents, producing 50,000 deaths annually and four times that number in morbidity or injury. It is also probably responsible, therefore, for 50 percent of the gun deaths and injuries."

H. Brill agrees that alcohol "is recognized as a disinhibiting, aggression-provoking substance that plays a role in some 60 percent of homicides either in the killer or the victim, an indication that when people drink together the stage may be set for murder." He also notes that "the barbiturates are less well known in this connection than is alcohol, but 'on the street' pentobarbital is considered even more likely to precipitate sudden violent behavior."

On the other hand, Brill points out that, although the public thinks that addictive and nonaddictive drugs similarly lead to aggression, the opposite is often true: "The contrasting effects of alcohol and opiates may be seen clinically in cases who alternate in dependence between alcohol and opiates. This shift is accompanied by a corresponding alternation between overt and dangerous aggression under the influence of alcohol and deep apathy with peaceful withdrawal while under the opiate. Other drugs seem to have a pacifying effect and produce anergia and loss of initiative. This occurs with the hallucinogens as a chronic effect after repeated use. In spite of statements to the contrary, heavy use of cannabis is described as having a similar effect. These drugs lower the drive to action, whether constructive or not. Paradoxical results occasionally occur when an acute paranoid episode may be precipitated. Cannabis has a direct short-term sedative effect which is probably different from the long-term tension reduction of the hallucinogens. The major stimulants are credited with a direct and acute effect on aggressive behavior, and abusers of these drugs have been implicated in more than their share of aggressive crime."

Contrary evidence about the use of marijuana and other psychedelic drugs comes from a study by Edwards, Bloom, and Cohen, who found that drug-dependent individuals tend to be significantly more hostile than those occasionally taking psychedelics. Such drug-dependent persons seemed to be predisposed to being hostile and were not toned down by their drug-taking. J. Black surveyed the use of amphetamines (or "speed") and reported: "Large doses create extreme suspiciousness and hyperactivity, which often combine to produce a hostile, belligerent temper."

Research on the effects of other drugs and chemicals on the production and reduction of anger is still in its infancy stage, but indications are that important results may be found. An investigation by Goodwin, Brodie, and Murphy of the use of the potent drug, L-DOPA, with depressed patients found that the majority of these individuals experienced increased anger when using it. It also caused a mild form of mania in depressed patients whose depressed mood remained unchanged. It is quite likely, in view of recent experiments with various drugs, that other substances will be found which augment or ameliorate feelings of anger.

Though heroin addicts are normally passive and unhostile when their habits are fed, they become notoriously aggressive when they are deprived and when they need money to finance their habit. All over the world, literally from New York to Hong Kong, there are innumerable reports of hard-core drug addicts turning to violence and murder in a frantic effort to maintain their addiction.

We have been examining, in this chapter, the important

effects of man's biology and physiology on his feelings of rage and on his expressions of violence; but we would also better mention some of the reverse effects: namely, the influence of his angry feelings on his physiological responses. There is considerable evidence that temporary or prolonged hostility has many physical effects on the average individual, some of which are beneficial—that is, arousing him to constructive action—and some of which are pernicious—that is, causing him to experience pain, malfunctioning, and disease. Thus, Donaldson points out that during anger and hostility the individual automatically shifts his functional organization to a pattern of heightened external adaptability, supported by heightened self-maintenance, heightened assimilation, and heightened excretion, with concomitant reductions in growth and reproduction. As a result of this shift in his ways of reacting, he is more likely to become prey to certain disease states, such as hypertension, peptic ulcer, irritable colon, diabetes mellitus, and other ailments. Some of these disease states may be viewed as a variant mode of vulnerability arising out of a weakening of the oversustained hyperfunctional state which is motivated by chronically sustained hostility. For reasons of physical health, as well as for individual and group stability, the study of the interrelationship between man's anger and his biological reactions would appear to be highly important.

To summarize the effect of biological factors on the creation of rage and the commission of violent crimes, including murder, we may say that although there is no conclusive evidence (as yet) that any specific biological deficiency or aberration, such as neurological hyper-irritability or some kind of brain defect, is an important etiological factor in this kind of antisocial behavior, there is impressive evidence that persistent criminals and murderers are usually seriously disturbed and that their disturbance is both biologically and environmentally caused. Many—perhaps most—of the people who kill their fellowmen seem to congenitally or genetically acquire the kind of temperament which makes it easy for them to think crookedly about themselves and the world, to believe that they absolutely cannot tolerate being thwarted by others, and consequently to have sporadic outbursts of extreme rage or paranoia in the course of which they slay someone. When these individuals' inborn temperamental leanings interact significantly with poor conditions of early upbringing and with special crises of their adult lives, they become criminally violent. It is likely that, if they were reared under ideal conditions and kept free from stressful circumstances during their lives, they would rarely get into serious difficulties. But it is also likely that some of them have a genius for *creating* troublesome living conditions and that they would tend to get into more than their share of trouble no matter how they were reared or in what kind of environment they resided.

Chapter 7

The Emotional Disturbance of Murderers

From the foregoing material on the emotional lives of various individuals who killed either one individual or two or more victims, it can be seen that indications of severe disturbance, often from early childhood onward, are common in murderers. We have combed the crime literature for detailed reports on most of the well-known murderers of the past century; and wherever we have found any appreciable amount of evidence about the psychological make-up of these slayers, it has invariably pointed in the direction of their being partly or fully psychotic. This is particularly true, as one would expect, of multiple murderers; but it is true of most one-choice killers as well.

Hundreds of detailed psychological reports on convicted killers who were tested and interviewed either before or after conviction exist in court and prison files. Unfortunately, few of these are available for publication. By rare coincidence, one of the most detailed reports of this nature was published in a professional journal, *Case Reports in Clinical Psychology,* by the senior author of this book two decades ago. The author, at the time of the original report, was Chief Psychologist of the New Jersey State Diagnostic Center at Menlo Park, a facility where many criminals, including murderers, were often examined in depth. The murderer in this case was an attractive twenty-six-year-old white female who had been in a state reformatory for two and a half years on a charge of manslaughter, after having shot and killed her father. She was examined at the New Jersey State Diagnostic Center, to decide whether she might be considered a good parole risk. As part of the diagnostic procedure, which was rather complete, she was given a social history interview, a psychiatric interview, a sodium amytal interview, a special interview on her love and sex history, an electroencephalogram, and several psychological tests, including the Wechsler-Bellevue Adult Intelligence Scale, Word Association Test, Abbreviations Test, Sentence Completion Test, Rorschach Test, Thematic Apperception Test, Description of and Associations to Paintings, Human Figure Drawing Test, a Personality Inventory, Expressive Movements Check List, and a Personality Rating Sheet. Full test data are given in the published report.

After this mass of material was considered, the final report on the patricidal woman included this comment: "The question of diagnosis is an extraordinarily interesting and provocative one in this case. The patient has been variously diagnosed as neurotic, psychopathic, and psychotic; and there is considerable evidence to support all three of these diagnoses.

"To support the diagnosis of neuroticism, there is the following evidence: (a) The patient has severe underlying anxiety, which tends to become overt whenever she is placed under sufficient stress. (b) She has distinct hysterical patterns of behavior, with several conversion symptoms. (c) She normally has good, if compulsive, control, as well as intellectual and emotional integration; but from time to time this control breaks down into somewhat disorganized, impulsive behavior. (d) When the patient does suffer a breakthrough in her personality defenses, she usually makes a spontaneous, and for a time fairly effective, recovery. (e) She is quite moody, with depressive tendencies; but her suicidal attempts are not too convincing, and seem to be patently designed to reawaken the protectiveness of others. (f) She neurotically keeps running away from minor and major difficulties of life, and consistently refuses to face herself or the consequences of her acts. (g) She is most immature emotionally, is immensely narcissistic, and shows little capacity for frustration tolerance. (h) She has deep-seated feelings of inadequacy, which she frantically keeps trying to cover up. (i) She is sexually inhibited, evasive, and frigid and is quite psycho-sexually immature. (j) She is fixated on childhood levels of behavior, and keeps employing typical neurotic defenses—*e.g.,* extreme rationalization, repression and evasion—to maintain her fixations. (k) She makes considerable use of neurotic gains, and rarely suffers the full consequences of her aberrant acts. (l) She suffers from traumatic dreams and nightmares about her father, which show that she has considerable unconscious guilt about killing him. (m) She is conventionally concerned about social disapproval and specifically disturbed about the possible stigma of being imprisoned.

"To support the diagnosis of psychopathy, there are these indications: (a) The patient has a consistent record of negativistic, primitive, hostile and antisocial behavior. (b) She has had distinct cruel and sadistic tendencies from her childhood. (c) On the surface, she shows little affect concerning her suicidal or homicidal acts, and does not appear to be guilty about any of her antisocial behavior. (d) She does not easily tolerate the monotony of everyday living, and seems to have a need to do exciting, dangerous, and somewhat rash things. (e) Her narcissism is so immense that she will construe any disciplinary acts as being unfair and unwarranted, and will rebelliously feel that the world is against her. (f) She is patently absorbed only in her own feelings and pleasures and is selfishly oblivious to the feelings of others. (g) Her goals and daydreams are of an extreme self-centered, unrealistic nature which are common to a good many individuals with character neuroses of an antisocial or psychopathic type.

"To support the diagnosis of psychosis, there are the following observations: (a) The patient is in some respects distinctly paranoid, and feels that others are out to trick or betray her. (b) She has grandiose notions of herself which are not in the least rooted in reality. (c) Her narcissism is so extreme that it may be viewed as a regressive flight from the present, back to the loving protectiveness of her childhood. (d) Her dreams and nightmares about her father partake of a hallucinative and extremely obsessive character. (e) Her affect is distinctly flattened, and her feelings for anyone but herself (and possibly her mother, who represents an extension of herself) are quite shallow. (f) Her control over her feelings is tenuous, and a breakthrough into the realm of over-impulsiveness and unreality is always imminent. (g) Her verbalizations and actions are frequently bizarre and peculiar. (h) She is irrationally blind to the behavior of her mother, and maintains a desperate, compulsive attachment to her mother that goes beyond the depths of neurotic involvement. (i) She is able to adjust only to a very small portion of her potential life space, and even then in a limited manner. She does not appear to have adequate physical energies or tolerances to stress to meet the normal demands of everyday living. (j) She usually manages to achieve some measure of integration from conflict and confusion; but the conflict and confusion are never essentially overcome, and remain basic, while the integration temporarily achieved is superficial, immature and shallow. (k) When faced with any difficulties, she tends to become confused and panicky, and to make an immediate withdrawal into herself. (l) Her narcissism is so extreme as frequently to lead into autistic behavior. (m) She has, in spite of her incarceration, gained no insight whatever into herself, nor does it appear that she will ever permit herself to gain any. (n) Her grasp on reality is so tenuous that totally unrealistic attempts at solving her problems, like suicide and murder, may well continue to be utilized by her as she encounters normal life difficulties.

"All things considered, the diagnostic impression is that this patient is an exceptionally narcissistic woman who never has achieved, and probably never will achieve, any appreciable degree of emotional maturity. She is fixated on such an early stage of development, and is so desperately attached to infantile ideas of her own inflated worth, that she dare not allow the realities of social living or of outside events to impinge upon the protective inner walls which she has compulsively constructed around herself. Basically and underlyingly, she is a psychotic personality, with paranoid, obsessive-compulsive, conversion and antisocial tendencies, who can only be expected to make a limited and tenuous future adjustment to life."

The material for this published diagnostic impression was gathered and the Diagnostic Center report on the murderess it describes was originally written in 1950, some two decades ago. Although this diagnosis is not quite the same as we would make today—since it does not emphasize the woman's tendency to think in a slippery manner and to make herself needlessly miserable about the problems and hardships that her environment presents to her—it probably is a sufficiently accurate description of the killer's psychological disturbances; and it does emphasize the many neurotic, psychopathic, and psychotic tendencies that a somewhat typical murderess displays. We would guess that, if adequate information were available on other slayers, they too would tend to exhibit a great many disturbed traits—and significantly more of these traits than would an equated group of noncriminals and of criminal nonmurderers.

Many other investigators have found that perpetrators of homicide tend to be exceptionally disturbed. Thus, A. J. Snider reports a controlled study by Dr. John M. MacDonald, psychiatrist at the University of Colorado, in which he studied (1) mental hospital patients who had made verbal homicidal threats and (2) a group of convicted murderers. He found that the latter group differed significantly from the former in that they more frequently were firesetters, had been cruel to animals, had police arrest records, had been arrested for assault, were alcoholic, and had attempted suicide. A similar study of convicted murderers and nonhospitalized members of the general populace would in all probability show even greater differences in these types of pathological behavior.

Ruotolo did detailed psychiatric interviews and studies of four confessed murderers and a fifth individual who fired point-blank at his victim's forehead but miraculously only grazed her scalp. He found that "in this series of murderers, the degree of alienation was invariably enormous."

The first slayer attempted suicide, had blocked thought processes, depression, confusion, and perplexity, and was diagnosed as "suffering from a schizophrenic reaction of the schizo-affective type." The second one had hallucinations and "his inappropriate affect, unrealistic suspiciousness, looseness of associations, blocking, and agitation led to the diagnosis of schizophrenic reaction." The third one was perfectionistic, hallucinatory, and paranoid. The fourth one attempted suicide three times, had an overweening pride system and an unrealistic fantasy about himself, and crumpled completely when his victims did not cooperate with his "new image" of himself. The fifth one demanded that he be absolutely "masculine," "passed judgment on himself and condemned himself to the unrelenting flagellation by his emergent self-hate," and found it "preferable to appear a callous killer than a cringing coward."

Ruotolo concludes: "All these murders were useless. Though each murderer was striving for a greater 'good' within his distorted scale of values, no permanent solution was attained. Their self-images were not well constructed edifices that could withstand the buffetings of time and the vicissitudes of events. Their personality makeups remained shaky structures anchored in sand. Murder was impulsively resorted to in order magically to produce an ultimate, permanent solution to *all* their psychic problems."

E. V. Yanouskaya studied fifty-eight males and five female paranoid schizophrenics and reported that not only were their homicidal acts related to their being psychotic, but that most of them had committed murder in the course of a specific "delirious experience." He concluded that this kind of "key" delirious state is of great importance when the murderer is schizophrenic.

Satten, Menninger, Rosen, and Mayman studied four individuals who had apparently committed "motiveless" murder. They not only generally found these individuals to be highly disturbed emotionally, but more specifically found them to have (1) poor impulse control, (2) blurring of boundaries between fantasy and reality, (3) shallow emotional reactions, and (4) a violent and primitive fantasy life.

Tuteur and Glotzer investigated five instances where mothers had murdered their children. They found all these mothers to be schizophrenic and felt that murders were committed when they were in a particularly acute state of schizophrenic excitement.

Butter and his associates tested Berg's deviation hypotheses: namely, that crimes are committed by those whose perception is deviant. He compared 200 college students to 26 killers and had his subjects rate ten pictures of faces on the basis of their assumed leadership quality. He found that there was no significant agreement between the judgments of the two groups, thus tending to sustain Berg's hypothesis of deviant perception on the part of murderers and other criminals.

A. W. Stearns reviewed four cases of adolescents who had murdered and found them to be very clearly different, in their emotional make-up, from a typical group of adolescents.

Romano and Paolella gave psychological tests to twenty incarcerated murderers and found two distinct personality types, both of them pathological. The first type is characterized by hyperthymia in emotional responsiveness, while the second type is characterized by coldness, detachment, and schizoid affect.

H. Gillier examined 59 males and 7 females in Scotland who were charged with murder. He found 18 of these alleged murderers to be psychopathic personalities, 14 psychotic, and 4 mentally retarded. The court's findings in these cases were even stronger than those of Gillier: Seventeen of these accused individuals were insane and unfit to plead; 33 had indulged in alcohol at the time of the killings; 22 were psychopathic; and 11 were schizophrenic. Gillier and the court found that in four of the cases where a mother had killed her child, all four were schizophrenic.

Blackman and his associates studied 43 murderers and found that most of them had conflicts concerning personal adequacy and conformity. Their subjects tended to be very labile emotionally and hoped for and despaired of obtaining intimacy with others. They concluded about the typical murderer: "It is just when . . . his relationships with other persons are at the point of becoming real or meaningful . . . that the conflict between his dependent needs and his fear of being again rejected creates an increasing sense of self-doubt, tension and repressed rage. At that time, even an insignificant insult from the social environment may lead to murder."

B. M. Cormier investigated the cases of eight wife killers. He found that most of these husbands were unable to effect a final separation from their wives, in spite of their own awareness of hostility to their wives and threats to kill them. He concluded that these husbands were so disturbed that they could see no possible alternative to getting out of their marriages but murder. This kind of rigidity and failure to see other solutions to a problem than an obviously poor solution is one of the main characteristics of severe emotional aberration.

T. C. N. Gibbens studied the records of 120 murderers who had been declared insane and 115 who had been declared sane. He discovered that both groups displayed, as their main personality trait, highly antisocial tendencies. Such tendencies are often indicative of schizoid individuals.

M. W. Kahn obtained data on the personality, intelligence, and social history of a group of fifteen murderers and twenty-four burglars. He concluded that "murderers are more likely than burglars to have personalities which are characterized by the potential for an impulsive breakthrough of ordinarily rigidly controlled sadistic hostility, and by fewer resources for other than direct expression of hostility."

Helfer and Kempe investigated a particular kind of physical violence that frequently leads to homicide but that is most often never entered as such in the records of crime—that is, the syndrome of the battered child. According to their findings, tens of thousands of children are severely battered in the United States every year (mostly by their own parents) and perhaps a quarter of this number are killed in the process. As might be expected, their detailed study of the parents of such children indicates that they are for the most part severely emotionally disturbed and they recommend that it is less important to punish than to give them proper treatment for their disturbances.

Wertham, writing in *A Sign for Cain,* believes that parents who batter their children frequently do so while under the influence of alcohol. It is most probable, though, that many do so when they are perfectly sober (as occurred in the case of a mother who committed infanticide, which we present in detail in Chapter 10 of this book). It is also likely that a large percentage of those who do so when they are intoxicated are alcoholics or near-alcoholics who frequently resort to liquor because of severe emotional problems.

J. L. Batt studied a group of twenty psychotic murderers and a control group of twenty-nine killers, none of whom were considered to be medically or legally insane. He found that most of the psychotic individuals were severe depressives and that the majority of the depressives were suicidal. His summary statement on the psychotic depressive slayer is as follows:

"It will concern a married woman, rather than a man, of about thirty years of age, who kills the person or persons of whom she is most fond, adopting a 'homely' method; who is also suicidal herself, and yet goes for assistance after the crime; and finally who has shown the symptomatology of a depressive psychosis before the incident with which we are primarily concerned."

Although it is to be doubted that Batt's group of nonpsychotic killers consisted of individuals who were truly nondisturbed, it seems clear that his psychotic group consisted of persons, largely women, who had a longstanding history of severe depression and who were impelled to kill largely because they were seriously disturbed and not merely because of the inciting circumstances surrounding their crimes.

D. J. West made an interesting study of 148 murders followed by the suicide of the alleged murderer and compared them to 148 murder incidents where the offender was found insane or sent to a correctional facility. He found that in England one of every three murders is followed by the suicide of the suspected murderer and one of every two murders by the attempted suicide of the suspect. He also found that, with the exception of the chronic criminals, there was no significant difference in mental illness between the two groups. In both groups, a high portion of the murderers manifested psychiatric disturbance at the time of the crime, the diagnosis being primarily a depression of either neurotic or psychotic dimensions. Of the forty-five women involved in the murder-suicide sample, it was felt that thirty-nine would have been tried under the insanity or diminished responsibility rulings in England. The six remaining women were not insane but were noted by their associates to be "odd or peculiar." West's impression was that the psychotic depressions found in these slayers were largely hereditary in origin.

George Bach interviewed 38 husbands who had killed their wives and 36 wives who had killed their husbands. He found that only six percent were psychiatrically "sick" individuals. But he found that an additional 20 percent "were narcissists with strong omnipotent expectations of being catered to, spoiled and adored, or being obeyed by all to whom they made their sexual pleasure available." He also found that almost all these spouse murderers "*were cognitively fixated* on how they should feel, what satisfaction they should get out of the relationship, what kind of a life they should build together, and their very rigid ideas of *how the other should be!*" [italics in the original].

He reports, again: "Our subjects were, on the whole, very secretive." Although 70 percent of his subjects stated that they abhorred conflict and aggression, he found most of these murderers to be overtly accommodating but underlyingly quite hostile: "They never really learned anything from their occasional hostility outbreaks, except that things were painfully dissonant with what each had *secretly* hoped would take place: some change for the better. They did not try to negotiate effectively for change and improvements. They did not know how to do it with each other alone, and they rarely confided any of their marital troubles, as it was important to both of them to present out front a *picture of marital success.*" In spite of Bach's finding only a small percentage of his subjects psychiatrically "sick," he seems to have found the vast majority of them to have, in our sense of the term, rather severely disturbed traits.

Cole, Fisher, and Cole studied 112 female slayers whose cases were scheduled for review at the California Institution for Women. They found that 50 percent of the women were under the influence of alcohol and 10 percent were using narcotics at the time of the killing; that 30 percent had prior criminal records of assaultive crimes and 36 percent had prior records of other types of crime; that 111 of the 112 were emotionally disturbed and "that only one subject in this study was considered to have an essentially normal, well-functioning personality"; that the main disturbed patterns of behavior included 18 masochistic women, 41 overtly hostile and violent women, 14 covertly hostile and violent women, 12 inadequate women, 20 psychotic women, and 6 amoral women.

R. Blackburn studied 38 extremely assaultive individuals, including many murderers, who were incarcerated at the Broadmoor Hospital in Crowthorne, England, and compared them to 25 moderately assaultive individuals. On the Minnesota Multiphasic Personality Inventory scales, the murderers or very assaultive subjects were significantly more overcontrolled, more introverted, and more conforming than were the moderates, thus confirming

McGargee's hypothesis that killers tend to be more basically constricted than nonkillers.

Lachman and Cravens examined 10 patients charged with homicide who were incarcerated in Bellevue Hospital, New York, who had also been examined before they committed murder. They found that 9 of the 10 had spent over a year in prison prior to their killings; and at least half had exhibited major behavioral problems before the age of ten, diagnosed as childhood schizophrenia in 4.

In almost every case there was everyday acquaintance with knives and pistols: "These items were normally at hand, and the patients were not only skilled in their use but accustomed to using them as the response to stress. In nine of the ten cases the crime was associated with the intemperate use of alcohol. . . . Four were also under the influence of drugs at the time of the homicide."

They also found that "mental status examination disclosed several characteristics in common. Less than average verbal productivity was associated with shallowness or flattening of affect. The latter was a feature showing little tendency to change after months of hospitalization. . . . Another common feature was the callousness displayed in response to topics of violence. . . . There was little change in diagnosis between the pre-homicide and post-homicide examinations of these men. . . . The abnormality of this group was in some measure reflected in their social adjustment. They resided in a social constellation that generally ranged from the aberrant to the chaotic."

Clearly, then, murderers usually are severely disturbed individuals; and there is reason to believe that they kill partly because of their personality deficiencies. As we have shown in this chapter, and as we indicate again in our later chapter on the psychology of assassination, they are generally individuals with severe feelings of inadequacy, with compensatory expressions of grandiosity, with exceptionally low frustration tolerance, with inability to relate warmly and consistently to others, with lack of self-discipline, and with various other strong tendencies to get themselves into continual difficulties with themselves, other people, and the world around them. It could well be that their personality problems are mainly the result of their early upbringing—since most of them are reared in execrable homes by unloving or ambivalent parents, who themselves are often severely aberrated. But it is our impression that this is not the entire reason for their ugly behavior, and that the majority of them have an innate predisposition to act badly and to create needless difficulties for themselves. This predisposition may have been inherited directly from their parents or may be the result of congenital problems—such as accidents that happen while they are in their mothers' wombs or in the process of being born.

Evidence confirming the possible influence of heredity is sometimes available whenever the full facts on the behavior of many murderers' parents are known. In the cases included in Dr. Reinhardt's book, we find that in just about every case where detailed information is given on the parents, one or both of them was a seriously disturbed individual. In Robert Bruhm's case, his father was the husband of his mother's sister; his father's two brothers were epileptic. His mother was "promiscuous and a heavy drinker. . . . She became a homeless derelict. When referred to the agency, she was living with four children in a deplorable condition in a two-room shack."

In the case of Melvin Davis Rees, his parents were "fine people" who were law abiding and did not get into any trouble, but his mother was a religious fanatic. In Carl Austin Hall's case, one of his brothers died in a mental institution; both his parents were exceedingly prim, proper, and ashamed to let anyone know what their family really was like; neither of his parents showed him any love when he was a child. Once, when a neighbor told his mother about a cute remark that Carl had made, "the mother turned a shocked face upon the child. She warned him to avoid 'any more such impudence.' "

In Masters and Lea's book, *Sex Crimes in History,* more evidence of tainted heredity in the cases of some of the murderers listed in the book is given. Thus, in the case of Albert Fish, who was executed in 1935 for the lust-murder of ten-year-old Grace Budd, and who was believed to have killed and eaten between eight and fifteen children, "almost every member of Fish's immediate family was mentally ill." In the case of Peter Kurten, who was executed in July, 1931, after being found guilty of nine murders and seven attempted murders, "His father was a drunkard who abused the members of his family, and who served a prison term for incest committed with one of Kurten's sisters. Several members of the family were or became alcoholics. . . . Two of his brothers served long prison sentences."

Karl Menninger, in *The Crime of Punishment,* points out that, after Charles Whitman climbed onto a campus tower at the University of Texas in Austin and began shooting everyone in sight, killing twelve people and injuring others, it was found that his father was "an authoritarian, a perfectionist, and an unyielding disciplinarian" who was quoted as saying, "I raised my boys to know how to handle guns."

Truman Capote relates that in the case of Perry Edward Smith who, with his partner Richard Hickock, was hanged for the slaying of four members of the Clutter family in Kansas, his brother Jimmy committed suicide and his sister Fern, after becoming an alcoholic, died by falling out of a window, and may have been a suicide too.

Additional evidence for the strength of a hereditary or congenital factor in murder is found in recent chromosomal findings. Thus, Casey and his associates found that, when individuals of subnormal intelligence have an additional Y chromosome in their make-up, this tends to predispose them toward overly aggressive and violent behavior. Several notable murderers in the last few years, such as Richard Speck, the six-foot-two Chicago drifter convicted of killing eight nurses, have been found to have an extra Y chromosome; and their lawyers have claimed that they were physiologically defective, were naturally prone to crime and violence, and therefore should be treated as hereditarily disturbed. Evidence in this connection is by no means yet clear-cut or indisputable; but it is at least another sign of the possible hereditary influence on some murderers.

In our own practices we have almost invariably found that when we discover the facts on the backgrounds of individuals who commit homicide, either one or both of their parents is an exceptionally disturbed individual, with a long history of anxiety, depression, or extreme hostility. Also, in the material we later present on assassins, it is fairly clear that often a parent was seriously neurotic or psychotic.

Our main hypothesis about the psychology of murder, therefore, would tend to be that killers are usually aberrant personalities and that they frequently inherit a predisposition to be pathologically inclined, to be insensitive to the hurts of others, and to be angry and sadistic, as well as being environmentally influenced. Their chief goal in life is often to show how great they are. Because they do not honestly and directly achieve this goal, they feel underlyingly inadequate; and they cover up this deep-seated feeling of inadequacy with abrasive, overrebellious, inconsiderate behavior which finally reaches murderous dimensions. A goodly number of them can be diagnosed as paranoid schizophrenics; another high proportion are otherwise psychotic or near-psychotic; and only a small percentage of them are truly sane.

Although it may be easy to maintain that a high percentage of murderers are disturbed, this generalization is far too vague to be of much practical use. How, exactly, do such individuals become emotionally aberrated? And how, specifically, do their proclivities for disturbance finally break out into overt activity of a murderous nature? In terms of our own theory of rational-emotive psychotherapy, we feel that murderers frequently undergo the following kinds of experiences and psychological reactions:

At point A, there is an Activator or series of Activating Events—usually, occurrences in the murderer's life which are unfortunate, frustrating, or unpleasant. Thus, he may be treated badly at home; or may fail to achieve adequately at school; or he is rejected, for one reason or another, by his peers. These Activating Events (or, in psychological language, stimuli) arise from (1) accidental situations afflicting the individual (such as poverty, rough neighborhood conditions, or loss of a parent during childhood); from (2) the biosocial inadequacy of the individual's parents and other close relatives; and (3) the potential murderer's innate tendencies to over-react or to under-react to certain kinds of life stresses, and thereby to make these stresses even more frustrating and difficult than they would otherwise be.

Once an unfortunate series of Activating Events arises at point A, the individual who later resorts to homicide tends to react to these Activators in two major ways at point B, which stands for his Belief System. At point rB (which stands for his rational Belief about A), he perceives the Activating Events, observes that they are unfortunate or dislikable to himself, and sanely tells himself or convinces himself something along the following lines: (1) "It's too bad that my family is so poor. But this kind of a handicap simply means that I'll have to adjust to living on a lower standard or to work harder to make money myself and improve my economic status." (2) "I wish my parents would pay more attention to me. But if they don't, I can still survive and be a relatively happy person." (3) "I realize that I'm not as physically attractive as some other people are. But I can still keep trying to find people who will like me, and if I keep trying I'll almost certainly find some."

Murderers, however, usually seem to have only a limited tendency to accept, to internalize, and to act on rational Beliefs. For the most part, they tend to favor highly irrational Beliefs (iB's) or philosophies and to tell themselves such things as: (1) *It's awful* that my family is so poor! I *can't stand* this kind of an existence! I'll have to do something, almost anything, to get more money quickly!" (2) "*It's terrible* that my parents do not pay more attention to me! They *should* love me more than they do! I can't be happy *at all* unless they love me much more than they seem to love me. I *must* get their or someone else's approval immediately!" (3) "*It is catastrophic* that I am not as physically attractive as some other people are! I'll *never* be able to find anybody I want, looking the way that I do! If So-and-so doesn't love me, I think I'll kill myself—and maybe kill her, too, for not being able to see what a fine person I really am!"

Potential and actual murderers strongly, fanatically believe, as the senior author of this book and his collaborators have shown in a number of publications, in one or more of the basic irrational ideas which are so common to individuals who display severe emotional disturbance. They particularly seem to believe these kinds of notions:

1. The idea that it is an utter necessity for an adult to be loved or approved by almost everyone for virtually everything he does.

2. The idea that one should be thoroughly competent, adequate, and achieving in all possible respects if one is to consider oneself worthwhile.

3. The idea that it is terrible, horrible, and catastrophic when things are not the way one would like them to be.

4. The idea that human unhappiness is externally caused and that people have little or no ability to control their emotional disturbances or to rid themselves of their negative feelings.

5. The idea that certain people are bad, wicked, or villainous and that they should be severely blamed and punished for their sins.

6. The idea that it is easier to avoid than to face certain life difficulties and responsibilities than to work at achieving self-discipline and changing certain undesirable aspects of the world.

Murderers—like most other individuals with disturbances—spend much of their time and energy condemning: (1) themselves for their own inadequacies and failures; (2) others for their shortcomings; and (3) the world for its difficulties. Their irrational Beliefs, or their unrealistic attitudes toward themselves and others, tend to rule their thinking and behaving.

Consequently, at point C—which stands for emotional and behavioral Consequences—most murderers make themselves needlessly upset. By convincing themselves that they *have to be* approved and that they *must* do well and by condemning themselves when they are rejected and when they do badly, they create severe feelings of anxiety, self-deprecation, and depression. By convincing themselves that others *should* do what they *want* them to do—and that they are terrible villains when they don't—they make themselves enraged, grandiose, over-rebellious. By convincing themselves that the world is *too* rough and that it *ought not* be the way it is, they make themselves self-pitying, undisciplined, and inert.

Although practically all of us have some of this disordered thinking and consequent emotional upsets, some of us have more than our share. Murderers are generally in the latter class. They intensely and rigidly cling to their hypothesis about how they, others, and the world *should* be, and thereby remain continually on the verge of disturbance. Often they do not actively erupt, but for a long time quietly and irritably sit on their feelings. But they seethe underneath; and sooner or later—particularly when a set of stressful circumstances or Activating Events arises—their disturbances boil over.

Unfortunately, many sociologists and psychologists are prone to look only at the stressful events at points A and C when they perceive that someone is upset, and upset to the extent of murderous potential. But we stoutly hypothesize: It is not A (Activators) but B (Beliefs) that people hold in regard to A that truly cause C (emotional Consequences). To understand murderers fully, we'd better get a pretty good picture of what has happened and is happening to them at A. But we'd better also look at what they are convincing themselves at point B. Then we will be able to see what truly moves them to their heinous deeds.

Chapter 8

Psychological Factors in Assassination

An assassination is, of course, a murder; but it is significantly different from most murders in several important respects.

First of all, we usually speak of assassination in regard to the slaying of some public figure, usually a political figure. Quite commonly, the assassin disagrees violently with his victim's views and thinks he is doing his country or the world some kind of favor when he commits his crime.

Second, even when the assassin does not object seriously to his victim's political ideologies or when he does not have any illusion that his deed will change the world significantly, he generally chooses to kill a president, a prime minister, a king, or some other outstanding person just *because* this person is outstanding. He may be intensely jealous of his victim's status; or may think it unfair that he ever achieved such status; or may feel that, if he chooses this kind of individual to slay, he himself will achieve great renown; or may for some other reasons deliberately select someone who is clearly in the public eye.

Third, the assassin generally has had no prior personal contact with his victim. He knows *of* him; but he really does not know him. And he sometimes has nothing personally against the individual he chooses to kill and only slays him because he is a *symbol* of something that he dislikes or that he thinks should be fought.

Fourth, the assassin frequently commits his act of murder publicly, in full view of hundreds or even thousands of people. This is partly because he would have great difficulty in achieving a private interview with the man he is determined to kill. But it is also partly because he *wants* to be seen doing his thing and is rather proud of the fact that he does it in front of so many witnesses.

Fifth, because of the circumstances of most assassinations, the assassin is obviously taking an enormous risk of being apprehended for his crime, often immediately, and of being severely punished for it. Sometimes he deludes himself that he is doing a fairly unrisky act and that he will get away with it. But often he seems to know that he will be apprehended—and he may even *want* to be taken into custody for his crime.

In significant ways, then, assassination differs from run-of-the-mill murder; and because of these differences there is reason to believe that, if many or most murderers are severely emotionally disturbed, assassins even more often have enormous personality problems. This is not to claim that every single assassin in history has been a psychotic; for it is likely that some slayers of prominent people have not been crazy. For example, the generals who plotted to murder Hitler some time before his death, and who came within a hair of succeeding, may have been reasonably sane individuals who found that living with Hitler as their leader was intolerable and that it was better to risk killing him than to continue under his leadership.

It should also be noted that, although many assassinations are senseless and do not bring about the specific political changes that the assassins fervently desire, some of them bring about significant changes in the social system. W. F. Buckley, pointing to the political and social events that occurred as a fairly direct result of the assassinations of individuals such as George Lincoln Rockwell, Imre Nagy, Malcolm X, Huey Long, Leon Trotsky, and Robert F. Kennedy, contends that "Assassinations more often than not *do* accomplish something—I think offhand only of the exception of Hendrik Verwoerd and maybe Diem in recent times. It is not surprising that they should, inasmuch as every man is unique, exactly irreplaceable. 'Why do they want to kill you?' somebody asked Malcolm X. 'Because I'm me,' he answered."

Nevertheless, a case can be made for the hypothesis that most assassins are acutely or basically psychotic at the time they kill. We shall examine some of the facts that tend to support or invalidate this hypothesis, especially using the data that have recently accumulated on the assassins of President John F. Kennedy, of Martin Luther King, and of Senator Robert Kennedy, but also employing information on less publicized assassins.

Although on the surface, assassination may seem to be a cold-blooded result of political partisanship, it is our contention that it rarely is. Perhaps in the old days of Czarist Russia, the anarchists and other revolutionary groups produced true political hotheads who just couldn't stomach the existing regimes and who calmly shot, blew up, knifed, or otherwise violently rid themselves of the high officials of these regimes, and who committed their murderous deeds in a reasonably objective manner, with little personal rancor or disturbance. But this can hardly be said of contemporary assassins—who almost always prove to be exceptionally deranged individuals. Some of them, in fact, appear to have few or no political motives. Lee Harvey Oswald, who seems almost certainly to have been John F. Kennedy's assassin (though it is possible that he had one or more accomplices, as various dissenters to the Warren Commission's Report insist), differed from his victim in political views, but there is no evidence that he killed President Kennedy primarily for this reason and there is considerable reason to believe that his personal jealousy of the president, especially when viewed in the light of his dismal life failures, was a much more important motive. Jack Ruby, who assassinated Oswald in the most dramatic circumstances possible—right in the middle of a police station, with the television cameras turned directly on Oswald—also seems to have had no real politico-economic motives, but probably was impelled to kill because he was distraught over Kennedy's death and over many things that were going badly in his own life.

We may even suspect that most members of revolutionary groups (such as the anarchists of nineteenth-century Russia) who openly advocate and sometimes dramatically carry out "political" assassinations, adhere to their creeds of violence not merely because of their social ideologies but because they *want* to kill. They may *say* that they are would-be or actual assassins because they passionately want to fight against oppression and that they have dispassionately figured out that political murder is an effective method of upholding the ideologies in which they believe; but we have to suspect that they are also driven to their deeds by less altruistic motives.

It is interesting to note that the word *assassin* is derived from the term *Hashishin.* The Hashishin were a special subgroup of the Ismailites, a fanatical, mystical-minded sect of Moslems who were powerful during the eleventh and twelfth centuries, particularly in Persia and Syria. The Hashishin were specially educated to commit murder, including the murder of high officials who opposed the Ismailite beliefs. They were said to have frequently resorted to the use of the drug, hashish, which is a powerful form of marijuana. According to one theory, they took the drug before going out to kill in order to help themselves become disposed to an absolute resignation to the will of their chief. Another theory is that they imbibed a beverage made from hashish in order to intoxicate themselves and drive themselves into a frenzy, so that they could then go out and murder.

In any event, as Joseph von Hammer-Purgstall informs us, the Assassins constituted a large group and were powerful leaders in Muslim politics for many years. "The crimes of the society of murderers, which has long ago exceeded the measure of humanity, had, at length, filled to overflowing that of retributive vengeance: after an existence of a hundred and seventy years, the tempest of destruction fell, with terrific fury, on the Assassins. The conquering power of Jengis Khan, thundering in the distance, had passed innocuously over their heads; but under the third of his successors, Mangu Khan, the whirlwind of Mongols swept over the eastern world, and, in its desolating progress, carried away, along with the khalifat and other dynasties, that of the Assassins."

Before their gory end, as Von Hammer-Purgstall makes clear, the Assassins committed every conceivable crime known to man, including the murder of numerous public officials in Persia and Syria. Although leadership in this group was often hereditary, its recruits were drawn from the general population; and it would seem quite clear, from all historical accounts, that both the leaders and the followers were frequently sadistic and deranged individuals, and religious fanatics to boot, who relished their murderous forays and often had no need of hashish or other drugs to motivate their deeds. A study of their history would indicate that, from earliest times, men who specialized in assassination have been both personally and politically motivated and that they have been, in most instances, highly unstable individuals.

From a study of murders in general and of assassins in particular, what can be said to be some of the main psychological factors that drive certain people to assassinate prominent figures? Here are some that we can tentatively list, together with some evidence that they are valid.

Impotence and self-hatred. Assassins often seem to be individuals who, though not basically stupid, have been so seriously disturbed all their lives that they have been highly inept in getting what they want. They often have poor interpersonal relations; they are unable to work steadily at interesting or well-paying jobs; and they characteristically get rejected by friends, acquaintances, members of the opposite sex, and even political groups or countries to which they would like to swear allegiance. All these traits—as will easily be recognized—were true of Lee Harvey Oswald.

Because of their inherently low estimation of themselves, we may surmise that potential or actual assassins keep failing at one task or another; then use their failures as "evidence" that they are worthless and must keep failing. Rather than conscientiously admit to themselves that they are woefully inadequate, and that they'd better do something to change their ways, they frequently build up defensive hostility against others, and insist that they are being persecuted by these others.

Consequently, they tend to hate bosses, officials, statesmen, and other authority figures, and contend that it is *those* "bastards" who are keeping them down. They are loath to acknowledge the hard work and resistance to dismay over physical and other handicaps that are characteristic of statesmen such as the Kennedy brothers and Martin Luther King—since such an acknowledgment would spotlight their own tendencies to groan and run away in the face of even minor difficulties. So they sometimes become insanely jealous of outstanding achievers, insist that the celebrants do not truly deserve their place of eminence, and bitterly resolve that something must be done to annihilate them and drag them from the positions they have "unfairly" won.

Typical of the impotence and self-hatred that Oswald felt for himself is that, as Kerry Thornley points out, "despair, it would appear, existed—but it was not despair with resignation. Rather, Oswald exhibited something quite prevalent in our culture today: frantic despair." Thornley is perhaps one of the most qualified persons to comment on Oswald, since he had close contact with him in 1959, four years before President Kennedy was murdered, when they were both assigned to El Toro Marine Air Station in Santa Ana, California. He was so struck then with Oswald's unusual personality that a year later he wrote a novel, *The Idle Warriors,* featuring a protagonist modeled after him. He later gave a long deposition to the Warren Commission about his association with Oswald.

Like so many despairing and self-deprecating people, Oswald apparently had to believe there were special reasons for his not succeeding in life. So he became defensively paranoid, and wishful-thinkingly got himself to "discern" that others were deliberately picking on him and blocking his way. As Thornley notes: "I don't think he was consciously, perhaps, aware of the fact that he went out of his way to get into trouble. I think it was kind of necessary to him to believe that he was being picked on. It wasn't anything extreme. I wouldn't go so far as to call him a paranoid, but a definite tendency of being persecuted was necessary to his self-esteem. That is, I understand, a common thing, and it certainly fits in with everything else I know about him."

The Warren Commission's Report, in its summary of Oswald's condition, concurs: "He used his Marxist and associated activities as excuses for his difficulties in getting along in the world, which were usually caused by entirely different factors."

William Manchester, the main biographer of Kennedy's death, felt that feelings of rejection and inadequacy were among the main reasons for Oswald's deed. Commented Manchester: "He was the diametric opposite of John Fitzgerald Kennedy, and he was aware of this. Significantly, he attributed the President's success to family wealth: Kennedy had all the breaks. Like many delusions, this one had a kernel of truth. One man had almost everything, and the other, almost nothing. Kennedy was spectacularly handsome. Oswald's voice hadn't yet lost its adolescent tone, he was balding, and he had the physique of a ferret. The President had been a brave officer during the war. Oswald had been court-martialed during his peacetime service. As Chief Executive and Commander in Chief, Kennedy was all-powerful. Oswald was impotent. Kennedy was cheered; Oswald, ignored. Kennedy was beloved; Oswald, despised. Kennedy was a hero. Oswald was a victim."

To add insult to injury, Manchester insists, Oswald was spurned by his wife, Marina, who preferred her friend, Ruth Paine, to him. "Even before Ruth's appearance, the Oswalds' marriage had become a disappointment. In Minsk, Lee thought he had found a beautiful dedicated Communist, who would forever be his submissive darling. He had expected her to scorn the world that scorned him and reject the materialism of a capitalist society. Instead, she hounded him for new gadgets and movie money, jeered at him because he was such a poor competitor in the capitalistic wage market and ridiculed him because he failed to gratify her sexual appetite—because, as she told him in front of others, he was 'not a man' in bed.

"There were many fights, and Marina, a quick girl with a knee, was the better fighter. It was Lee who was shut in the bathroom as punishment after one quarrel, Lee who sank to his knees in the dark and wept bitterly as the great darkness of his private nightmare enveloped him."

Robert L. Oswald, Lee's brother, concurs that he was driven to the brink of despair by his feelings of inadequacy and failure: "The discouragements and disappointments beginning in his childhood, continuing through the school years and the years in the Marines, the death of his dream of a new life in Russia, the boring jobs back in the United States which made it impossible for him to support Marina adequately and gain some recognition as a man, even the fact that he hoped for a son and had two daughters instead—the whole pattern of failure through most of his 23 years led to the outbursts of violence in April and the final tragedy in November, 1963."

Dr. Heinz L. Ansbacher and his associates, in presenting an Adlerian interpretation of Oswald and his deed, also stress that "in Lee's case there was an accumulation of factors conducive to the development of increased inferiority feelings. He was of slight build. He had had no father, and had a step-father for only a short time. The innumerable changes of home, school, and neighborhood constantly put him at the disadvantage of being a newcomer and outsider. Lee also suffered from an impairment of his hearing, when he had to have a mastoid operation. . . . Most probably he also felt the pinch of economic inferiority: 'I saw my mother as a worker, always with less than we could use.' "

However arrogant and "superior," then, Oswald appeared to be on the surface, he apparently always had deep-seated feelings of self-deprecation; and much of his swaggering and violence may have resulted from an attempt to deny or cover up these inadequacy feelings.

James Earl Ray, the assassin of Dr. Martin Luther King, W. A. McWhirter records, was a highly self-conscious child "whose nose ran all winter, who missed anywhere from 25 to 30 percent of a school year, flinched when a teacher dared so much as to reach out an arm, and sat painfully aware that to the other students in the Ewing, Missouri elementary school he was just another member of the family 'out there on the side of that hill without enough to eat.' " He spent two years in the army as an enlisted man, but was unable to make it; and he was discharged for "ineptness and lack of adaptability" and turned to a continuous life of crime. Instead of having regular girlfriends, he was reported to have frequently visited prostitutes; and the London "police also found a hypodermic syringe in the toilet drain" indicating that he was probably addicted to drugs.

L. S. Clemens did a survey of all the slayers of American presidents—John Wilkes Booth, Charles Julius Guiteau, Leon F. Czolgosz, and Lee Harvey Oswald—and of three would-be assassins—Richard Lawrence, John Nepomok Schrank, and Guiseppe Zangara—who failed in attempts on the lives of a president, president-elect, and presidential nominee. He found that "they were loners . . . all of them. . . . They were also failures—in work, in play, and in life." Although Booth was something of a matinee idol, that was only in the hinterlands. In spite of his great talent, his lack of discipline stopped him from being a great artist. Guiteau wanted a post as consul from President Garfield. "It was his failure to win it that drove him to assassination. Prior to that he had been a failure as a lawyer, as an evangelist, and as an insurance man. His life was a sordid record of skipped bills, petty thefts, and lonely hikes after he had been thrown off a train as a nonpaying passenger." Schrank, Lawrence, Zangara, and Czolgosz at times worked productively; but all of them stopped working and entered a period of almost total idleness some time before they turned to assassination. Clemens believes, and apparently with some reason, that their dismal failures in life, and their consequent feelings of inadequacy, were important factors in driving them to try to do away with powerful presidential figures who obviously were just as successful as they were not.

P. Tompkins believes that feelings of inadequacy played a significant part in the assassination of Admiral Darlan in Algiers on December, 1942, by Ferdinand Eugene Bonnier, a twenty-year-old son of a law reporter. Because he was the child of divorced parents and because his schooling had been retarded by fragile health, Tompkins hypothesizes, this assassin had a great ego stake in joining the plot to kill Darlan; and for him to have weakened and withdrawn from the plot before his deed was committed "would have been to destroy his whole self-image."

I. D. Levine holds that feelings of impotence and self-deprecation played a strong part in Ramon de Rio Mercader's assassination of Leon Trotsky. States Levine: "As a boy, he was willful. Although smaller than his schoolmates, he got into incessant fights with them. He was particularly concerned with proving his bravery and never hesitated to fight boys much bigger than he was. He believed that he was something of a child prodigy, but in school he was not studious and relied on his native intelligence to get good marks. . . . He was anxious to prove his ability to perform any task or succeed in any test set before him. . . . His extreme competitiveness and desire to succeed at everything he attempted made him make wild guesses when he obviously did not know the right answers." He also had a "consistent pattern of self-punishment" and told this story about his childhood days: "Once when my mother scolded me for having eaten some apples, she told me that the next time I would be punished and that she would stand me facing the wall. One day when she was not at home I ate some apples and then put myself facing the wall. When my mother arrived, she found me standing there."

Lack of frustration tolerance. Political or economic change of a profound character almost invariably takes considerable time to achieve. Even long *after* significant revolutions—such as the American Revolution and the Russian Revolution—have occurred, numerous vestiges of the old regime survive; and it is only as a result of constant vigilance and action by the revolutionists that many of their aims are finally achieved.

Political assassins, however, usually are individuals with low frustration tolerance and lack of prolonged discipline, who want—or, rather, demand—what they want when they want it. Which means: immediately, pronto, *right now!* As Fredric Wertham points out in *A Sign for Cain,* there is a general tendency for the sadistic and murderous individual to champ at the bit and to demand quick, phenomenal solutions to complex problems: "In acts of violence, there is often something that is supremely arrogant. The persons are habitually disposed to lift themselves not by work or thought but by some quick action against others, to something that is higher in their own eyes."

However worthy their causes may be (or may seem to be in their own biased eyes), assassins are frequently unwilling to keep *working* to achieve the goals they seek; and they impatiently, and to a large extent mystically, believe that they will be able to attain them at one fell, dramatic swoop. Sudden assassination of their foes is therefore their frequent (and usually quite unrealistic) choice.

In Oswald's case, it is fairly clear that he was a short-range hedonist who rarely saw difficult projects through, even when he believed in them. Although he was fairly intelligent and although he valued reading and education, he shirked his school work as a child and never quite finished high school. He never held onto jobs in a steady fashion; and he didn't even stick things out when he went to the Soviet Union and tried to become a citizen there.

Thornley significantly notes that Oswald, though a seeker after a better philosophy of world order, evaded responsibility in that respect, too: "Had he been willing to exert the effort, Oswald could have worked out for himself a rational view of the world. At times, according to his notes, he attempted to formulate what he called a 'third alternative.' That he did not continue this effort, and that he spent his time instead in conspiring to do violence to those with whom he disagreed, is the fault of no other person than Lee Harvey Oswald."

Even Oswald's vaunted political views, Thornley insists, were partly rationalizations for his taking the easy way out and making a great name for himself *without* resorting to any persistent effort: "He was concerned with his image in history and I do think that is why he chose the particular method he chose and did it [identified with the Communist cause] in the way he did. It got him in the newspapers. It did broadcast his name out. I think he probably expected the Russians to accept him in a much higher capacity than they did."

Like ever so many individuals with low frustration tolerance, Oswald was a classical injustice collector. To quote Thornley again: "He was always speaking of the injustices which had been perpetrated against him. . . . And it was the fact that he had lost his clearance and gone out of his way to get into some degree of trouble, that went to support this. For example, we would stand at mast in the morning, and Sergeant Spar would call the roll and he would say 'Oswald' and Oswald would step out of the ranks and Spar would send him off to mow the lawn or something. Oswald did get special treatment. As I say, he had brought it on himself, but he made the most of it, too, as far as using it as a means of getting or attempting to get sympathy."

This is one of the usual ironies with people with low frustration tolerance: They hate working to get the usual rewards of life (including being unpersecuted by others) so thoroughly that they go out of their way (or work very hard!) to defy authority. Then they *really* get more frustrated because of their misguided efforts and they actually wind up doing *extra* work (such as mowing the lawn as a penalty for insubordination in the Marines); and, finally, they squawk loudly about how unfair the world *truly* is, and point to their self-instigated persecutions to "prove" their point. Once they convince themselves that it is the world that is discriminating against them (as it finally is) and that there is no *reason* for this discrimination (which is nonsense), they do not have to go very far to the next step: "Since the goddamned world is so unfair to me, it is only right and proper that I do something drastic to get back at it!" Some deed of violence on their part is consequently easy to consider and execute.

Heinz Ansbacher and his collaborators concur with Thornley that Oswald had low frustration tolerance and was primarily interested in getting away with things easier than life normally would allow. "In all probability," they note, "Oswald read and grasped primarily the deterministic, materialistic side of Marx, as these concepts are better known and could more easily explain to Oswald the enigmas and disappointments of his life. . . . As for work," they observe, "he never held a job for any length of time, and the work he tried was relatively unskilled."

Charles J. Guiteau, the assassin of President Garfield, intruded on the president several times, trying to obtain a public office from him. He became so nasty and insulting in the process that Garfield became more and more convinced of his unfitness for office, and finally had him expelled from the White House. Thereupon, mortified at his failure to obtain the appointment that he wanted, and determined to have revenge for his "unfair" eviction, Guiteau decided to revenge himself against Garfield, and finally shot and killed him. Even though Guiteau's frustration in not obtaining an official position was largely self-caused—since hardly anyone would have trusted him after the negative manner in which he acted toward Garfield—his frustration tolerance was so low that he apparently convinced himself that he was unfairly handled, and he made himself angry and violent.

Admiral Darlan's assassin, Bonnier, was a delicate and sensitive youth, but he was also intolerant of many frustrating circumstances and tended to be overly impulsive.

Dr. Carl Austin Weiss, Jr., who assassinated Senator Huey P. Long on September 8, 1935, in Baton Rouge, was disturbed over Long's unfair treatment of some of Dr. Weiss's friends and relatives and stated that he could not stand this kind of unjust behavior. When he was in the midst of a heated discussion, with some of his fellow physicians, about Huey Long and the unfair way in which he continued to act, he could not bear continuing the conversation and S. Opotowsky reports suddenly "bolted from the room and as he did so a surgeon noticed that big tears roamed down Dr. Weiss' face."

Trotsky's killer, Ramon de Rio Mercader, had such low frustration tolerance that he often refused to think before he acted. "It is ridiculous for a man to spend his days thinking about what he is doing," he told his examiners after the assassination. "I do not do this. I like to act and to solve my difficulties while I am acting." Two psychologists who examined him concluded that he was "a man of great energy in a tremendous hurry, possessing little concern for form. . . . The prisoner described himself as irascible, impulsive, vengeful, excitable, rebellious and dominating."

P. Dawnay points out that, even as a criminal, James Earl Ray was a resounding failure: "In 1949, he was convicted of burglary in Los Angeles and was arrested in 1950 for vagrancy. In 1951 he was charged with driving an automobile without a license, and in 1952 he collected a two-year sentence for robbing a Chicago cab driver of $11. Later he collected another two-year sentence in Kansas for forging postal money orders. Finally, in 1959, he received a twenty-year sentence for robbing a grocery store in St. Louis. It is the typical record of the small-time, unsuccessful crook. Ray was clearly a man whose standing even among criminals must have been exceedingly low." There is reason to believe that Ray brooded over this low standing and that he thought he finally would compensate for it and hit the criminal jackpot by assassinating Martin Luther King, Jr.

Sirhan B. Sirhan, Senator Robert F. Kennedy's assassin, seems to have been continually thwarted in his ventures, and consequently to have developed severe feelings of inadequacy. He was never able to succeed in college, as he had planned to do; he failed miserably in his attempt to become a famous jockey, and received a serious head injury in the process; and he never got very far with his devotion to the study of the occult. After he had been dismissed from school and was unable to find a satisfactory job, he reported in a National Broadcasting Company interview in June, 1969, "I had nothing. I had no identity. I had no hope, no goal. . . . I simply gave up. There was no more American dream for me. I couldn't buy it any more. I wasn't an American, and I was an Arab, sir, and that's my greatest setback in this country, especially after the Arab-Israeli war. Everybody in America loved a winner and the Israelis won, sir, but I was a loser, and I did not like it one bit."

Sirhan was so obviously overwhelmed with feelings of inadequacy and shame that he could hardly believe much of the testimony about himself during his murder trial. At one point, he got so disturbed at the presentation of some of the evidence against him that he became enraged, said that he wanted to change his plea to guilty, and demanded to be executed. As L. Fosburg reports: "This change started when the prosecution first mentioned his personal diaries early in the week and culminated Friday when a defense witness listed his below-average scores in school on countless achievement tests. In both instances Sirhan protested the use of any evidence, by either side, which he considered intimate and humiliating. The notebooks, lying on the table in front of the three prosecuting attorneys, were full of boyish dreams and political ramblings, fantasies about girls, and a constantly repeated obsession with killing Robert Kennedy.

"The threat of having the personal scribblings or his school grades made public was so terrible that he preferred to change his plea to guilty immediately. This, he thought, apparently, would preclude the necessity of anybody knowing about them."

On several occasions, Sirhan broke out into inappropriate and raucous outbursts; and finally Superior Court Judge Herbert Walker, who was conducting his trial, during a lecture on his behavior, warned him that if he was not quiet he would "be put in chains" and be forced to wear a face mask. Asked by Sirhan's lawyers about the possibility of forcibly restraining him, the judge remarked: "He is just like a child. He gets worse and worse and we have to stop him someplace."

In all these cases, we find a fairly typical picture of the kind of individual who is highly disturbed and who frequently comes for psychotherapy: namely, the kind of person who builds up false expectations of how the world *should* treat him; who goes out of his way in many instances to insult and inflame others, so that they do finally lose patience and treat him somewhat coldly or unkindly; and who thereby "proves" (at least to his own satisfaction) that reality is definitely the way it *ought not* (by his own unrealistic definition) to be. One of the main ways in which this kind of frustration-intolerant individual is going to be able to right the "wrongs" which have been done him is, with equally trigger-happy unrealism, to harm or to kill those who are more favored than he—and who often have worked very hard (as most assassinated public figures tend to do) to earn favor.

We'd better not assume, in regard to low frustration tolerance, that the matter is entirely individual, since it has many important social aspects as well. As we have emphasized throughout this work, deviant (as well as so-called normal) behavior is the result of a two-way process: that is, the interaction or transaction between an individual and his make-up and the social context in which he is reared and lives. The kind of low frustration tolerance, therefore, which leads or encourages some people to become assassins has important sociological or culturally learned roots.

In this connection, Philip G. Zimbardo, a professor of psychology at Stanford University, contends in an interview with David Burnham that "Americans are being transformed into potential assassins by the powerful social pressures of big-city living. In formulating a unified theory on violence and vandalism, Dr. Zimbardo points to 'the sharp increase in murder during the last few years, the estimated total of 40,000 American youngsters who each year are beaten and tortured by their parents or their brothers and sisters, the 230 violent urban outbreaks of the last five years and the assassinations of Medgar Evers, Malcolm X., the Rev. Dr. Martin Luther King, Jr., President John F. Kennedy and his brother Robert F. Kennedy.

"He further noted that in 1967 vandals in New York City smashed 202,712 school windows and 360,000 pay telephones and did $750,000 worth of damage in the parks and $100,000 worth of damage to the transit system. 'What we are observing all around us, then, is a sudden change in the restraints which normally control the expression of our drives, impulses, and emotions.' . . . Dr. Zimbardo suggested that many of the old restraints in American life, imposed by such institutions as the large family, were being dissolved by a process he called 'deindividuation.' . . . 'Conditions which foster deindividuation,' he said, 'make each of us a potential assassin.' "

The National Commission on the Causes and Prevention of Violence, in its report on assassination, also highlights the importance of environmental conditions in reducing the frustration tolerance of some individuals who become assassins: "Though an assassin is mentally deranged, the violent rhetoric of our politics and our constant flirtation with actual violence may be factors that bring him at least half-way to his distorted perception of what actions are right and legitimate."

Magical thinking. Many people who vigorously oppose a certain politico-economic viewpoint—whether that view be extremely right-wing, left-wing, or even centrist—are strongly inclined at times to wish for the death of the outstanding spokesman for the view that he despises. But since most political oppositionists are reasonably sane, they calculate that it would be foolish to directly or indirectly try to effectuate their murderous inclinations. Obviously, they could easily fail in their attempts; and even if they succeeded, they would endanger their own lives. Obviously, too, they would not kill the entire party or movement they oppose by silencing one or more of its leaders; and, in fact, they might well publicize and aid the cause they abhor by creating public martyrs for it.

By resorting to assassination, political oppositionists are normally able to see, they would mainly bring down on themselves the wrath of officialdom—and very likely of the shocked populace itself. They would thereby do their cause more harm than good. Consequently, sane proponents of extremist politico-economic views frequently *think* how nice it would be if they could eradicate their opponents in one huge blood bath—but they practically never take overt steps to carry out such a wishful notion.

Political assassins, on the other hand, are not equally stable, and frequently seem to believe that they and their supporters *can* get away with the bloody deeds they at first fantasize and then carry out. They are often deluded, at the moment they commit their misdeeds, that there *will* be a massive public uprising in their favor; that the individuals they assassinate *will* be universally condemned rather than raised to martyrdom; and that they, the murderers, will *not* be caught and punished.

Thus, many months before he finally killed Lincoln, John Wilkes Booth evolved a fantastic plot to abduct the president, to take him to Virginia, and to turn him over to the Confederate government, which would then supposedly be in a strong position to bring the Civil War to an end on its own terms. Guiteau, Garfield's assassin, quite magically seemed to believe that if he became insistently obnoxious enough in hounding Garfield to appoint him to public office, he would be successful in his quest for an important political job.

After Ferdinand Bonnier, Admiral Darlan's murderer, had been captured, notes P. Tompkins, he expressed the opinion "that a mysterious hand would come that might free him. . . . He said, 'I am calm, London has been advised'. . . . Romantically, he spoke of a simulated execution like that of Cavaradossi in *Tosca* before a firing squad with blank cartridges arranged by a modern Scarpia who would then allow him to slip away to Tangiers." As might be expected, this magical thinking led him to no better end than Cavaradossi found in the opera.

Leon Trotsky's murderer, Ramon de Rio Mercader, apparently believed he would positively affect his police guards and examiners by impressing them and the rest of the world with the great political act which he had performed and which he thought history would justify. He insisted that he had done the working class of the world an immense service by destroying one of its false leaders; and he advised his examiners to read Lenin, whose writings were those of a true revolutionary genius and would presumably fully justify his slaying of Trotsky (whom Lenin actually trusted) and his siding with Stalin (whom Lenin mistrusted).

Ansbacher and his associates believe that Lee Harvey Oswald's long flirtation with communism was a kind of magical thinking on his part. Oswald himself described his reading Marx, when he was in high school in New Orleans, as being "like a very religious person opening the Bible for the first time." It is probable that he could not relate to other people or understand what his life was all about, and that therefore he convinced himself that he had found a magical solution to all his problems in the communist ideals. It was perhaps after he had become somewhat disillusioned with the Soviet Union and communism, and saw no way out of his dismal life with his wife, Marina, that he again turned to a magical solution to his problems: the killing of President Kennedy, which would presumably make him famous and lead to all kinds of important consequences.

Robert F. Kennedy's assassin, Sirhan Bishara Sirhan, apparently became so convinced that he could not succeed in life with his limited abilities that he became a firm believer in various kinds of magic that would help him get what he wanted. He convinced himself that he would make a killing at the race track and thereby show others how great he was; and he became greatly involved with mysticism. As Fosburgh notes: "He would go to the race track in the day time, or work on a local ranch exercising the horses, and return to his bedroom at night. There in the dark and silence, he would read thick tomes and stare for hours at candles and diagrams, trying to increase his power of concentration. 'I thought it would make me a better person,' he explained last week." Although he did not exactly believe that he had unequivocal powers by which he could magically influence world events, he did believe that, if some natural catastrophe occurred to someone he hated, such as one of the officials of Israel, his thoughts and wishes about that person's coming to harm would somehow help that natural event to occur.

A significant percentage of assassins, then, appear to make their wishes father to magical kinds of thought. Even when they realistically acknowledge that they may not be able to escape earthly retribution for their murders, they seem to believe that they will be rewarded in some later celestial existence—in a heaven that is somehow ruled by their own kind. At the very least, they think that their memories will be ennobled on earth and that they will be gratefully remembered by their countrymen for eons to come. Occasionally, as in the case of Charlotte Corday, the assassin of Marat, they achieve some measure of benevolent fame after their demise; but the vast majority of them go down in history as publicly disgraced screwballs—which is hardly the role that they expected to be assigned to their shade. This kind of magical thinking, which usually leaves assassins with enough perspicacity to carry out their death-dealing blows but not enough sense to make good escape plans, is probably the reason that such a high percentage of them are caught so quickly.

Extreme moralism and hostility. Although assassins are normally considered immoral—since they commit the one act, murder, which is almost universally condemned—they seem to be unusually moralistic or blaming. They not only condemn the basic ideologies of their politico-economic opponents, but they severely castigate these opponents for *having* such ideas. This excoriation of an individual for espousing certain creeds or engaging in various behavior patterns is an act of extreme bigotry, of course, and has little connection with healthy opposition to philosophies which we may think are mistaken. It is a carrying of the argument *ad hominem* to exceptional extremes. As pointed out in the basic writings of rational-emotive psychotherapy, such as those by Albert Ellis, Robert A. Harper, and Paul Hauck, it is essentially a metaphysical, irrational way of thinking and behaving.

Granted that a man (such as the head of a political party or government) may be wrong in certain of his views and specific actions (as his opponents frequently think he is), he is a fallible human being and has an inalienable right to be wrong. To refuse to grant him this right is to demand unrealistically that he be perfect and infallible.

Moreover, since virtually every individual is capable of changing his ideas and actions and since he will think an incredibly large number of ideas and perform a vast number of actions during his lifetime, it is inaccurate to say that he is perfectly wrong, even though some of his philosophies and deeds, at a given period of his life, may be. By labeling *him,* rather than his views or performances, "wrong," "crazy," "immoral," or "horrible," we mean that he is globally, absolutely, for all time mistaken or vicious—and this is a metaphysical notion that there is really no way of proving or disproving.

A man is obviously more than and different from what he thinks or does at any single moment. To condemn him, in toto, for how he behaves is to contend that he cannot possibly change his behavior and is to evaluate him in a dogmatic, bigoted way. Furthermore: To condemn a person because he behaves badly is, by logical extension, to condemn one's *own* self whenever one happens to perform incorrectly. No human being, therefore, remains safe from eternal damnation and potential assassination if any man takes it upon himself to condemn another for his mistakes.

Even if it could be unerringly proven that a political figure were entirely wrong about his beliefs and actions (which, obviously, it can never be, since later history may prove him to have been correct), to condemn him, in toto, for being wrong is to be as wrongheaded as he is. To be human *is* to err; and unless each of us is given the inalienable right to be errant, and is protected from personal denigration and punishment for so being, freedom to think for ourselves becomes a mockery, and arrant bigotry and obscurantism begin to prevail.

The typical political assassin is unable to see this. He fails to distinguish between a person's being wrong and his being blamed, punished, and devalued as a human being for making mistakes. The assassin dogmatically and authoritarianly *wants* to blame; *demands* that his own views be considered absolutely right and everyone else's utterly fallacious; *insists* on making himself the final arbiter of human destiny, while placing all those who dissent from his views on an infinitely lower, dehumanized, and preferably nonexistent level. He is an unregenerate moralist and hater; and as a result of his childish grandiosity, he is usually severely emotionally disturbed.

That Oswald was, from his childhood to his death, an exceptionally moralistic, hostile individual, seems well attested by the facts of his existence. Several times during his early years he got into trouble with school and other authorities; and a full decade before he was accused of murdering Kennedy he was suspected of being psychopathic by a psychiatrist who examined him. Kerry Thornley doubts that Oswald was truly dangerous in his youth and at the time he knew him in the Marine Corps; but he gives several indications of his hostility at this time. Thus, in response to Albert Jenner, Jr.'s, questioning him when he appeared before the Warren Commission, Thornley admitted that Oswald "had gotten into difficulty with a staff sergeant and had poured beer on the person of a staff sergeant and gotten into some kind of altercation. . . . As a result of that he was court-martialed and had been subjected to the loss of clearance."

Again, according to Thornley, "He seemed to be a person who would go out of his way to get into trouble, get some officer or staff sergeant mad at him. He would make wise remarks. He had a general bitter attitude toward the Corps. He used to pull his hat down over his eyes so he wouldn't have to look at anything around him and go walking around very Beetle-Bailey style."

In regard to Oswald's relationships and his camaraderie with others in his Marine Corps outfit, Thornley tells us that these were "almost nil. . . . He got along with very few people." As an example of Oswald's bellicosity, he notes that on one occasion, when he remarked to Oswald, "Comes the revolution, you will change all that"—meaning Oswald's views of military organization—the would-be revolutionist screamed at him and "he never said anything to me again."

Typically, Oswald exhibited lifetime patterns of surliness and unfriendliness; and it is perhaps noteworthy that at the time Kennedy was shot, he was at serious odds with his wife and appeared to have no close friends. As Ansbacher and his associates note: "When friends gave gifts for his baby, he could not accept them, as he was incapable of joining in any give and take; he impugned the friends' motives as humiliating charity, apparently being unable to see how others could get positive pleasure in giving and sharing. . . . On a questionnaire Lee completed, he could not list a single close friend. One of his teachers thought him to be a belligerent, hostile boy who would lash out at anyone who offended him. Throughout school, there is the recurring theme of the boy being alone, and hints of his hostile feelings. Later, in the Marines, he is said to have been a hothead but that he could not hold his own in fist fights, possibly because of his small stature."

Again: Oswald was rejected when he offered to work with an anti-Castro Cuban exile group. He then distributed pro-Castro leaflets, got into a fight with the anti-Castroites, and was fined for disturbing the peace. Oswald also seems to have been hostile toward truly successful individuals; and Condon insists that his "indicated murder of Mr. Kennedy seems motivated only by his resentment against the most successful man in the world."

Manchester tells us that by the age of eleven Oswald "had become truculent with men and inadequate with women—and quick to rage at both." Bettelheim states: "The example we think of immediately today when we talk of hate and haters is Lee Oswald. From the evidence I have seen, he fits into the classic pattern of hate even though he was apparently not a member of any of the various hate groups on the American scene."

Like Oswald, Jack Ruby, who publicly assassinated Kennedy's alleged murderer, had a lifetime history of hostility and overrebelliousness. When he was eleven, according to the Warren Commission Report, he was examined at the Institute for Juvenile Research in Chicago and it was found that he was "quick-tempered . . . disobedient. He frequently disagrees openly with his mother, whom he considers an inferior person. . . . He also claims that he can lick everyone and anybody in anything he wants to do." A *New York Times* report (October 10, 1966) tells us, "He was always hot-tempered, and was called 'Sparky' when he was a boy because of his temper. Being called by his nickname provoked more than one fight itself, according to a sister, Mrs. Eva Grant. . . . Ruby never married, although he had an eleven-year romance with a Dallas divorcee, who says she refused to marry him because of his hot temper, among other things. One of Ruby's clubs, the Carousel Club, featured strip-tease dancers and had other burlesque features. A number of his former employees told the Warren Commission . . . that Ruby was a bad boss, that he frequently refused to pay them, and that he used obscene language toward them and sometimes struck them. Ruby was his own bouncer at his clubs and frequently beat patrons whose conduct he disapproved of. He was arrested several times in Dallas on assault charges."

Hartogs and Freeman also record evidence of Ruby's consistent hostility: "In 1941, at thirty, he suffered a concussion during a brawl. In 1955, at forty-four, while running the Silver Spur he got into a fight with three customers, and a woman clouted him over the head with a half-gallon jug of wine. . . . Dr. Walter Bromberg, well-known psychiatrist, who is clinical director of Pinewood Psychiatric Hospital in Katonah, New York, also examined Ruby for the defense. . . . He said the murder was committed under the surge of conscious hate and unconscious conflicts."

Dr. Martin Towler, neurologist at the University of Texas in Galveston, examined Ruby for the prosecution; and he noted that "despite an outwardly friendly and ingratiating manner, this patient seethes with hostility. Much of the time he is able to keep it under control, but his controls are brittle and when they break, the hostility erupts with volcanic force."

Thomas D. McMillon, the police officer who put handcuffs on Ruby right after he shot Oswald, testified at Ruby's trial that he heard him say as he pulled the trigger, "You rat son of a bitch, you shot the President!" Ruby then told the police: "I hope I killed the son of a bitch. I hope I killed the son of a bitch!"

Hartogs and Freeman also note that "Ruby fought regularly with his sisters and brothers, physically assaulting Eva at times, then making up. . . . Ruby was an Orthodox Jew who fought at the slightest provocation on religious grounds."

The *New York Times* gives still more details on Ruby's bellicosity: "Jack Ruby, the man who shot Lee Harvey Oswald in Dallas in November, 1963, has been described by his friends as a semi-illiterate hothead. Although outwardly a gregarious, nattily dressed individual, he lived in a gloomy apartment cluttered with old boxes and newspapers. And a close friend said he brooded in the privacy of his rooms. He loved animals, especially dogs, but could not establish a close relationship with more than one or two humans.

"Many of his acquaintances dodged him because he would lash out at them in vile language or suddenly strike them with his fists. Ruby was an accomplished brawler, and would not hesitate to tangle with men six inches taller and 50 pounds heavier than his 5 feet 9 inches and 175 pounds. Nor would he back away from disputes with men smaller than he or with women. 'Jack was always fighting,' said one of his sisters."

The convicted killer of Martin Luther King, Jr., James Earl Ray, was, according to his principal at the Ewing school, "a rebel. He rebelled against authority and his approach to most of his teachers was very bad." He violated almost all school regulations, was dishonest, had a repulsive appearance, and was seldom if ever polite to others. He was an unmanageable bully. Later, when he lived at the St. Francis Hotel in Hollywood, the drinking crowd in that area recall him "as an obsessive racial bigot, an abrasive patron who belted screwdrivers, dozed on the bar stool and bickered with anyone around. Everyone at the Rabbit's Foot Club remembers 'Galt's' [an alias of Ray] big dispute. A young woman had the temerity to tell him that Negroes were 'good people.' This so enraged Galt that he grabbed her arm and hauled her to the door, shouting: 'I'll drop you off in Watts and we'll see how you like it there!' " (*Time* Magazine, April 26, 1968.)

His acquaintances, *U.S. News* reports (April 4, 1968), found him to be "alternately moody and quarrelsome in his behavior." Harold Swenson, the warden of the Missouri State Penitentiary where he spent some time, called Ray "extremely dangerous, cold-blooded and ruthless" (*Time* Magazine, April 26, 1968).

Sirhan B. Sirhan was not only exceptionally moralistic and hostile about Senator Robert F. Kennedy, whom he assassinated, but about almost everyone who seemed to block his major wishes and goals. He wrote in his notebooks on May 18, 1968, nineteen days before he shot Senator Kennedy, "My determination to eliminate R. F. K. is becoming more of an unshakeable obsession." D. Robinson reports: "The rest of the page bore the phrases 'R. F. K. must die,' 'Robert F. Kennedy must be assassinated.' The last phrase was repeated about 20 times."

L. Fosburgh adds: "Sirhan Bishara Sirhan testified today that several weeks before the assassination of Robert F. Kennedy he saw the Senator on television helping Israelis to celebrate their independence and became so enraged that he wanted to kill him. 'I became burned up,' he told the stunned courtroom. And it was then, he added, that he wrote over and over in his notebooks, 'R. F. K. must die, R. F. K. must die.' 'At that time, sir, if he had been standing in front of me, so help me God, sir, he would die,' the 24-year-old Jordanian immigrant said to his defense counsel, Grant B. Cooper."

A few minutes later (Fosburgh states), "Mr. Cooper reminded him of a photograph of joyous Israeli soldiers that he had seen and asked him how he felt about it. 'At the time, sir,' he replied fiercely, 'if I saw those guys in person, I would have blasted them. I'd have killed them, the God damn Zionists.' "

Lest it be thought that Sirhan's moralism and hostility were triggered only by the Israeli situation and by Senator Kennedy's aid to the Israeli cause, it should be noted that in 1962 and 1963, a half decade before he killed Senator Kennedy, Sirhan had studied a book entitled *The American People* and underlined passages dealing with the assassination of President William McKinley. In the margin, alongside the marked section, he had written in pencil, "Many more will come." When given an alcohol test, soon after the assassination, to see how he would react, he was, according to Dr. Eric H. Marcus, a Los Angeles psychiatrist who was appointed by the court to study him, "a sort of wild beast. . . . He mumbled '20 years is long enough for the Jews' and 'Kennedy doesn't have to help them.' He was fierce and angry." Several times in the course of his trial, whenever testimony was given or a judicial ruling was made that displeased him, he displayed angry outbursts and acted like a thwarted young child.

Admiral Darlan's killer, Bonnier, was a "natural rebel," according to Tompkins. Of Darlan's political activities, Bonnier remarked: "Certain people spoke before me of this fruitless *demarche* and said: 'Darlan must disappear.' So I said to myself: 'Then I will undertake to make him disappear. . . . Clearly the Ten Commandments forbid killing, but there are moments when one must go so fast that the death of one who stands in the way of the general good is a necessity."

G. Catlin tells us that the Hindu extremist, Nathuram Vinayak Godse, who assassinated Mahatma Gandhi, "had persuaded himself that murder was a righteous act of indignation against him who by charity betrayed Nathuram's right to hate their enemies, the Sons of Islam. Nathuram Godse was a partisan and a zealot. For him zealotry excused murder."

The extreme moralism and hostility of Ramon de Rio Mercader, Trotsky's assassin, is shown from this observation of I. D. Levine:

"In addition to visible scars, there were reminiscences of acts of self-injury. Once, while playing a game, he made a bad play and kicked himself so hard that he injured his knee. He recollected that, when he was a soldier, he had had a disagreement with a subordinate and had taken out his anger by kicking the ground and severely injuring his ankle. Again, he had a disagreeable encounter with a superior officer. Finding this man's impertinence almost unbearable, he went away and 'took the anger out' on himself. This practice of kicking and wounding himself when angry with others is similar to the behavior of three-year-olds who are frustrated in their attempts to express their rage by kicking or otherwise injuring the omnipotent adults who restrain them, and therefore indulge in temper tantrums in which they scream and kick the floor. . . .

"When angry, he repressed all motion except for the trembling of his fingertips. The lines of his face deepened; the eyes became fixed and staring, penetrating and very brilliant; the lips were pressed closely together and the nostrils would flare. The sudden access of anger was accompanied by involuntary trembling and extreme pallor. When profoundly disturbed by questioning in any area which Mercader felt very dangerous to him, he would fumble with his cigarette, burn his fingers, drop ashes or sparks on his clothing or papers. This state of anxiety was accompanied by a tendency to compulsive talking so that the words seemed to pour from his mouth without volition, there was frequent repetition of phrases and often the sense was lost."

The foregoing facts about the hostility of Oswald, Ruby, Ray, Sirhan, and other assassins do not mean that every negative, truculent person is likely to become a murderer. Potentially, yes; but in all likelihood, no. For there is something final and far-reaching about taking another person's life that stops even the most angry individuals in their tracks and that makes them think more than twice about dispatching the objects of their rage. Even when an angry person does kill, he frequently has immediate profound regrets and insists that his act was unpremeditated and nonvolitional, and that now that he is again in control of himself he would never think of committing such a heinous deed.

In the case of assassins, however, who publicly and with malice aforethought slay an outstanding person, there does tend to be a long-time history of extreme resentment. Theirs is usually no spur-of-the-moment incitement to homicide. Frequently, as in the case of Garfield's murderer, Guiteau, they plan their murders days, weeks, or even months in advance; and they sometimes, as in Guiteau's case, make more than one abortive attempt before they succeed. There is every reason to believe that, if they had totally failed as assassins, they would have continued to find new objects of hatred for the rest of their lives. Their actual homicide tends to be one of a long series of hostile acts occupying almost their entire life span; it is merely a dramatic denouement, and in a sense a logical conclusion, to their generally hostile way of thinking and acting.

Grandiosity. The political assassin is frequently an individual who feels that he *has* to be outstanding and who deludes himself that he actually is or will be as a result of his killing a public figure. His feelings of inadequacy and impotence often stem from his need to be great and infallible—and from his partial recognition that he never will be, and that others will discover him to be something of a fraud. The more he demands greatness, the more consciously or unconsciously inferior he tends to feel. And the more he senses his inferiority, the more he believes that he has to achieve fame in order to prove that he is not *really* worthless.

Oswald's grandiosity was displayed in a number of ways during his short lifetime. Ansbacher and his associates contend that his "goal was to be superior to everyone. One way of striving toward this goal was to depreciate those who were actually his superiors. As a marine, his second court-martial was for using provocative words toward an officer. A former officer recalled Oswald as a trouble-maker and officer-baiter; he enjoyed stumping an officer with a question about some obscure situation, just to show off his own superior knowledge."

These same authors note: "One of the few fields into which Oswald put real effort was marksmanship, and he became a fairly good shot with a rifle in the Marines. We may assume that for him a gun was the means to be above others, to gain superiority by absolute power over others."

Oswald's wife, Marina, testified to the Warren Commission that "he wanted in any way, whether good or bad, to do something that would make him outstanding, that he would be known in history. . . . He had a 'sick imagination.' He engaged in fantasies about his future greatness, such as predicting that in twenty years he would be 'prime minister.' " Oswald also induced Marina to photograph him, in a triumphant pose, holding his 6.5 Mannlicher-Carcano carbine and carrying his .38 Smith and Wesson revolver in his hip pocket. He held a Trotskyite newspaper in front of his chest, as though he represented a conquering revolutionary.

Lee's brother, Robert, said Lee really had no understandable political motivation in shooting President Kennedy. Instead, he "tried to gain the world's attention through violence and destruction. . . . I am convinced that Lee could easily have chosen as his victim someone entirely different politically from John F. Kennedy."

When questioned about the possibility of Oswald's engaging in a widespread conspiracy to kill President Kennedy, Dr. Renatus Hartogs pooh-poohed this idea. Said Hartogs: "Oswald never would have shared with anyone the prestige of being the assassin of the President. . . . Paranoiacs like Oswald are loners. They neither need nor want a conspirator to share or dilute the responsibility for their crimes." Hartogs is one of the few psychiatrists who ever had first-hand knowledge of Oswald, since he was the one who examined him at the age of thirteen, when Oswald was already getting into serious school and social difficulties. He continued:

"The man in the tower in Texas, the one who killed the nurses in Chicago, and the boy who killed the women in the beauty school were all people who wanted to act alone—they, like

Oswald, did not want to share with anyone. . . . In my opinion, after reading all the books and the report itself, Kennedy's death was not a political assassination designed by a group of conspirators but a brutal murder conceived, planned and perpetrated by the morbid inner-world forces of a single insanely destructive power-operator."

D. Abrahamsen strenuously objects to the theory that Oswald had fellow conspirators and describes him as a person who "was unable to be part of a conspiracy" because he was so intent on showing the world how powerful he could be in his own right, even if everyone were against him. He was a solitary figure, "craving to be in the limelight," Abrahamsen insists; and he was "a conspirator against his own parents, his own family—against himself." Criminals in general, according to Abrahamsen, frequently must show their parents and the world that they are not insignificant and that they are able to take revenge upon those who reject them; they are consequently, in a grandiose manner, preoccupied with taking revenge. Oswald was typical in this regard.

Jack Ruby was another grandiose individual. He seems to have spent most of his life trying to prove how great he was—usually by fighting viciously with others and by trying to put them down so he would appear to rise on the other end of the competitive seesaw. He was apparently afraid to admit his actual age, and during his life he used a half-dozen or more different birth dates. He actually seems to have believed that he was a self-appointed martyr when he killed Oswald: He felt that he was beautifully avenging the death of President Kennedy and at the same time graciously saving Mrs. Kennedy the added grief of having to return for Oswald's trial in Dallas. When he was in jail both before and after his death sentence in March, 1964, he refused to cooperate with his lawyers, who claimed (apparently with good reason!) that he was insane when he shot Oswald. Instead, one of Ruby's principal interests was to prove that he was not insane—and that he was quite justified in assassinating Oswald.

James Earl Ray, the murderer of Martin Luther King, had grandiose illusions, according to pre-assassination acquaintances, as well as some of his lawyers and close associates who knew him after the crime. William Bradford Huie, an Alabama author who bought publication rights to Ray's life, who collaborated with Ray for many months when he was in jail, and who at first was convinced that the assassin was part of a large plot to kill King, later checked Ray's stories and concluded that he was the lone assassin of the black civil rights leader and that he committed the crime to gain "status" among criminals and their guards, for whose respect Ray consistently hungered. Said Huie:

"He hungered for the drama of a trial. He sustained himself with a fantasy in which he took the witness stand 'before the world' and performed masterfully. He surrendered this fantasy and agreed to plead guilty, I feel sure, only after he decided that, despite his guilty plea, he will now be an important person in prison, and that he will yet win freedom in some dramatic manner. . . .

"Ray thinks he fired the first shot in a social or racial conflict, a second Civil War, which will eventually result in his being freed. He therefore feels fulfilled: he believes he is liked, respected, even admired. And he is confident that political developments in the United States will cause him to be freed in two to four years."

Percy Foreman, who for a while served as Ray's attorney, concurred with Huie: "I think Ray believed Dr. King was a Communist; that his crusades had opened the Pandora's box of riot; and that, though he preached nonviolence, by indirection he created Black Muslims, Black Panthers and Invaders. Ray thinks that the war between the races is imminent, and he wanted to fire the first shot. The shooting of Dr. King, to him, was the Pearl Harbor of that war."

Foreman also thinks that Oswald, Ruby, and Sirhan were killers who were largely motivated by grandiose publicity-seeking: "Why did they kill? They each wanted the world to hear of them. They wanted credit. Top billing. Headlines. Front-page pictures. A by-line. Self-realization. A shortcut to fame. To exercise the ego. To them, notoriety and fame are synonymous. What other men study, plan, and struggle a lifetime to achieve, these killers thought they could win with lead. . . . For a few hours, I represented Oswald's killer, Jack Ruby. He was a frustrated showman, successful only at showing off the backsides of itinerant girls. To perform before 50 million television viewers was a chance he couldn't resist."

Dr. Eric H. Marcus, a court-appointed psychiatrist who examined Sirhan B. Sirhan several times in his cell after he killed Senator Robert Kennedy, who carefully examined Sirhan's notebooks, and who interviewed his mother, Mrs. Mary Sirhan and his thirty-year-old brother, Adel, testified during Sirhan's trial that the assassin saw himself as the "savior of society" when he fired the fatal shots. Dr. Marcus said that the Jordanian-born killer was so mentally ill that, in a manner typical of megalomaniacs, "he planned to destroy the current political leaders of the country and even to start World War III. . . . He decided he knew what was best for the country."

J. Shearing reports that Charlotte Corday, who stabbed Marat, the leader of the French reign of terror during the Revolution, to death in his bath, as a child "had no one to disturb her ingenuous passion for sublimity and heroism. . . . The child began to dream of herself as devoted to some great sacrifice, some splendid abnegation, some tremendous service to a high ideal. She mused over heroism as some girls muse over love; she felt in herself the pride, the courage, the fortitude necessary to accomplishment of a famous deed. So exactly did the tragedies of Corneille suit her temper that she exclaimed: 'I am of the race of the Emilias and the Cinnas!' "

Charlotte's extremist tendencies seem to have penetrated practically all aspects of her life. As Shearing continues: "She became very devout in her religious observances. . . . Everything mediocre being distasteful to her, she strove to raise her religion to sublime heights, she wished to be not only a Christian, but a saint, a martyr; to the rites of the church she brought the emotional heroism of Corneille, the stoicism of Plutarch's worthies. . . . Often her musing, her concentration on these heroicisms, these ideals, would result in ecstasy."

One of Ferdinand Eugene Bonnier's main motives in assassinating Admiral Darlan was that he was assured he would be a national hero. Among his military companions, Tompkins notes, he "found himself in his proper element. The morale was high, and the air breathed . . . was that of fairy tales and glory, of sacrifice and poetry, in which all were predestined heroes."

R. G. Caldwell observes that Guiteau, President Garfield's assassin, felt "in some strange way that he had a great political mission to perform." Following his crime, a letter was found in his pocket in which he wrote: "I have just shot the President . . . his death was a political necessity. I am a lawyer, a theologian, and a politician. I am a Stalwart of Stalwarts."

Trotsky's murderer, Mercader, had an "attitude of superiority" which led him into trapping himself with the psychologists who examined him after the assassination. He found these psychologists' interest in himself most absorbing and thought he could easily dominate and deceive them. Even as a small boy, he was proud and taciturn; and he would invariably try out his accomplishments in private before showing them to his family, as he was terribly afraid of failing at anything in public.

In a study of 137 male subjects who did not actually make any assassination attempts but who, from 1945 to 1965, made threats or gestures of assassination serious enough to lead to their arrest and/or their psychiatric evaluation, Weinstein and Lylerly found that these individuals tended to be "socially isolated persons who adapt to stress by symbolizing their problems in a political idiom and who identify with the President in terms of violence and death." Would-be assassins, these authors hold, are personally disturbed rather than truly politically active, but they construe their projected assaults on presidents as heroic acts which will save the country, will bring themselves fame and approval, and will solve their own problems.

In this respect, these individuals who threaten high-placed political figures are like the nineteen-year-old youth who was accused of attempting to murder the Australian opposition leader, Arthur Caldwell. According to Karl Menninger, he told the police after his capture, "I realized that unless I did something out of the ordinary, I would remain a nobody." Grandiosely inclined assassins stubbornly refuse to remain nobodies—even if, to become a somebody, they have to murder.

Chapter 9

The Emotional Disturbance of Assassins

Although it may be contended that many assassins are not unique in having serious feelings of inadequacy, low frustration tolerance, persistent hostility, and displays of grandiosity—since innumerable nonmurderers also exhibit these traits and perhaps all "normal" human beings possess them to some degree—it cannot as easily be held that severe emotional disturbance, or what is commonly labeled "mental illness," is rampant among the general populace in Western civilization. The fact remains, however, that, if we objectively examine the lives of political assassins who were personally involved in the killing of outstanding public figures, and who were not paid gunmen or members of a political organization who were specially appointed to carry out a murderous deed, we find that almost all of them are characterized by severe emotional instability or outright psychosis.

Lee Harvey Oswald's extreme disturbance was obvious from an early age, as indicated from reports by A. H. Newman, the Warren Commission, and others. He was a "loner"; was resentful of discipline; was bored and restless in school; shirked his studies, although he was well above average intelligence; felt that he and his family were persecuted by society; was fanatically devoted to communism but unable to gain acceptance by the Russians when he decided to give up his United States citizenship; was distressed about losing his hair (which he irrationally attributed to the cold Russian winters); was unable to hold some jobs because of his incompetently performing work that could have normally been easily grasped by someone of his intellect; acted so suspiciously that causes that he favored refused to have any connection with him; and generally behaved in a withdrawn, irresponsible manner.

More concretely, we have the first-hand evidence of Thornley, who replied to the question of Mr. Jenner, one of the Warren Commission investigators, "Do you think he was emotionally unstable?" with an unequivocal "I think so." "That," Jenner continued, "is an opinion you gathered from your association with him in the Marines?" And Thornley, again without cavil: "Yes."

When Jenner asked Thornley, "To what did you attribute this inability of his to maintain reasonably cordial or at least service-family relations with his fellow Americans?" the latter's reply was: "Well, at the time I just thought: well, the man is a nut. . . . I just thought: something is wrong with him; maybe something is bugging him today; maybe he is crazy; I don't know what. . . . Later, I did reflect on it, and that, combined with his general habits in relation to his superiors, and to the other men in the outfit, caused me to decide that he had a definite tendency toward irrationality at times, an emotional instability."

William Manchester, after reviewing all the evidence on Oswald and Kennedy, tells of the day, right before the date of the assassination, when Marina Oswald told Lee that she could manage without him and that she was going to find an asylum with Ruth Paine, her trusted friend: "That was the breaking point. He had nothing left, not even pride. In Marina's later testimony, 'He stopped talking and sat down and watched television.' She glanced in once and saw him staring at an old film of a World War II battle. Apparently, he was intent upon the flickering screen. In fact, he was going mad. Madness does not strike all at once. Lee Oswald's disease had been in process all his life. Unquestionably, his mother's influence had contributed to his weakness. Nevertheless, the impact of his confrontation with his wife on November 21 appears to have been decisive, and it seems equally clear that the total eclipse of his reason occurred shortly before 9 p.m. that evening, a few minutes after Jacqueline Kennedy had finished her brief Spanish speech in Houston, and while she and the President were making their way out across the crowded lobby."

In his thirteenth year, when Oswald was brought into Youth House in New York City because of chronic truancy from school, the Chief Psychiatrist, Dr. Renatus Hartogs, diagnosed him as "personality pattern disturbance with schizoid features and passive-aggressive tendencies" and the social worker called him "a seriously detached, withdrawn youngster." When Dr. Hartogs reviewed the Oswald case a decade later, he was more than ever inclined to believe that Lee was an exceptionally disturbed individual who had delusions of grandeur, who was seriously sexually repressed, who was obsessed by overwhelming fear and fury, who was incapable of a lasting relationship with a woman, who was megalomaniacal, and who failed to achieve even a semblance of maturity.

Priscilla McMillan, who lived with Marina Oswald for six months in 1964 and who has devoted more than five years to studying the Oswalds, points out that Kennedy's assassin "probably did not care enough about killing President Kennedy to have made the short bus trip from Dallas to Fort Worth to do it. He would not have walked across Dallas to do it. Oswald murdered the president because circumstances afforded him the opportunity. In his disordered scheme of things, the fact that he worked in the Texas School Book Depository, along Kennedy's route, signified to Oswald that his star fated him to do the deed."

She also notes that this same disordered scheme of things led him to make at least four suicidal gestures during his life. There is much reason to agree with her that President Kennedy was not really that important to him. Less than a year before, he had tried to kill Major General Edwin A. Walker, too. *Correcting his own internal disorder* was what really seemed to matter to Oswald; and he vainly tried to do just that, in his own peculiar way, until the very end.

From all the data that are now available on Oswald, it would appear that, although he was never hospitalized for mental illness, and might never have been institutionalized had he not decided to assassinate Kennedy, he was at least a borderline schizophrenic and was seriously aberrated from his early childhood onward. While most of the psychiatric opinions on Oswald emphasize the dreadful circumstances of his childhood, it is doubtful whether these alone produced his severe emotional aberration. Some of the most traumatic life experiences, as Renaud and Estess found in a study of one hundred normal American males, result in nonpathogenicity; and many children reared in fine, stable homes by loving parents turn out to be criminals and murderers. Early environment, therefore, although important in conditioning human beings to become emotionally healthy or unstable, is not the whole story. There are significant biologically based factors as well; and it is probable that individuals like Oswald are (as we shall note in more detail below) constitutionally predisposed to be unduly influenced by their poor childhood surroundings and to make the worst, rather than the most, of the unfortunate conditions in which they are raised.

From what we have noted about Jack Ruby's bellicosity and grandiosity, it may be suspected that he, like Oswald, was an exceptionally disturbed individual from his earliest years. That is the opinion of most of the psychiatrists who testified for both the defense and the prosecution at his murder trial. Dr. Walter Bromberg reported that Ruby had a "brain disease, a subtle one." Dr. Martin L. Towler stated that Ruby had "a rare form of epilepsy of the psychomotor variant pattern." Dr. Manfred Guttmacher, medical officer of the psychomotor Court of Baltimore, testified that he thought that Ruby had suffered "a rupture of his ego. . . . I think he was struggling to keep his sanity during this period. I think that he had an unusual degree of involvement in the whole tragedy. . . . He came upon the perpetrator of the tragedy . . . there was disruption of his ego, a very short-lived psychotic episode in which the hostile part of his makeup, which is very strong, became focused on this one individual."

Dr. Frederic Gibbs, a leading authority on epilepsy, examined Ruby's brain-wave tracings and concluded that he suffered from "psychomotor epilepsy" which drove him into "rage states." Dr. Towler reported "there is a distinct paranoid flavor in his relationship with people. He sees insults and criticisms when none was intended. He exhibits some distrust of his lawyers and his psychiatrists. His hypochondriacal trends, his food fads, and his narcissistic concern over his body weight and his baldness are frequently associated with abnormal suspiciousness." Dr. Louis J. West, head of the Department of Psychiatry at the University of Oklahoma Medical Center, described Ruby as suffering from a "paranoid state," said that he was "obviously psychotic," and that he needed hospital treatment.

Dr. Robert Stubblefield, chairman of the Department of Psychiatry, Southwestern Medical School, University of Texas, in a letter reproduced as one of the exhibits in the Warren Commission Report stated that Ruby "has had and has now an acute psychiatric illness, with paranoid depressive features" and that he "should be under the supervision of a psychiatrist, preferably in a psychiatric hospital, until the prisoner recovers sufficiently to proceed with his appeal with rational understanding." Dr. Renatus Hartogs compared Ruby with Oswald and found many psychiatric similarities between them, including the facts that Ruby was obsessed by overwhelming inner fear and fury during his childhood, was an impulsive individual who was driven by his fantasies, was constantly quarreling with members of his family, was overconcerned with food, was incapable of a lasting relationship with a woman, was a megalomaniac, and was a failure at achieving even a semblance of maturity.

Sirhan B. Sirhan, who murdered Senator Robert F. Kennedy in the midst of a large public function, and did so in circumstances which practically guaranteed that he would be caught and convicted for his crime, has a history of severe emotional disturbance that would be difficult to duplicate even in the histories of many institutionalized psychotics. At his trial, a long procession of reputable psychiatrists and psychologists, on the basis of extensive tests and interviews with Sirhan and with other members of his family, unequivocally testified to his highly disturbed state of mind considerably before and just prior to his shooting Kennedy.

According to *New York Times* reporter, D. Robinson, Dr. Martin Schorr, a clinical psychologist, stated that he exhibited "paranoid and schizophrenic tendencies," that his tests indicated that he was more paranoid "than 95 out of 100 people," that he showed "marked reduced intellectual function under stress," that he was "severely, markedly disabled," and that he had "not only had impulses for homicide, but for suicide."

Dr. Roderick Richardson, another clinical psychologist, told the court that Sirhan "did not have the 'mental capacity' to premeditate the murder of Senator Robert F. Kennedy. . . . 'My general feeling is that Sirhan for at least one or two years before the crime was unable to fathom his actions,' Dr. Richardson said. 'He sees himself as a soldier of his nation and as such he goes beyond normal behavior.' "

H. Dudar reports that Dr. Eric H. Marcus, a psychiatrist, "found Sirhan too mentally ill to reflect meaningfully and maturely on the gravity of his contemplated act. . . . Two factors heavily influenced his conclusions, the psychiatrist said. One was the results of the psychological tests. The second was the notebooks. They are, reported Marcus, the ravings of a psychotic—'typical of the notebooks and diaries and letters insane people write who have threatened Presidents and are now hospitalized.' Marcus said he has a package of letters written by insane murderers now in a state institution and the contents are not very different from 'the irrational ramblings' of Sirhan's notebooks. . . . Marcus said the prosecution psychiatrist found the defendant suffering a paranoid illness, probably paranoid schizophrenia. 'This I agree with.' "

Dr. Bernard L. Diamond, who hypnotized Sirhan in his jail cell and got him to re-enact the killing of Senator Kennedy, testified: "He acted in a blind rage. The shooting . . . was a reflex action, an outgrowth not only of chronic psychosis but a very abnormal state that began when he became confused and vague by all the lights and mirrors" outside the pantry where the shooting occurred. Diamond, in an interview with T. George Harris, has also stated: "The expert witnesses were not in serious disagreement over the diagnosis, only over the conclusions to be drawn from it. Ten of the eleven psychologists, anthropologists, and psychiatrists who examined the raw data were in substantial agreement: chronic paranoid schizophrenia."

Dr. Seymour Pollack, one of the first psychiatrists to see Sirhan after the assassination, was the only witness whom the prosecution could get to say that the killer was not too mentally ill to have premeditated the death of Senator Kennedy and that he did have the mental capacity to plan and carry out the murder. Although he had originally described Sirhan as a "psychotic person," Pollack claimed in court that "he is a psychotic person, but he is not clinically psychotic"—by which he meant that he did not have maximum evidence of mental impairment. *New York Times* reporter Douglas Robinson, however, reports: "Dr. Pollack acknowledged that, in his opinion, Sirhan had a paranoid personality, but he said that this alone did not mean he was psychotic. He later described the defendant as a 'borderline psychotic' whose behavior patterns were more on the normal side of the border than on the psychotic side. . . . He agreed with a suggestion by Mr. Cooper that Sirhan's 'brakes were not in good order' and that the 'glue' that held him together 'was not of good quality'. . . . At one point, Dr. Pollack disclosed that Sirhan once told him in an interview in his jail cell that he expected to be 'sent to prison for only a couple of years' for the killing of Senator Kennedy. . . . Dr. Pollack agreed that, on this matter, the defendant did not display [meaningful and mature] judgment."

It was also Pollack who pointed out what we previously noted in this chapter about Sirhan's magical beliefs: namely, that he believed that "were Dayan to be killed by a bolt of lightning or had Senator Kennedy, say, died in a plane crash, his wishes in some way would have influenced their destruction." It is fairly obvious, from Pollack's testimony, that he thought Sirhan to be a distinctly psychotic individual, but felt that he wasn't quite psychotic enough to be ruled legally insane under the laws of the state of California, and therefore he gave the court some very guarded testimony.

Another clinical psychologist, Dr. Leonard B. Olinger, agreed with Dr. Pollack that Sirhan had been mentally capable of planning and carrying out the fatal shooting of Kennedy and that he was not really too paranoid. But Dr. Olinger described Sirhan as a "person with borderline schizophrenia with primarily neurotic schizophrenia" and as a "pseudo-neurotic schizophrenic." All told, then, nine psychologists and psychiatrists testified that Senator Kennedy's assassin was outright psychotic and paranoid, and two testified that he was basically psychotic, or at the very least borderline schizophrenic. We have to agree with Dr. Diamond that this amounts to a rather rare unanimity of opinion in the annals of psychological testimony; and it would seem to be more than clear that there is ample evidence, from the trial itself, and from the rest of Sirhan's behavior before and after the slaying that he was always highly disturbed.

Thus, we find that Sirhan dwelt endlessly on the injustices of the Jews to Arabs in Israel, and presumably identified Kennedy, who supported Israel to some extent, as anti-Arabian. According to reporters T. Smith and R. Windeler, he was a secretive individual who gave up his ideas of being a journalist, a diplomat, or a teacher to pursue a career as a jockey. When he was an exercise boy, he fell off a horse, landed on his head, and possibly suffered brain damage. He was a loner, who did not participate much in the Arab activities in his community, though his sympathies were very much with the Arabs. Although college educated, he was addicted to race-track betting, and frequently lost all the money he had in his pockets when he went to the track.

The pastor of his church described him as "a clever boy—very quick—but unstable and very unhappy." He seemed to have some of his father's violence in him. "He was thin and nervous and inclined to sudden bursts of temper. At other times he was oddly quiet, for long periods." A former high school classmate reported that he was "despondent about his failure to do better and a feeling that life was taking him nowhere, that he was not going to make a mark." Although he stopped going to church, he was said to be an avid religionist; and some acquaintances said he was a Rosicrucian—a member of a fanatical, mystical sect.

We also learn that a diary, handwritten in a spiral notebook, was seized at Sirhan's home, and that an entry of May 18, 1968, read: "Kennedy has to be assassinated before June 5, 1968." June 5 was the date of the Six-Day War between Israel and the Arab states in 1967, and Sirhan apparently smoldered over the fact that Israel easily won this war. One of his neighbors, Alvin Clark, additionally reported that Sirhan "hated Kennedy because he hated everyone with money." We learn, again, that there is evidence that Sirhan premeditated his shooting of Senator Kennedy, in that he practiced rapid firing on a range which did not permit this kind of practice and did so only a short time before the assassination took place.

Robert Blair Kaiser, a free-lance writer who had special access to Sirhan and who contributed part of the earnings on his book, *R. F. K. Must Die!* to his defense, agrees with psychiatric opinion that Robert Kennedy's assassin had severely disturbed traits—especially the overweening desire to become famous at any cost. Kaiser reports that Sirhan told him, "They can gas me. But I am famous. I achieved in a day what it took Kennedy all his life to do." In order to cement his fame, Kaiser believes, Sirhan resisted all defense attempts to have him declared insane, and therefore not responsible for his crime. He tried to change his plea from not guilty to guilty during his trial, and heatedly told the judge: "I killed Robert Kennedy willfully and premeditatively and with twenty years' malice aforethought." When Judge Walker told him, "I know of nothing in the law which permits a defendant to enter a plea of guilty and ask for his own execution," Sirhan replied, "I do," in a loud, emphatic voice. This, Kaiser contends, is because Sirhan felt that pleading emotional disturbance might save him from the gas chamber but it would not keep his feelings of grandiosity and his need for fame intact. Relates Kaiser: "He'd rather go to the gas chamber than have anyone 'fucking around' with his mind."

The well-known psychiatrist, Thomas Szasz, in reviewing Kaiser's book wonders whether Sirhan was really "mad" and points out that "man has an insatiable appetite for meaning and significance. People will thus often believe, and sometimes do, anything—no matter how absurd or abhorrent—so long as the belief or act renders them and their lives more interesting and more important."

What Szasz does not face here is that when an individual has such an overweening desire—or, really, *demand*—for significance that he is driven to (1) become famous at all costs, (2) assassinate a well-loved public figure in order to achieve this goal, and (3) welcome dying in the gas chamber when he could probably get a long-term prison sentence, he probably has a high degree of "madness." For the terms "madness" and "an insatiable appetite for meaning and significance" that includes homicide and suicide are, for all practical purposes, synonymous. Kaiser (along with most of the psychologists and psychiatrists who examined and testified about Sirhan) and Szasz really seem to agree, though their language may be different.

In a good many ways, then, Sirhan's life was a steady history of childish temper tantrums, unrealistic goals, preoccupation with vindictive thoughts, schizoid withdrawal, fanatical religiosity, and persistent refusal to accept and adjust to reality.

James Earl Ray, the convicted assassin of Martin Luther King, had a school record marked with absence and misbehavior. He was convicted several times, between 1949 and 1967, of burglary, armed robbery, car theft, and forgery. He was notably withdrawn much of the time, especially when the conversation got personal. He lacked coordination. According to P. O'Neill, he "took amphetamines on and off" and was "an ingrown, emotionally stunted lover." He "seemed governed by a curious, even touching unreality." He was exceptionally bigoted, unreliable, and disturbed.

In William Bradford Huie's book, *He Slew the Dreamer,* he points out that Ray was little more than a small-time hoodlum who had an immense need for an ego trip; that he desperately wanted to gain status among his criminal peers by making the F.B.I.'s list of the Ten Most Wanted desperadoes; that he was motivated to kill King because of his extreme racial bigotry; and that even after his conviction and sentencing to a ninety-nine-year term for the assassination, Ray continues to view himself as a hero and to believe that public opinion will eventually elect someone such as George Wallace to the presidency, that the public will then clamor for his release, and that he will be set free in a blaze of TV-covered glory.

Marat's assassin, Charlotte Corday, resolved to kill the French political leader, Shearing tells us, when she heard that the Girondists had been expelled from the convention. "Convinced that this duty and the sacrifice had been divinely laid upon her, she had achieved the task of detaching herself from all earthly considerations and at the same time of making careful preparations so as to involve no one but herself in the consequences of her deed. . . . She had no doubts as to her fate. 'One cannot attack a savage beast without being bitten,' she had said in Caen. She had not even wished for fame, for glory; she had hoped to be destroyed and never be made known."

Even in her younger days, "her ideas became early set; no one had much influence over her once her mind was decided. . . . This child of fourteen was already inclined to extremes." Nor was her fantasy life impaired: "Her manner was grave and serene; she disclosed herself to none, and the hard reality of life did not interrupt her dreams." She "deliberately trained herself to endure suffering in silence. One of her friends saw her dragging herself along the walls by the abbaye, her face covered with blood, half-fainting from pain and shock. She had fallen in leaving the church, but refused to admit that she was hurt and smiled at her frightened mother who exclaimed: 'Ah, this poor child is too hard on herself! She never complains and I have to guess when she is ill—she never tells me!' "

Charles Franklin, in his picture of Charlotte Corday in *Woman in the Case,* gives more evidence of her lifelong pattern of serious emotional disturbance: "She welcomed death. And with this death wish . . . she combined an exaggerated fear of any infringement of her modesty. . . . She also had a strong desire to be a saint and a martyr, to be immortal, to be remembered, to be the heroine dying for her country. . . . Francois Chabot, who was an unfrocked priest and a friend of Marat, took charge of the questioning. She replied to him with an arrogance and courage which astonished them all.

" 'How was it that you were able to strike him to the heart at one blow? You must be well practised.'

" 'The anger in my own heart showed me the way to his,' was her quick, uncompromising reply.

"The questioning was nearly over, but Chabot did not want to let her go. He stood over her, looking down at her bosom, full of hate and desire, and spotted a piece of paper which was inside her bodice.

"He suddenly thrust his hand right in between her breasts and plucked the paper out.

"Charlotte Corday was prepared for death, but to her this indecent hand touching her was worse than death. She leaped to her feet with blazing eyes, and unable to protect herself because of her bound wrists, made a backward movement against the wall so violent that it broke the laces of her bodice.

"As the bodice burst apart, her firm full breasts were revealed for a second for all in the room to see. Then she collapsed on the chair, bending double to hide her nakedness, flushing hotly in an agony of shame."

Felice Orsini, an Italian revolutionist around the middle of the nineteenth century, attempted the assassination of Napoleon III on January 14, 1858. Although he failed to kill his intended victim, the bombs which he set off did annihilate ten persons and wounded one hundred and fifty. M. Rougeau investigated Orsini's life and wrote a small book on his psychopathology. He found Orsini to be a person who had a boundless pride, considerable hostility and marked defiance against the world, social maladjustment, exceedingly poor judgment, and paranoid tendencies to over-reach himself. In spite of the failure of his assassination attempt, Orsini was in many important respects typical of the near-psychotics and psychotics who actually succeed as assassins.

John Wilkes Booth, Lincoln's assassin, was commonly believed to be emotionally unbalanced. According to Pitman, Booth as a child was "a wild young lad, handsome in appearance like all the Booths, but, also like them, erratic and unpredictable." In 1864 he concocted a crazy scheme to kidnap Lincoln and hand him over to the Confederate government; and his distorted enthusiasm to abduct the president grew into madness and the eventual decision to assassinate him. He became so psychotic as the time of assassination grew near that he was not even sure what year it was: " 'Merrick, is the year 1864 or '65?' 'You are surely joking, John,' he rejoined, and on being told resumed writing."

At this same time Merrick also noticed something very troubled and agitated about Booth's appearance, quite at variance with his usual quiet deportment. Booth's behavior before, during, and immediately after his assassination of Lincoln would indicate that he was at the very least suffering from a temporary psychotic state; but his previous history, as well as that of various other members of his family, would lead us to suspect that he was never entirely sane and that for a long time he was at least prepsychotic.

A graphic indication of Booth's severe disturbance just before he assassinated Lincoln is shown by this description of the oath he and some of his fellow conspirators took the night before the deed took place. Emmett McLoughlin quotes this account from *The Great Conspiracy,* published by Barclay and Co., Philadelphia, 1886:

" 'The oath! the oath! bring out the crucifix, Mrs. Surratt.'

" 'You will pardon me, Mr. Booth, but that must not be in my house.'

" 'And why not, madam?' replied Booth, 'we are engaged in a holy cause.'

"Awed by the tone of command in which these words were spoken, and the fiery glance accompanying them, the sculptured representation of the savior was placed on the table, and Booth lit three candles he had brought with him, and extinguished the gas. The starry flames of the candles alone prevented utter darkness; and cast a pale gleam on the countenance of the conspirators.

"Booth advanced to the table, and seizing the cross, exclaimed in a low, but deep and earnest tone, 'I do solemnly swear by the passion of our Lord and Savior Jesus Christ.'

" 'Mr. Booth, I entreat you, go no further,' said Mrs. Surratt.

" 'Peace, madam,' he replied sternly. 'The oath shall be taken! Is this child's play, or have we come here merely to have a little sport? The oath shall be taken, and by all in this chamber; no one leaves till he has sworn to obey. Where are your protestations of loyalty to the South, have they all vanished, have they all melted into thin air? I say again that the oath shall be taken. Disobey me at your peril!'

" 'I shall now take the oath, and you, madam, will be silent. If you utter a word or make a movement, you shall die.'

"Herold and Atzerodt produced loaded pistols, and Booth pronounced these words.

" 'I do solemnly swear, by the passion of our Lord Jesus Christ, by his agony in the garden, by the sorrow which pierced his soul when Peter denied him, and by the spotless purity of his Holy Mother, that I will aid and abet, by all the means in my power, the plot which has just been planned; and I further swear by all that man holds sacred, both in this world and the next, that should any one attempt to reveal the plot or any part of it, that I will pursue him with the most utmost vengeance, no matter how closely connected with me.' He then kissed the crucifix."

Charles J. Guiteau, President Garfield's assassin, was said to have been from earliest boyhood an erratic, self-willed, cruel individual. After he had failed at his law practice and at writing and marketing religious books, R. H. Conwell relates, "he floated about from city to city unsuccessfully swindling landladies and hotels and whoever would trust him. His plausible manner and knowledge of religious literature gained him admission to the clergy and churches, and nearly all of them suffered more or less from his dishonesty. . . . Being laughed at, hooted, and driven out of the field as a religious lecturer, he turned his attention to politics, and, by his great assurance and falsehoods, secured engagements and money in the campaign of 1880, in New York, Pennsylvania, and Illinois. . . . Some persons excused his eccentricities and dishonesty by the thought that he was insane, and his father, before he died, seemed to think that his son's persistent lying and swindling was the result of a diseased brain."

C. E. Rosenberg quotes Dr. Edward C. Spitzka, a young neurologist who wrote about Guiteau immediately after Garfield's assassination and who testified at his trial. Said Spitzka: "A thorough study will convince an impartial and competent jury of medical examiners, before whom such a case should be laid, that Guiteau is not only now insane, but that he has never been anything else, that his crime was the offspring of insanity, and that in every act he will betray the characteristic features of querulent monomania. They will also conclude that, inasmuch as his insanity is not the result of his own vices, but based on defective organization inherited from a diseased ancestry," he is not really responsible for his crime. Spitzka also stated: "The marked feature of this man's insanity is a tendency toward delusive opinion, and to the creation of morbid or fantastical projects . . . there is a marked element of imbecility of judgment."

Rosenberg concurs with Spitzka's diagnosis; and H. F. Graff, in reviewing Rosenberg's book, agrees: "In a psychiatric diagnosis of our own day Guiteau would probably be described as a paranoid schizophrenic—and be hospitalized for possible treatment."

Our view is that Guiteau was a so-called psychopath or sociopath; and, as Cleckley has fairly convincingly shown, psychopathy of this nature is nothing more than a mask for insanity. Either borderline psychosis or outright psychosis can certainly be suspected in Guiteau's case.

Prendergast, who shot and killed Carter H. Harrison, mayor of Chicago in 1893, was, according to W. J. Abbott, "a half-mad seeker after places under the city administration, an illiterate fellow . . . with a craving for notoriety. . . . In a period of moody wrath over his failure of appointment, he shot down the mayor whom he held responsible. . . . He was a man of blunted moral sense, overweening egotism, and with a fancied grievance [who] thought himself doing the State a service by the assassination of the Mayor. Throughout his trial, which resulted in his execution, the murderer steadfastly refused to plead insanity, firmly declaring his conviction that the people would justify him in what he had done."

Richard Lawrence, who attempted to shoot President Andrew Jackson, Weinstein and Lylerly report, was "an unemployed, destitute house painter whose pseudo-community was the Kingdom of England and America. He claimed to be King Richard III and charged that Jackson had taken his money and usurped his throne." There seems to be little doubt that he was psychotic.

Giuseppe Zangara, who attempted to kill President-elect Franklin D. Roosevelt and killed Mayor Anton Cermak of Chicago instead, was, according to Weinstein and Lyerly, an immigrant Italian laborer who "had long suffered from pains in his stomach which he attributed to the hard labor exacted from him by kings and presidents. While still in Italy, he had wanted to assassinate King Victor Emmanuel but did not have the opportunity. In the winter of 1932, he had first planned to assassinate President Herbert Hoover in Miami, but did not follow him north because the cold weather aggravated his symptoms. He then shot at Mr. Roosevelt, as he apparently considered that the President-Elect fell into the category of kings and presidents. In later statements, while maintaining his hatred for kings and presidents, he disclaimed any desire to harm emperors, rich men, and bosses!"

As this evidence shows, he, too, was almost certainly psychotic.

Ramon Mercader, Leon Trotsky's assassin, was exhaustively studied by Dr. Jose Gomez Robledor, head of the Department of Social Medicine at the National University of Mexico and Dr. Alfonzo Quiroz Cuaron, professor of criminology in the School of Law and Social Sciences at the University of Mexico and Director of the Mexican Reformatory for Boys at Tlalpan. After spending 972 hours in their investigation of Mercader's personality, their final report, comprising 1,359 pages and entitled *Organic-Functional and Social Study of the Assassin of Leon Trotsky,* included these statements:

"Complete inability to make close human contacts. . . . Even if there was an element of shamming in his behavior [while imprisoned] it was clear that Ramon was going through a phase of massive repression. He spent almost the entire time in bed, often with his face down and the sheet pulled over his head. . . . [In regard to sex] his answers showed superficiality and emotional dissociation. . . . He is shown to be fearful and self-destructive in his inner self. But to conceal from the world that self he builds a façade to protect himself from his own attitudes: he drives himself, he disciplines himself, he is compulsive, and he takes great risks."

Although the assassin of Jose Antonio Remon, the president of Panama, who was cut down by machine-gun bullets in 1955, was never officially convicted, it is generally believed that Ruben Oscar Miro did this deed, because he reportedly developed an assassination scheme and even admitted the killing. L. L. Pippin tells us that Miro was "a popular but inept lawyer with a long family history of mental instability; and was thought by his first cousin, 'Tito' Arias, to be 'crazy.' " Pippin continues: "Perhaps symptomatic of the derangement of Miro was the way he plotted against the Remon regime. . . . Almost all of the plotting was done openly—in streets, in cafes, and at parties. The maladjusted lawyer . . . was a supposed psychopath."

Violet Gibson was not an actual assassin: Her plan to kill Benito Mussolini on April 7, 1926, did not succeed. But she certainly tried. According to E. Ferri, who did a character study and life history on her, she was severely disturbed in several ways. He notes that "facts concerning Violet Gibson's former life were soon made known, such as her internment on former occasions in asylums in England, where she was found to be subjected to homicidal ideas and to attacks of acute violent mania; and her suicide was stubbornly attempted in a convalescent home in Rome; and a preceding attempt at homicide, when she used a knife (an unusual weapon for criminal women) to try to kill a young girl.

"Her idea on this last occasion was that of repeating the sacrifice of Abraham, which was sufficient to convince anyone that they had to deal with an abnormal, unbalanced, and infirm mind."

Miss Gibson was studied by Professors Sante De Sanctis and Augusto Giannell, both of whom had considerable experience with diagnosing mental hospital patients. They conclude that "she was in a state of mental infirmity . . . and was thus deprived not of her perception of right and wrong but of her freedom of will to act. We have thus to deal with a case of 'lucid insanity' or of 'conscious madness.' "

While awaiting trial for the attempted assassination of Mussolini, Miss Gibson wounded a fellow prisoner and showed a renewed inclination to commit suicide. Her entire life seemed to be a continuous succession of violent and psychotic episodes.

A would-be assassin named Ilyin fired at a group of Soviet cars on January 22, 1969, in an apparent attempt to kill some famous Soviet astronauts or leading officials. He actually killed the driver of a limousine carrying four astronauts and wounded a motorcyclist who was escorting the car. The Soviet Supreme Court, after making a thorough investigation of Ilyin, declared him insane and ordered him confined to a special mental hospital. B. Gwertzman notes that the Russian newspaper, *Izvestia,* reported: "Having studied materials of the investigation, and on hearing conclusions by experts and witnesses' testimony, the court found that Ilyin committed socially dangerous actions in a state when he was not answerable for his actions. . . . But considering that Ilyin is a socially dangerous person, the court decided to isolate him from society and send him for compulsory treatment at a special psychiatric hospital."

L. S. Clemens, reviewing the cases of the assassins of four American presidents (Lincoln, Garfield, McKinley, and Kennedy) and the attempted assassins of three other presidents (Jackson, Truman, and Franklin D. Roosevelt) and a presidential nominee (Theodore Roosevelt), noted that, of these, only the attempted assassins of Truman (Oscar Collazo and Griselio Torreselo) "are free of the suspicion of insanity, or a psychopathy that crippled personality." He also reported that two unsuccessful assassins, Richard Lawrence (who tried to kill Jackson), and John N. Schrank (who tried to kill Theodore Roosevelt), "ended their days in mental institutions. Lawrence 16 years after the death of his intended victim, Schrank 20 years after the death of his and 38 years after the event for which he was committed." He further observed that "only one of the nine made plans for escape after the deed was done, although only Collazo and Torreselo apparently expected to die."

Biological factors in the emotional disturbance of assassins. As noted above, it is easy to find poor environmental conditions in the childhood of many assassins and to conclude that they became murderous because of the loss of a father, jealousy of an older brother, neglectful treatment from a mother, the influence of neighborhood gangs, etc. Especially in the cases of Lee Harvey Oswald and Jack Ruby, where such negative environmental factors were indubitably present, it is tempting to conclude that they were the direct or indirect causes of the murderous impulses of the adult assassins.

The trouble with all such conclusions is that they are contaminated by other factors. For most execrable influences on children are the result of their parents' miserable behavior. And what most psychologists usually fail to ask is: "Assuming that this assassin's mother rejected or neglected him or otherwise reared him badly, *why* did she do so? Could it not be that she, too, was an exceptionally disturbed individual, and that, in addition to being environmentally conditioned by her teachings or behavior, he inherited some of her tendencies to over-react to the stimuli impinging on him?"

In the case of assassins, it is almost impossible to show, at the present time, whether environmental or hereditary factors were most significant in determining their murderous behavior. The chances are that neither one nor the other was the paramount influence but that a transactional intermingling of both conditions was the "real" cause. In any event, we would be foolish to ignore the importance of genetic predisposition in their disturbed thoughts and actions, since there is some evidence that one or both their progenitors were just as or more disturbed than they were.

Jean Stafford, the well-known novelist, went to interview Mrs. Marguerite Oswald some time after her son's death, and in her book, *A Mother in History,* records some bizarre views held by her subject. Mrs. Oswald suggested the likelihood that President Kennedy was dying of an incurable disease and that her son, Oswald, might have helped put him out of the way in order to perpetrate a mercy killing. Miss Stafford reports Mrs. Oswald as saying:

" 'We teach our boys to kill in war and we don't think a thing about it, yet if these same boys kill someone on the street they are lawfully put in jail or else electrocuted, which is right. So why wouldn't it be just a normal thing to have a mercy killing of the President?'

"She uttered the word 'normal' without a suggestion of inverted commas, and I think this is exactly what she meant; as for 'mercy killing,' she made that sound as commonplace as the use of aspirin to bring down a fever."

Mrs. Oswald continued: " 'If my son was an agent of the United States, this should be known. I wonder why Chief Justice Warren had tears in his eyes when President Johnson asked him to head up this commission? I wonder why.' She meditated, reading her palms. 'Did Chief Justice Warren have to whitewash something the public don't know about? Did he know my son was innocent? Who *used* my son? This is the question I must find the answer to. Research and research, until I can bring the truth to light. My son was killed on cue, and this I can prove. The television cameras were ready, and the TV directors gave the order. As I understand it, some very important men in the networks got into trouble, lost their jobs and everything. But that's beside the point. What I want to know is who used Lee Harvey Oswald?' "

Ansbacher and his associates note that "Mrs. Oswald certainly neglected Lee. . . . However, it is also sure that she pampered him, at least in the sense that she let him have his own way and excused him from responsibility for his actions. Whenever Lee came into conflict with others, or with law and order, she consistently released him from any obligation to comply with what was expected of him; denied any wrong on his part, and/or placed the blame for his behavior squarely on others. When he was a youngster she took his word against that of an adult complaining about his holding up the phone and using profanity on their party line. She once condoned his truancy by saying, 'He used to come home and say, "I already know all the stuff they're teaching. Why bother with that?" Then he'd go off to the library.' When he was investigated by the Children's Court of New York City, at thirteen, Mrs. Oswald refused to take him to a psychiatric clinic, as recommended; she kept saying he wasn't any problem, and she didn't understand what the fuss was all about. She told the probation officer: 'My son is not going to report to you. . . . He's given his word that it is not going to happen again. I was not going to have a boy of that age and caliber going to a probation officer.' Much later, when he couldn't find a job, she claimed it was all because the papers had blown up the matter of his defection. And last of all, she placed the blame for his final deed on the security officers who had not held her son under complete surveillance!"

Jean Stafford continues her inimitable portrait of Lee Harvey Oswald's mother: "Mrs. Oswald, pouring hot water over instant coffee, was saying, 'I can absolutely prove my son innocent. I can do it any time I want by going to Washington D.C., with some pictures, but I won't do it that way. I want to get my story before the public, so young and old all over the world will know the truth. Why don't I go to Washington?' With this question, she turned to face me, arms akimbo. Embattled, but at the same time an imperturbable strategist, she answered it: 'Because they've been so ugly to me, to me and my boy. I'll write a book and the title of it will be *One and One Make Two* or *This and That.* Oh, I could write three books or five books! I could write books and *books* on what I know and what I have researched.'

" 'Now, maybe Lee Harvey Oswald was the assassin,' she pursued, stirring the coffee. 'But does that make him a louse? No, no! Killing does not necessarily mean badness. You find killing in some very fine homes for one reason or another. And as we all know, President Kennedy was a dying man. So I say it is possible that my son was chosen to shoot him in a mercy killing for security of the country. And if this is true, it was a fine thing to do and my son is a hero.'

" 'I had not heard that President Kennedy was dying,' I said, staggered by this cluster of fictions stated as irrefutable fact. Some mercy killing! The methods used in this instance must surely be unique in the annals of euthanasia.

" 'Oh, yes,' she went on with authority."

Dr. David Abrahamsen, in his detailed study of Oswald and his psychological capability of murder, devotes considerable attention to the character of his mother. He finds that, like her notorious son, she committed a good many delinquencies, such as failing to notify the authorities when Lee was on probation as a truant and leaving New York City with him and moving back to New Orleans. He concludes that: "In Marguerite Oswald's emotional make-up we find many of Lee's traits, in particular her rigidity, unrealistic and narcissistic self-idolatry and attention-seeking, withdrawal, hypersensitivity, possessiveness, disrespect for authority, false pride, exploitation of people, cruelty, impulsiveness, and acting out regardless of consequences."

From the foregoing information, it can easily be seen that Lee Harvey Oswald's mother was hardly a fully functioning, mentally healthy individual in her own right, and that some of his personality traits which significantly overlapped with hers perhaps are traceable to genetic as well as environmental influences. It is entirely possible that, had he been separated from his mother at birth and never been reared in her presence, he would have been a completely different kind of person; but this hypothesis cannot be validated.

In the case of Jack Ruby, apparently both his parents were seriously disturbed. His father was an unemployed carpenter for the last thirty years—yes, thirty years!—of his life; and he seems to have been an inveterate alcoholic. Alcoholism is one of the most common indicators of severe neurosis or borderline psychosis.

Ruby's mother lied to and beat her children, including Ruby

himself. She was totally incapable of coping with them and their delinquencies. She was extremely quarrelsome. She had various delusions, including one she had for years that she had a fishbone stuck in her throat. Although she claimed that her marriage to her husband was unhappy from the start, she had many children by him, eight of whom survived. She insisted that her sons were conspiring against her and influencing her other children to be impatient and cruel toward her.

She attended psychiatric clinics for many years, but became so unmanageable and hysterical, screaming and shouting day and night, that she had to be committed to Elgin State Hospital. One of her clinic psychiatrists made a diagnosis of paranoid condition; the admitting psychiatrist at Elgin State Hospital diagnosed her as "paranoid state with involutional changes" and stated that "the prognosis is poor because of the poor personality of the patient and the long duration (24 years) of her mental abnormality." Dr. R. Hartogs, who studied the Ruby family history in detail, concluded that "even though Mrs. Rubenstein's actual breakdown did not occur until she was sixty-two, there seems plenty of evidence that far earlier in life she was highly disturbed emotionally. She appears to have always remained a thwarted, demanding, lonely woman. She found her eight children a burden, admitted she did not like them."

Charles J. Guiteau, the lawyer who assassinated President Garfield, was an unusually disturbed individual, as we have seen, who had some highly peculiar religious views. Although his father admitted that Guiteau was disturbed, and even thought that he might have had a diseased brain, the facts show that the father himself held some peculiar religious opinions and that much of his behavior was eccentric. There is a strong possibility that in his case, too, hereditary disposition as well as environmental circumstances (including the death of his mother when he was an infant) contributed to his criminal tendencies.

John Wilkes Booth came from a brilliant and erratic family of actors. His father, Junius Brutus Booth, was the first of the notable actors in this line and made quite a name for himself at Covent Garden and in support of Edmund Kean at Drury Lane. He came to the United States in 1821 and continued to give outstanding performances as Othello, Iago, Richard III, and Shylock. Unfortunately, he was subject to periods of insanity in his later life; and it is possible that John Wilkes Booth inherited some of his psychotic tendencies.

Leon Trotsky's murderer, Ramon de Rio Mercader, had a mother who was severely disturbed and is reported to have said of herself: "If anything happens to me, because if I am assassinated by those for whom I murdered, by those for whom I made my son into a murderer . . . they must know that Caridad Mercader is not simply Caridad Mercader, but the worst of assassins . . . yes . . . the worst. Because not only did I travel throughout Europe tracking down Chekists [Soviet Secret Agents] who had defected or diplomats who had abandoned paradise, so as to assassinate them pitilessly . . . I have done even more! . . . I made—and I did this for them—an assassin of my son, of Ramon." Levine quotes from an unsolicited letter by Enrique Castro Delgado, who personally knew Mercader and his mother, saying that in 1959 she was living in Paris "more disturbed than ever."

According to Ferri, Violet Gibson, who attempted to assassinate Benito Mussolini, suffered not only from paranoia but from a religious mania. Her family history showed several cases of alcoholism, apoplexy, and probable insanity.

T. Smith observes that Sirhan Bishara Sirhan, Robert F. Kennedy's assassin, had a mother who was zealously religious and "whose view of life was as rigid as her ideas of salvation." Her pastor said that she was harsh to her children and that "she was terribly narrow-minded and religious in religious matters." A cousin reported that "Sirhan was always with his mother. . . . She never let him out of her sight. She always seemed to be afraid to let him go out by himself." Being a teetotaler and a strong moralist, she protested strongly against her other son, Adel, becoming a musician in an Arab night club.

Robert B. Kaiser, a journalist who was a member of Sirhan's defense team when he was on trial, spent some time with Mrs. Sirhan. He reports that, in the face of the overwhelming evidence against him, she "clings to the faith that somehow, some way, her son will be acquitted. . . . The family members keep themselves closely informed about the legal procedures connected with

Sirhan's defense. In addition, Mary Sirhan keeps the June 14 issues of *Time* and *Newsweek* on a buffet table in the dining room and the special Kennedy issues of *Life* and *Look* on the coffee table in the living room. She picks up the magazines now and then and talks to the face of Robert Kennedy on the *Time* cover, telling him how sorry she is. Kennedy, moreover, talks to her. 'It's O.K., Mary,' she says he says. 'I forgive you. It's O.K.' "

Sirhan's father, Bishara, could not get along with his wife or family and did not communicate with them at all when he left for Jordan after they had been living in Pasadena for some time. He had terrible fights with his wife, beat his children severely, and drove his two oldest boys to desperation until they moved out and lived by themselves. He made charms and amulets for his appreciative neighbors and apparently believed fully in their effectiveness. The family pastor noted that he "had frequent violent fits and was given to breaking what little furniture they had, and beating the children. He thrashed them with sticks and with his fists, whenever they disobeyed him. Toth and Smith went to great pains to interview many of the Sirhan neighbors to discover how the parents and children of the family generally behaved. They report : " 'They were a confused family,' says Mrs. Jubran. 'No one knew what was between Mary and Bishara.' She often heard Bishara shouting at his wife. 'The father did not allow Sirhan to go out of the house. All of them were afraid of the father. He turned the house into a jail for them . . . the father always made Sirhan afraid. The boy was not well in his mind. He was a complicated boy. . . . Another neighbor, Mrs. Laila, recalls that Bishara used to lock Ayda [Sirhan's sister] in their room and her friends would have to bring food to her. Once, she says, Bishara chained her to the grilled window."

The general instability of the Sirhan family may also be noted from an incident that happened while Senator Kennedy's assassin was on trial. One of his older brothers, Saidallah, was injured in an automobile accident. According to D. Robinson, "another Sirhan brother, 37-year-old Sharif, was arrested in the night when he forced his way into the intensive care unit where his brother was lying at the Pasadena hospital. The police said he had shoved a nurse who tried to quiet him as he began shouting that Saidallah

Sirhan was being 'mistreated.' Sharif Sirhan was later freed on $125 bail."

James Earl Ray, the accused murderer of Dr. Martin Luther King, came from a family whose parents and siblings seem to have been far from stable. His father died in 1951, most probably of chronic alcoholism. The parents did not take care of their children very well, and placed them routinely in foster homes. When Ray was in the army he would send money home, asking his parents to deposit half of it for him in the bank and to keep the other half; but his sister says that his parents spent it all (*Newsweek,* April 29, 1968). Ray's next eldest brother served prison time for burglary. His sister has been fanatically religious and has kept in her room a huge red, white, and blue wooden cross, lettered "rugged cross." She once walked it down Main Street in Quincy, Illinois.

Additional evidence on the emotional disturbance of assassins comes, interestingly enough, from the case of an individual who technically was only a murderer, and who ostensibly committed a crime of passion. Actually, he shot a very well-known public figure, before a huge theater audience, pointing a gun only two feet from his victim's face and firing three times in slow, rhythmic succession. The assassin was Harry K. Thaw and his victim the famous architect, Stanford White. Supposedly Thaw killed White because, as he said to a member of the Madison Square Garden security force who rushed over to him after the shooting, "He deserved it, he ruined my wife." The facts of Thaw's trial showed much the opposite: that Evelyn Nesbit, his wife, had been "ruined" by both him and Stanford White long before she became Mrs. Thaw. As Richard O'Connor notes in recounting the famous case: "There was no mystery but the eternal psychological one. It all turned on Harry Thaw's alleged motive for killing White, that the latter had 'ruined' his wife. And if there is one unsolved mystery concerning the case, it is whether this was true."

Thaw was as close to being an assassin, in the usual sense of this term, as anyone can get. He planned to kill White, he did so publicly, he knew he would be apprehended, and he picked as his victim a highly honored and revered figure. Consistently enough, the picture of Thaw's psychological disturbance from childhood onward is typical. From O'Connor's report we learn the following facts about him:

"Almost from birth, Harry had been a problem child. . . . He was subject to frequent tantrums, and even as an infant often went sleepless. . . . Signs of mental aberration only increased during his youth. Charles Koehler, an instructor at Wooster University where Harry was sent at the age of sixteen, recalled that he often 'walked in a zig-zag manner . . . his capacity for concentration was weak . . . frequently asked irrelevant questions.' . . . At least once, during a European tour early in his youth, he was committed to a private sanitarium following a suicide attempt. . . . Even when he was well into his twenties, his mother said, he would weep bitterly for no apparent reason, and would 'settle into gloom and absent-mindedness.' "

When Harry K. Thaw's father died when he was only eighteen, "the boy had already given such unmistakable indications of imbalance that the father stated in his will that 'with great regret and reluctance and solely from a sense of duty, I hereby cancel and revoke any and all provisions of my said will directing payment of money or property to my said son, Harry Kendall Thaw.' "

Thaw advertised for young girls to train for the stage, ages fifteen to seventeen, and apparently used two whips to "train" them. "In later life, too, Thaw gave plentiful evidence of sadistic tendencies." In studying the Thaw trial, Dr. John H. Cassity, chief psychiatrist at Bellevue Hospital, concluded that he was incurably insane. At his second trial, the jury found him not guilty by reason of insanity and he was confined in the State Asylum for the Criminal Insane at Matteawan, New York. His family tried to get him released on many occasions but for a decade did not succeed, in spite of paying large sums to psychiatrists to testify in his behalf, because at each hearing he talked semi-coherently and acted badly.

When Thaw was finally released from custody, nine years after he assassinated White, he kept getting into difficulties. "In 1917, he was arrested on charges of having kidnapped and whipped a teen-aged boy. Again he was committed to an asylum, this time in Pennsylvania, with his mother, finally disillusioned, requesting that he never again be turned loose. But he was released seven years later, just in time to attend the notorious 'nude in a bathtub' party given by Broadway producer Earl Carroll, the tabloid sensation of 1924. In the following years Harry was in and out of the court on breach of promise proceedings, for having started a row in an Atlantic City nightclub operated by Evelyn, for having beaten up a speakeasy hostess, and other unsavory activities. His life was troubled, pathetic, sensation-seeking to the day of his death in February, 1947."

Confirmatory evidence of Harry K. Thaw's severe emotional disturbance is given by G. Langford, who points out that Dr. Charles J. Wiley, a specialist in mental disease, noticed irrational behavior on Thaw's part when he was in a streetcar a year before he murdered White; that the family physician for the Thaws, Dr. Charles F. Bingamon, testified that as a boy Harry had been of a "neurotic temperament"; that Dr. Britton D. Evans of the Greystone Park Mental Hospital in New Jersey visited Thaw in the New York City Tombs after the murder and found that he "exhibited the condition of a man who has just passed through an explosive and fulminating condition of the mind. He exhibited those symptoms observed in persons of unsound mind who suffer the delusions of exaggerated personal importance. . . . I discovered proof of a delusion of persecution"; and Dr. Allen McLane Hamilton, who examined Thaw immediately after the murder, found him disorganized, irrelevant, and clearly insane.

Although Thaw was not a political assassin, his murder of Stanford White had a real assassinationlike quality; and the pattern of his life and the degree of his emotional disturbance characteristically mirrored that of so many other assassins.

From the foregoing information, it seems clear that many political assassins, especially those who are part of United States history, are exceptionally disturbed individuals who kill more for personal than for political motives. Confirmation of this view has been voiced by Dr. Donald W. Hastings, chairman of psychiatry and neurology at the University of Minnesota Medical School. Dr. Hastings made an extensive study of the psychological makeup of presidential assassins and found that all but two of the nine murderers and would-be murderers of American presidents were psychotic. The two exceptions, he states, were "fanatics," Oscar Collazo and Griselio Torresola, who in 1950 tried to kill President Truman because they thought it would help Puerto Rico. The other seven psychotic assassins were all paranoid schizophrenics.

Dr. Lawrence Z. Freedman, research psychiatrist at the University of Chicago School of Medicine, quoted by *New York Times* reporter, J. E. Brody, also holds that presidential assassins are "emotionally disturbed social isolates, acting on their own, without any rational expectation that they or the party and cause with which they identified themselves could benefit from the slaying." Dr. David Rothstein, who made a study of federal prisoners who were jailed because they threatened the life of a president, found that they, too, were schizophrenics. Drs. A. E. Weisz and R. L. Taylor of the Stanford University Department of Psychiatry reviewed the literature on presidential assassinations and found that almost all the assassins have been young men with delusional thought processes who tended to lead alienated and socioeconomically deteriorated lives.

Long before the assassinations of President John F. Kennedy, Martin Luther King, and Senator Robert F. Kennedy took place, Robert J. Donovan, writing in his book, *The Assassins,* commented that "by and large the true story behind the assassinations and attempted assassinations of American presidents is that the assassins not only were lone operators, but were, most of them, suffering from mental disease, who pulled the trigger while in the grip of delusion."

Donovan notes that although Collazo may have been sane, "all the others—Lawrence, Guiteau, Czolgosz, Schrank, and Zangara—were unmistakedly victims of mental disease. . . . 'Our country,' wrote Booth in his diary after the assassination [of Lincoln] owed all her troubles to him, and God simply made me the instrument of His punishment.' 'God has called me to be his instrument, so help me God,' Schrank wrote as he prepared to shoot Theodore Roosevelt. 'His removal is an act of God,' wrote Guiteau in explaining his purpose in assassinating President Garfield. . . . None of the assassins repented his deed. To a man they felt their acts had been justified. Zangara went so far as to say that his only regret was that he had failed to kill Franklin Roosevelt. Others maintained they had done their duty. Some considered themselves martyrs."

The evidence, then, is fairly convincing. With few exceptions, public assassins of outstanding political figures tend to be psychotic. They generally have long histories of emotionally aberrated behavior; they often suffer specific life crises just before they kill; and they murder in a senseless manner as far as their political beliefs and aspirations are concerned.

Chapter 10

Treatment of a Mother Who Committed Infanticide

This is the case of Joyce, a young married woman who was committed to a state hospital in the northeastern part of the United States because, at age eighteen, she killed her six-month-old daughter. Three years earlier, she had been raped by her brother-in-law and had been forced to give away her first child, also a girl, for adoption. She had bitterly resented this fact, as well as her parents' allegation that she had really seduced her raper and that only she was responsible for her plight.

Prior to the loss of her first child, Joyce insisted, she had been a happy, carefree individual, an outgoing person with many friends. Her parents gave quite a different picture, seeing her as an inordinately demanding, love-hungry girl who had consistently mean spells, and who was exceptionally jealous of her two older twin sisters, both of whom had been born crippled and who needed more attention than she did. Everyone in her family agreed, however, that after she was forced to give up her illegitimate daughter, whom she desperately wanted to keep, Joyce began to withdraw from people. She lost all interest in going back to high school. She felt, despite no confirming evidence, that everyone in the large city in which she lived was talking about her and making fun of her for giving in to her parents about the adoption. "When I came home and went back to school, even some of the Puerto Rican kids used to say, 'Where did your baby go?' They used to laugh and snicker at me in class, so that one teacher had it in for me. My family never gave me a chance. I guess no one wanted anything to do with me because I'm such a bad person!"

A year and a half before she killed her second daughter, Joyce was married to Carl, one of her childhood sweethearts. He knew all about her previous history but was "kind and understanding" and loved her in spite of "everything." They were both happy that she became pregnant within a few weeks after their marriage; but she had a bad pregnancy and had to stay in bed much of the time, utterly exhausted, with severe pains in her stomach, and often got quite hysterical. She would alternately laugh and cry over nothing, and felt unable to stop this distressing behavior.

Following the birth of her second daughter, Joyce felt that she was very happy. Nonetheless, she couldn't forget the loss of the first daughter and the fact that she did not even get a chance to hold the baby before it was taken away for adoption. She had vile fits of temper, was distraught when she could not get the new child to breast-feed, and tried to cut her wrists because she felt she was not a good mother. "I would wake up with awful nightmares, feeling that I had failed her, my husband, and everyone. As the months went by, the situation got worse. Finally, I woke up from another nightmare on Monday morning, fixed the bottle for her, and gave her a bath. She slept until 2 P.M. and then started crying, crying, crying. I felt dizzy—just like I felt several years before, when my mother had slapped me very hard and I blacked out and had to be taken to the hospital to see if there was anything seriously wrong with me. I just couldn't take anything then; I was beside myself, and I hit the child hard and her head hit the side of the bed."

With that, she became quite emotionally upset; and she could only later vaguely recall what happened. "Everything was like a dream—I can't remember clearly." She put the girl back to bed and went out to eat with her husband. While eating, she suddenly panicked, feeling that something had gone wrong with the baby. She rushed home, and when her husband saw that something really was wrong, she made up a fantastic story about a burglar breaking in their house that afternoon, her trying to protect the child from him, and the little girl getting mauled and bruised during the fight. They took the baby to the hospital and found she was dead. "I didn't mean to hurt her. I didn't know what I was doing." She admitted, however, that since she had been apprehended for the crime and felt that it was all over with, she stopped being nervous as she had been for months before the child's death.

When questioned during the admissions interview at the hospital, Joyce said that she had had a very rough time with the baby —who was colicky, who vomited incessantly, and couldn't eat well. Consequently, she had been out of the house only a few times since its birth. She had been constantly fearful that something would happen to the baby—that someone would take her away. Because of her fears, she went to extremes in caring for the child and keeping the house clean, lest anyone should say she wasn't taking care of her properly. She was a compulsive housekeeper: "I couldn't even go to bed at night unless everything was done. Or sometimes I'd go to bed and then have to get up again because I remembered that I'd forgotten to do something and knew I couldn't sleep till it was done." No matter what she did, her mother and stepfather criticized her, so that she wasn't sure whether she was doing things the right way or not. She became unsure of making decisions of any kind, fearing that she would make a mistake.

Because of her fears of making a wrong move, of being criticized, and of having horrible nightmares, Joyce became afraid to leave the baby alone, even for a short while. "I would never go any place without her. I couldn't trust her to the care of a babysitter. Nobody could care for her the way I did."

When hospitalized, Joyce felt as if everything that had happened to her was all a dream and wistfully hoped that she would wake up and find everything all right. "I keep thinking I'll go home and find my husband and baby waiting for me." In a more pessimistic vein, she said she was afraid that she would never leave the hospital, that nobody would want her, that nobody cared what happened to her. She was concerned that her husband would forget her and worried that he was going out with other women.

Joyce said her parents had showed all their interest in her twin sisters. "I was sensitive and they always made me feel bad. As a child of four or five, when I made a noise my stepfather used to pull his belt strap off and whip me. Sometimes he would hit me quite hard, oftentimes beating me with his hands, or anything he could pick up." Her stepfather, a cab driver, worked long hours and her mother and sisters watched television all day. Whenever she tried to talk to her mother and seek her advice, she only received complaints about her mother's aches and pains.

According to Joyce's husband, she was reasonably well and content until after the birth of their daughter. After that, she would call him to supper when he came home; but she would not have the supper ready, or even the table set. She would then insist that everything was on the table. A month before the child was killed, he came home from work and was told that she had fainted that day, while holding the baby in her arms, and that their daughter had suffered a scalp wound in the process. He didn't know, in retrospect, whether she had actually dropped the baby during a fainting spell or whether the scalp wound was caused by physical abuse.

Joyce was considered by the hospital staff to be amenable to psychotherapy and was seen for her first session shortly after her incarceration. All told, she was seen for fifty-nine sessions, over a period of thirteen months. For the first five months, the therapist employed psychoanalytically oriented methods with her. Because of his gradual disenchantment with this method, he switched to rational-emotive psychotherapy. As is often found with this kind of change in therapy, Joyce began to make much more rapid and far-reaching progress with the rational-emotive approach than she had made with the psychoanalytic methods; she was ultimately given an absolute discharge from the hospital.

During her early psychotherapy sessions, Joyce admitted that for weeks before committing her crime, she had uncontrollable feelings of "meanness" toward her daughter. On the day of the murder, she first tried to suffocate the baby by placing a pillow over her face; and when that didn't work, she severely spanked her. Finally, she hit the child's head against the side of the bed.

Soon after she was apprehended, Joyce thought she heard her baby crying for her—which may or may not have been a psychotic hallucination—and also felt that she was a different person, dissociated from her usual self. She felt so empty and guilty that she thought of taking her own life.

She at first claimed that her previous hysterical fits—when she felt "shaky, trembling, angry, indifferent, just not myself at these times"—came on gradually, after the adoption of her first daughter. "I grieved so much over the loss of her. . . . I was worried about what kind of home she would be in." On further questioning, she revealed that she had similar fits as a child and that at the same time she felt as if there were "a packing pressure against my head. Sounds similar to a seashell. Kind of like an airy pressure." These episodes stopped for a while but then resumed after menstruation started and would generally occur about two weeks before her periods. At the same time, she would also feel quite depressed.

The more material that was gathered about her childhood, the more Joyce insisted on its traumatic effects. Her story was consistently the same: The only person who might have really loved her, her father, died when she was less than a year old. Her mother and her stepfather neglected and abused her steadily. Her crippled twin sisters, a year older than she, were consistently pampered and favored at her expense and themselves plagued her continually.

While having no particular contact with her family when she was at the hospital, she had periodic bouts of intense anger and "meanness" every four weeks, apparently coinciding with the onset of ovulation. At these times, she felt like breaking out the windows of the hospital and running home; she thought that life was not worth living; she was overwhelmed by desires for love, care, affection, and attention.

About four months after therapy began, Joyce went home for a weekend visit, since she was between her periodic outbursts and the staff of the hospital thought it safe to let her try a few days with her husband. She found some letters he had written to another girl, indicating that he had had intercourse with this girl but not indicating whether this event had taken place during her absence or some time before they had become seriously interested in each other; and she raised a great fuss. "I was pretty well shocked when I saw the letters. In fact, I got hysterical and screamed and screamed; and so he kept hitting me and I just kept screaming and screaming. And I told him to let go of me and I tried to run out the door and he shut the door and he pushed me back." Someone, hearing the melee, called the police. When they arrived, she accused him of all kinds of skulduggery and signed a warrant to have him arrested.

Joyce's story of what happened during the five days with her husband was not clear; but it would appear that both were quite suspicious of each other. From what she had previously heard, she believed that he had been going out with other girls; and from what he had heard or imagined (according to her story) he believed that she had been having wild sex parties at the hospital. They had both been upset; there had been angry words and some mild blows between them; finally, her finding the letters had led to a real blow-off. Although he claimed that the letters were to an old girl friend, with whom he had gone before he became seriously interested in Joyce, she was inclined to believe otherwise; and she was moralistically shocked by his alleged "running around" and by the letters, which gave clearcut evidence of his having various kinds of coital and noncoital relations with the girl to whom they were written. A rational-emotive therapist would have not taken her shock and resentment at her husband's assumed extramarital behavior as natural, but would have quickly shown her how, even if the "facts" as she construed them were true, she was still upsetting *herself* by unrealistically expecting her husband to behave much differently than he was behaving, and by moralistically condemning him for his mistakes. If this had occurred, it is possible that Joyce would have been led to *challenge* her assumptions that (a) her husband was no damned good and that (b) she was a ninny for staying with him. She might have even discovered, in the course of forgiving him for his "bad" behavior, that much of his "wickedness" had never occurred at all or had partially occurred and been exaggerated by her.

Unfortunately, the therapist at this time was following the psychoanalytic procedure of letting the client ventilate her hostility; and he did not challenge her condemnation of her husband or her upsetting herself about his deeds. Consequently (as often happens in psychoanalysis) Joyce became more incensed as she related her version of her differences with her husband, and became increasingly determined to divorce him.

A month later, after Joyce was on her way to divorcing her husband, the therapist read *Reason and Emotion in Psychotherapy* by Albert Ellis and *A Guide to Rational Living* by Albert Ellis and Robert A. Harper, and began to intersperse some rational-emotive methods with psychoanalytic methodology. Thus, most of the twenty-fifth psychotherapy session was spent with the therapist's reflecting Joyce's feelings about her husband and her dead daughter. He got her to see that her main problem had been trying to please others and that she had been defining herself as a worthless individual when she had not succeeded at getting others to approve her. He then tried to get her to see that she either blamed herself for her mistakes, and thereby made herself anxious and guilty; or else she blamed other people, insisted that they had led her up the wrong path, and thereby became very hostile. He tried to show her that *any* kind of blaming, or condemning an entire *person* for her human *mistakes,* is unnecessary and almost always leads to bad results:

Therapist: You're not going to be any good to yourself if you continue to punish yourself.

Joyce: Uh huh.

Therapist: There's apparently a link here that gives us the reason you might want to punish yourself. I wonder if it might go something like this: You took your child's life and you did something wrong; and since you did this something that was wrong, uh, you're not a good person, you've got to punish yourself.

Joyce: Yeah.

Therapist: But that's nonsense.

Joyce: It really is, too. It's nonsense to try to punish myself for it.

Therapist: Because, first of all, you *are* a good person. You are a worthwhile person. There's a lot for you to live for.

Joyce: I can think of it that way now; but I couldn't before.

Therapist: In the sense that you're saying to yourself that you made this mistake and that you're not a good person, it would appear to me that at the same time you're saying you *should* be a certain kind of person. Perhaps, you might be saying something like, "I *shouldn't* make mistakes!" What about that?

Joyce: I don't say that any more.

Therapist: Do you feel that this is something you might have —you did say to yourself in the past?

Joyce: Yes. Because I thought I was better than anybody else, that I was perfect; and I was going to prove to everybody else that I was perfect.

Therapist: And you thought you should be perfect?

Joyce: Yeah.

Therapist: And since you made a mistake and, therefore, since you weren't perfect, you were saying that you weren't any good and that, therefore, you should punish yourself. And, of course, this is illogical! Obviously, you can't be a perfect person; you will never be, and neither will anyone else. What you should be saying to yourself is: "I made this mistake; it was wrong for me to take my child's life. It's too bad; I'm very sorry that it happened. But I'm not a perfect person and I do make mistakes." You know, my interpretations to you may be all wrong. I'm wondering if you are really believing all I say. I'm also wondering, on another level, if you perhaps feel that you have to please me by saying "Yes" to me and to the interpretations I offer you.

Joyce: No. I do find myself, now, thinking that I made a mistake and that I'm not perfect. I think twice about it; I mean, I'm real conscious of it. Like, uh, something came up last Thursday and I got bawled out by the Aides. And I kind of thought———. Well, like what we've been discussing. I thought, well I'd better get used to doing some things wrong. I'm not perfect and I'm going to make mistakes. So the heck with it! I mean, I make mistakes, too. But there's been others before me that's probably done the same thing; so I shouldn't worry about it. And I said to myself, "Yeah, it's kind of stupid, to make that mistake. But I make mistakes, too. And just as long as I realize I made a mistake and try not to do it again, that's the main thing."

Therapist: You realize you made a mistake; and you try not to make the same mistake again.

Joyce: Um hum.

Therapist: But suppose you *do* make the same mistake again?

Joyce: You just make it again—that's it. Then you say you're not going to keep making it, or at least you hope not to.

Therapist: You can make the same mistake one million times and you're still a good *person.*

There are several notable aspects of this exchange which distinguish it enormously from the much more passive reflection of Joyce's feelings which the therapist had been psychoanalytically doing a few sessions previously: (1) The therapist shows Joyce that it is unwise for her to keep punishing herself, to keep making herself guilty for her wrong deeds, including the killing of her child. (2) He demonstrates that her guilt flows from her concept of herself as a totally bad *person;* and that this idea of herself as a bad individual in turn stems from her perfectionistic notion that she *should* not make any serious mistakes. (3) He indicates that this is an unrealistic notion because, as a fallible human being, it is impossible for her to be error-free. (4) He points out that she does not even have to please *him,* and that she'd better not accept his interpretations for fear of making mistakes with him and having him dislike her. (5) He asserts that he can accept Joyce as a person even if she makes a million mistakes; and that likewise she can accept herself as a worthwhile individual just because she is alive, and not because she does things remarkably well.

Because Joyce is relatively unsophisticated, the therapist does not attempt to give her a higher-level, more philosophic version of rational-emotive therapy. If he did that, he would attempt to show her not that she is a good person because she exists and has a lot to live for, but that she is really neither a good nor a bad person, and that she doesn't have to rate *herself* at all. She'd better rate her performances—accept the fact, for example, that her act of killing her child was wrong and unfortunate and to be avoided in the future. But she, a total human being, is actually unrateable: since she is too complex an entity, and too much of an ongoing *process,* to be given a single global rating, or a report card. Therefore, she'd better learn to assess her *deeds* or *performances* objectively, and to try to correct them when they are wrong or inefficient; but she'd better learn not to assess *herself.* Not believing that Joyce is yet up to understanding and using this more subtle kind of philosophic analysis, the therapist gives her a shorthand version of rational-emotive therapy and tries to get her to see that if there is such a thing as a good person or a bad person (which, technically, there really isn't, since these are definitional or tautological terms, akin to Platonic ideals, and have no clearcut empirical referents), her goodness consists of her aliveness and her potential for enjoying herself in life: It does not consist of her constantly behaving perfectly.

Joyce apparently responds well to this line of reasoning, even though the therapist only started to use it in the session previous to this twenty-fifth session. She probably believes that her present or past mistakes are not too bad because she can correct them in the future; and she does not clearly see, as yet, that even if she *always* made serious errors she would still not be (except by self-definition) a worthless individual. But the therapist feels that if he continues to deindoctrinate her from her self-castigating attitudes, she will ultimately accept herself unconditionally.

Having gotten Joyce started on accepting herself with her errors and fallibilities, the therapist tried, in the following session, to get her to accept other people with their failings and thereby to minimize her hostility. When she admitted that she still held a grudge against her husband, her mother and father, and her uncle, all of whom had tried to make up her mind for her and get her to do things their way, the session continued as follows:

Therapist: They made some mistakes, didn't they?

Joyce: Yeah.

Therapist: Parents aren't perfect!

Joyce (laughs): Nobody's perfect. I expected them to be.

Therapist: You sure did!

Joyce (laughs).

Therapist: Yeah. Well———.

Joyce: I expected it from everybody. Sometimes I think, by my holding a grudge against them, I think they still should be perfect—think that they should be different than they are.

Therapist: Say that again. Sometimes—what?

Joyce: By holding a grudge against them, I think that they, I still think at times that they should be perfect or that they should be different than they are.

Therapist: That's right! That's just what I was getting ready to say. Which all comes down to the fact that you don't really believe that they can make mistakes, or that people can make mistakes, or that people are, uh, fallible. You don't *believe* that, do you?

Joyce: Well (giggles) I wanted them to be like other parents and they weren't. Other young people say the same thing about their parents. And really, in a way, all parents do what they think is best. One parent might stop his child from using his new car—and all that, you know.

Therapist: The point is, however, that you really don't *believe* this yet: that your parents are fallible. Because, if you did, you wouldn't be holding a grudge against them. Isn't that right?

Joyce (quietly): Yes.

Therapist: O.K. It takes time to believe this, even when you sometimes see it. It just doesn't hit you overnight, of course.

Joyce: I hold a grudge against my husband. I think he should be perfect. When someone else says something about what he's done, then I think, "Well, he's not perfect. He can make mistakes." But when he does something to annoy *me,* I can't tell myself that. I can't think, "Oh, well; so he's not perfect." But when he does something to someone else, I can.

Therapist: You mean, don't you, that you *don't* stop and say to yourself, when he does something to annoy you, "Oh, well; so he's not perfect." You *don't*; but you *can.*

Joyce (giggles): I don't know if I can.

Therapist: Will you stop and *think* about it?

Joyce: Well, he isn't perfect———(long pause). He's not the way I want him to be: everything perfect, you know; heaven on earth.

Therapist: I wonder why you want to feel that everything should be perfect.

Joyce: I don't know because, even though it may be wrong, I've felt that way for years.

Therapist: Um hum. It's not so important to understand why you *want* things to be so perfect. Practically all of us do. I think what is important is for you to recognize that this is something that you have been *demanding* of yourself and other people; and *demanding* things of people is a philosophy of life which is irrational simply because they just aren't *made* that way. They *do* make mistakes; and they *are* fallible, because that's the imperfect way people are. And they probably always will be!

Here the therapist emphasizes that Joyce's holding a grudge against her husband and her relatives does not stem from what happens to her at point A—that is, their behaving badly toward her—but from her interpretations or philosophy of life at point B—namely, her insisting that they should not act in this manner, that they ought to be perfect. He shows her that, although at times she tells herself that, "Yes, parents and other people are fallible, and I shouldn't expect too much from them," her real belief, most of the time, is that they should be *in*fallible—especially in their relations with *her.*

By emphasizing this point in many different ways, the therapist hopes to induce Joyce to change her perfectionistic *demands* on people into much more realistic *desires* or *preferences* that they act well toward her. As partial proof that he is reaching her, she then is able to discuss her uncle's seduction of her when she was six years of age. For a few years afterward, she allowed him to pet with her, because he was her uncle and she thought that she had to give in to him. She finally told her mother about it, who spoke to the uncle (her brother) in an angry manner and put a stop to it.

This is a fairly typical occurrence in rational-emotive therapy. Once the therapist shows the disturbed individual that she does not have to condemn herself or others for various types of wrong behavior which have been committed, she no longer feels she has to avoid thinking or talking about (and hence repressing) the events connected with this behavior; so she is able to recall and discuss them with relative ease. As the therapist showed Joyce that she could tolerate poor behavior by her relatives and that she didn't have to blame herself for foolishly going along with it for a period of time, she was able to bring up how she had allowed her uncle, for apparently several years, to pet with her against her inclination, until she finally had the courage to tell her mother what had been happening and to bring this unwanted sex participation to a halt.

This twenty-fifth session with Joyce ends with the following significant exchange:

Joyce: My uncle, the one I had this sex with for several years, was always the one that told me that I made mistakes and that I wasn't supposed to make mistakes. He told me that I wasn't supposed to do this or that; that I knew things were wrong that I did and that I should have had better judgment.

Therapist: Um hum.

Joyce: I got tired of listening to his criticism of me. So then I tried to do everything—.

Therapist: Go ahead.

Joyce: Oh, I was saying that, when my uncle told me I shouldn't be doing this wrong or that wrong, I thought I should be perfect (long pause).

Therapist: Uh huh. So I would think you've been telling yourself ever since that you should be a perfect person.

Joyce: I've grown up thinking that.

Therapist: Uh huh. I know you have! Well, Joyce, this might be a nice place to stop for today. We'll take up from here next week. I notice you haven't been smoking lately.

Joyce: Well, I guess I'm not as nervous as I was.

Therapist: You appear much more relaxed to me.

Joyce: I feel more relaxed.

Therapist: It's the first time I've seen you, you know, not smoking. Good!

During the next few sessions Joyce continued to improve and was able to go through with a divorce from her husband with unusual equanimity. Even when her ex-husband, who apparently still wanted her back, kept calling her on her visits home, and when her parents got upset by his calls, she remained calm about his behavior and their disturbed reactions to it. She began to get along much better with the other inmates of the hospital and to become less obsessively worried about things which formerly preoccupied her. She was surprised at some of her imperturbability. At the end of the twenty-eighth session she remarked, "It's amazing; it's really good that I've been able to excuse my father's reactions. It's really remarkable how I've gotten over many of the things people say and haven't gotten upset."

Like most people with deep-seated feelings of self-hatred and hostility toward others, however, Joyce tended to lapse from time to time—especially when she went home for a visit and several unpleasant things happened in a row. During the thirty-sixth session she started to complain that her mother incessantly kept after her to do various things and jabbered away at her when she didn't fulfill these demands. The therapist tried to get her to accept her mother the way she was, but had little success. Nonetheless, he continued:

Therapist: But what is upsetting about her behavior? (Pause) What do you tell yourself about it that upsets you?

Joyce: Well, I think it's plumb nutty!

Therapist: Well, sure it may be plumb nutty. But that's the way nutty people *are:* they act in a nutty manner! But if you were able to, if you just acknowledged the fact that she was nutty, and let it go at that—and say, "Too bad. There goes my kooky mother. She's off her rocker!"—if you would let it go at that, then you wouldn't be upsetting yourself, would you?

Joyce: Well, it's not that easy to do all the time.

Therapist: That's true. It's not that easy to do all the time. So you have to keep watching yourself and keep working on it. Hard work! Until it becomes automatic for you to believe it. Now what is it you're telling yourself about her nutty behavior that upsets you?

Joyce: It bothers me and I don't like it.

Therapist: No, you're saying more than that to yourself. If it *just* bothered you and you *just* didn't like it, you wouldn't be making yourself that upset. You go a little farther than that in your head, don't you?

Joyce: I don't know.

Therapist: Well, aren't you saying that: (1) "My mother is acting in a nutty manner and I don't like it; it's irritating; it's annoying." And aren't you adding: (2) "And she *shouldn't* be acting the way she is acting! The gall of her to treat me this way! I don't have any time to myself. I can't do the things I want to do. And *because* I don't like the way my mother's acting, she *shouldn't* act that way!" Isn't *that* what you're saying to yourself?

Joyce: Yeah, I guess. But she *could* act halfway normal once in a while!

Therapist: Yes, but you mean because she *could,* she *should*—which is an unrealistic demand on your part. Sure, she could theoretically act halfway normal; but she *isn't* halfway normal; she's nuts! She's got her problems. She's kooky. But you haven't got yourself to *accept* her yet for the kind of a person she is. She could be a lot of things; but she *isn't.* And you're demanding that she not act the way she *is* acting. It's very easy for her to act the way she is acting. Because she *is* the way she is. Now what can *you* do to help yourself become less upset when you're with her and she acts that way? (Pause)

Joyce: Accept her the way she is?

Therapist: Right! and *how* are you going to concretely help yourself to accept her the way she is?

Joyce: I don't know.

Therapist: Well, you have to say to yourself, you have to challenge, forcefully challenge your own beliefs: the things that you tell yourself to upset yourself to begin with. When you first find yourself getting upset, or when you already are upset, or even after you have been upset for awhile, you can then say to yourself: "Why did I get myself so upset? Because I told myself, 'My mother *shouldn't* be acting the way she is acting.' " And you can then challenge that self-reiterated belief. You can ask: "Why *shouldn't* she be acting the way she is acting? Disturbed people *do* act in a disturbed manner; and it's not her behavior, or what she says to me that is upsetting me. It's my *telling myself* that she *shouldn't* be behaving the way she is. *That's* how I keep upsetting me." So you keep challenging your own nonsense. For there is, of course, no reason why she shouldn't be acting the way she is. She's obviously off her rocker in some ways; and you can calmly accept that fact. You say, "So what? It's *too bad* she's acting the way she's acting. It's irritating, I don't like it. But what's the *horror?* That's the way she *is.* Tough!" If you follow this procedure, you won't be making yourself upset. You've done it before with her, haven't you?

Joyce: Yeah.

Therapist: Prevented yourself from becoming upset?

Joyce: Sometimes I don't pay any attention to her because—.

Therapist: You don't take her too seriously. For I think when you say, "Sometimes I don't pay any attention to her," you really mean that you do understand fully what she is doing but you don't take her too seriously for doing it.

Joyce: I just don't pay any attention to the things she does.

Therapist: Yes; well, all right, why can't you do that *most* of the time?

Joyce: Because some of the time I don't feel like it.

Therapist: Yes, and those are the times when you just don't try. You just don't work at challenging your own nonsensical sentences. And that's why, at those times, you upset yourself. For you don't *have* to take her behavior seriously at almost any time that she's acting crazily. For her behavior certainly is crazy now and then, just as your father's is. This doesn't mean that both of them are crazy *persons,* any more than it would mean that you were entirely a nut because *some* of your behavior is nutty. We want to get you to be able to distinguish between a person's *performance* and the whole *person,* and not to confuse the two. An individual can demonstrate all kinds of nutty behavior, but that doesn't mean that he as a person is a complete nut and that he can't be listened to or trusted at all. The fact that some of your *acts* may be wrong or inefficient does not mean that *you,* as a whole, are bad.

The therapist, sticking closely to the rational-emotive approach in this dialogue, illustrates the following points: (1) He agrees with Joyce that her view of her mother may be *quite* accurate (though he is not sure it is, since she may be grossly exaggerating), but insists that *even* if this is so, Joyce has no reason to make herself upset. (2) He shows her how it's going to take hard, persistent *work* for her to see and to *change* her unrealistic demands on her mother; and that only after she has done a considerable amount of such work is she likely automatically to believe the truth that her mother does behave poorly, but that there is no real reason that she *shouldn't,* though there are reasons why it would be nice if she *didn't.* (3) He demonstrates to Joyce that she isn't merely being annoyed or frustrated by her mother: She is foolishly insisting that her mother *ought not* be annoying; and it is this latter insistence, rather than her mother's annoying qualities, which are really upsetting her. (4) He concretely shows Joyce how she can not only get herself to see, but also actively to challenge her own irrational beliefs at point B, so that, without necessarily stopping her mother's irritating behavior at point A, she will be able to derive much different reactions (that is, emotional equanimity) at point C. (5) He reiterates what he has previously tried to get Joyce to see (and what he endeavors to get practically all his clients to see) that a healthy emotional attitude arises when the individual distinguishes between another individual's *performances* and this other's *person* or *self.* Although the former may be legitimately disvalued and abhorred, it is illegitimate to overgeneralize and to condemn the latter.

Joyce reluctantly agreed with some of the therapist's teachings at this point; but she persisted in blaming others, especially a friend of her mother whom she thought was a terrible telephone gossiper. Rather than dismiss this point lightly—since it is a cardinal rule of rational-emotive therapy that rage at other people is almost invariably wrong and self-defeating and that if the client can be shown how to stop this kind of raging she can make a basic change in her own personality—the therapist used it for most of the rest of the session in an effort to get Joyce to accept reality. Their dialogue ran as follows:

Joyce: So she's one of those telephone gossipers. It goes all over town what's happening next.

Therapist: Yes; well, that's her problem. Why doesn't she have the right to gossip?

Joyce: Why, I don't think she has.

Therapist: Well, why not?

Joyce: She's a nosy old hag!

Therapist: So what? Why doesn't she have the right to be a nosy old hag?

Joyce: I don't see why she does have.

Therapist: Uh?

Joyce: I don't see why she does have.

Therapist: Well, that's *your* theory. *You're* the one who says she doesn't have the right. And let's see if you can prove to me, right now, that she doesn't have the right to be a nosy old hag.

Joyce: Well, she's got the right to use the phone, like anybody else; but that doesn't mean—Oh, I guess there ain't no law against being a gossiper.

Therapist: That's right, there isn't. Except by *your* definition!

Joyce: That's because I don't like her.

Therapist: Yes. But if you just stopped there and just said you didn't like her being a gossip, you wouldn't be making yourself upset. But you're going a little farther than that. Now, what are you saying to yourself to go beyond that and to make yourself angry at her?

Joyce: That I don't like her and I don't like the way she is, and I don't want to be pestered by her.

Therapist: No, you're saying more than that. You're saying, "She *shouldn't* be the way she is. That goddamned bitch has no *right* to be gossiping and talking about me!"

Joyce: I guess she really does.

Therapist: Of course she does! And it's damned easy for her to gossip like that—because that's the way she is.

Joyce: But she wouldn't like it if somebody did it to her.

Therapist: She probably wouldn't. But that merely shows that she's got a problem.

Joyce: Well, she's supposed, she's supposed to be a very good Christian. She always claims she is. So you'd think she'd live by the Golden Rule.

Therapist: It's her privilege to subscribe to any religion she wants—and to not live up to it, if that's the way she is.

Joyce: She's certainly something!

Therapist: Maybe so. But just because she acts crazily, in your eyes, why do you have to upset yourself about her asinine behavior? What does it mean when she gossips about you?

Joyce: Well, it certainly doesn't make things any easier for me.

Therapist: No. But how does it really make things harder?

Joyce: It just does.

Therapist: How?

Joyce: Well, the more she can think about to gossip about me, the more she tells people about me.

Therapist: So what?

Joyce: The more it spreads around, the worse it gets.

Therapist: So?

Joyce: It goes from one to another; and everybody adds a little more to it; and when it's all done, it's really something.

Therapist: And?

Joyce: By the time it gets back to me, why it's as heavy as a rock.

Therapist: Well, okay; what about it? What's the worst that could happen as a result of this gossip being as heavy as a rock? What do you feel is the worst that could happen?

Joyce: I don't think it's fair.

Therapist: Huh?

Joyce: I don't think it's fair!

Therapist: Yes, but that's the way the world is: Things aren't always fair; there are a lot of injustices.

Joyce: And if I was to live back in my home borough, it wouldn't make things very easy for me.

Therapist: Yes, but you don't have to live in the same borough again. But let's assume that you did live there, what then?

Joyce: Well, it could lessen my chances of making very many friends. It could make it hard for me to get a job.

Therapist: Yes, it *could.* But even suppose it did lessen your chances of getting a job. Would that be catastrophic?

Joyce: Well, I think it would be a mess.

Therapist: Well, why would it be such a mess?

Joyce: Well, because I don't like to be all alone. I like to have someone to talk to.

Therapist: Oh, come now! Would you really have to be all alone, just because she talked about you? And would you die if you were?

Joyce: No. But I don't like to sit around and do nothing all the time—or sit around and work all the time.

Therapist: Yes, but you *could* live by yourself, if you had to. And there's no evidence that her gossiping will leave you absolutely friendless.

Joyce: No, but it may make a lot of difference. And I don't want to live that way, because I think I deserve a chance of having friends and everything, just as well as everybody else does.

Therapist: I'm sure you do; but you're merely assuming that if she talks about you absolutely no one will befriend you—which is certainly quite an assumption! You're really afraid that people will think you're a shit—is that right?

Joyce: Yes.

Therapist: And if other people think you're a shit, you'll have to think you're one too?

Joyce: I guess so.

Therapist: Well, how does other people *thinking* you're a louse *make* you one?

Joyce: Well, if you weren't a louse, you'd probably have friends; and people wouldn't be talking about you and wouldn't think that you *were* a louse.

Therapist: That doesn't follow. People could easily talk about you—especially gossipy people like her—no matter *what* you did. And how does people *talking about* you or *thinking* you're a louse really *make* you one?

Joyce: Well, maybe after a while you begin to believe it. Because you don't get anywhere in life, you don't have any friends or anything. Why, you can believe it, I think.

Therapist: Ah, but that's the real problem. *You* believe it.

Joyce: Well——.

Therapist: Isn't that right? Don't you believe you're a louse?

Joyce: I used to believe I was!

Therapist: But you don't believe it any more? Well, apparently you *do.* If you're getting so upset over this woman's gossip and if you're feeling that she's going to convince other people you're a louse, then you probably agree that if she and they think you're one, you really are. Isn't that right?

Joyce: Yes.

Therapist: But again: How does other people *thinking* you're a louse *make* you one? You explain to me the process by which their thoughts magically create your lousehood.

Joyce: Well, they might treat me like one.

Therapist: Yes, they may treat you like a worm; but does that mean that you *are* one?

Joyce: No.

Therapist: No, of course not!

Joyce: But if you get treated like one, you feel like one.

Therapist: Oh? And *why* would you feel like one, if you were treated like one?

Joyce: Because you were treated like one.

Therapist: Oh, no! It's not because you are treated like a worm that makes you *feel* like one. That's point A. At point A somebody, we'll say, like this gossipy woman, is treating you like a worm, treating you unjustly. Let's assume that this is a fact; that A really exists in the outside world. And at point C, you feel wormy. You feel like a louse. Now, how does that follow? How does the fact, at point A, that someone's treating you like a louse, make you actually feel like one, at point C? Can't you see: It's not their treatment of you that makes you feel that way—because that's impossible. How can *their* thoughts get inside your head and your body and make *you* have feelings? Obviously, instead, it's what you're telling yourself, at point B, *about* their treating you like a louse at point A. It's only your *agreement* with them, at point B, that really makes you feel the way they want you to feel.

Joyce: Well, how could you go on feeling that you were anything worthwhile if everybody treated you like you were a worm? I mean, after a while you just kinda, kinda break down—they break you down to thinking you really are a worm.

Therapist: Yes. You begin to *believe,* after a while, if you let yourself believe, that another person's bad opinion of you makes you the way he thinks about you. He thinks you're no good; you believe that he is right; and then, by believing in his nonsense, you upset yourself. In other words, you begin evaluating your worth as a person in terms of the way *he* evaluates you. But actually—if you stop and look at it for a moment—*how* does his evaluation of you make you *anything?*

Joyce: It just does.

Therapist: But how? How does it?

Joyce: Well, if everybody's going to kick you around, you're going to feel like you're not wanted and you're no good.

Therapist: Why *must* you? You *may* feel you're no good because they treat you as if you are. But does their treatment of you really *mean* that you're the kind of person they think you are?

Joyce: No, I guess it doesn't have to.

Therapist: Well, then, why do you believe this bosh?

Joyce: I don't know (pause). Because I've been shoved around since I was a little kid. That's where I first learned to believe it.

Therapist: Okay, you learned to believe it a long time ago. Your parents, your culture, all kinds of communications—such as books, the movies, your school teachers—told you you were no good if people didn't like you. And, being young and foolish, you unthinkingly accepted this crap and believed it. "If another person disapproves of me, that means I'm a no-good shit. I'm a worthless person if someone treats me as a worthless person. If people don't like the things I do, that must mean that I'm a slob!" This is what you sopped up as a child—this nonsensical value system about yourself. And today it's still your belief in it, your uncritical acceptance of these nutty values, that makes you feel you're no good and creates your upsetness. It's not what *other* people are now doing to you or saying to you that bothers you; it's the negative way you *interpret* their deeds and sayings. But there is another point of view you could take, instead. You don't *have* to believe that you're worthless because another person treats you as if you are. You don't *have* to accept his definition of you and make it your own. You could, instead, take his definition of you for what it really is: a theological construct that has no empirical referent. For there is no evidence that just because he *thinks* you are a total slob, you really are; and there is much evidence that no humans, not even those of us possessing the worst traits, are totally worthless. For we almost invariably have *some* redeeming virtues; and even if we didn't have any, we could always accept *ourselves,* and find some kind of joys in life, no matter how flawed or inept we were. So even if everyone in the world treated you as a slob that wouldn't necessarily *make* you one. It would mean, at most, that *they* had no use for you; but you could still have quite a bit of use for yourself. It is terribly frustrating, of course, if others think very little of you: a real pain in the ass, in fact! But it still doesn't *make* you a louse—except by your own stupid acceptance of their definition.

The therapist's work with Joyce seemed to keep paying off well. Immediately after this last session, she was independently evaluated by another psychologist at the hospital, who found that "her thinking was clear and pertinent to topics broached (no available data suggested that she was, or had ever been, 'psychotic'). She maintained a pretty even mood tone throughout (apparently calm and untroubled on the surface level) whether we discussed her relationships with parents, death of her child, or hospital living."

The evaluating psychologist quoted Joyce as saying, "Psychotherapy helped me greatly; it made me realize that things in the past can't be changed—that I must make a new life for myself." Having the usual contemporary bias in favor of relationship therapy, this psychologist wondered whether the pronounced progress made by Joyce largely resulted from her relationship with her therapist. To check his hypothesis, the therapist tried to ascertain, in the following session, whether she had any strong feelings about him as a person, especially in view of the fact that she had just sent him a Valentine's Day card.

Joyce insisted that the card, which was a humorous one, was not meant at all seriously; and she indicated no personal interest in the therapist. When he pressed still further, to see if she had any kind of romantic attachment to him, she said flatly that she did not. There were no other evidences, throughout the entire course of her treatment, that Joyce had any strong positive transference with the therapist, nor that the gains she made in therapy resulted from the relationship she had with him. When she did begin making real progress, which occurred shortly after the rational-emotive method began to be employed with her, it seemed to be correlated, first, with the philosophic discussions she had with the therapist; second, with her interactions with other inmates in the hospital; and third, with her learning how to handle her emotional reactions to her parents, relatives, and close associates when she was on home visits. This last sign of progress also seemed to be related importantly to her work with the therapist, because objective surveys by outsiders showed that her reports of her mother's and stepfather's poor handling of her and of themselves were quite accurate. The social service department of the hospital, in one of its routine reports on Joyce's family, stated that "her family situation is exceedingly poor—both parents being quite sick and more than likely borderline (if not actually) psychotic."

Typical of Joyce's progress in handling her problems with her parents is this dialogue which took place at the beginning of her forty-sixth therapy session:

Therapist: Well, how have things been going?

Joyce: Pretty good; just fine. I went home this weekend. While I was at home, I ran into a lot of the kids I went to school with and things went over pretty good.

Therapist: And your parents?

Joyce: We got along fine. There wasn't any real disagreements on anything. They had some trouble with my sisters, but I got along with them. And I got along with everybody—had a pretty nice time.

Therapist: How do you feel about your stepfather now?

Joyce: Well, he's still the same oddball he was; but you've just got to learn to get along with him and take him for what he is. You can't change him. You've just got to accept him for what he is and learn to tolerate his weird ideas and thinking and some of the crazy things he says. Just kinda laugh them off, you might say, and not let them bother you.

Therapist: How do you go about laughing it off now—not letting it bother you?

Joyce: Well, half the things he talks about, he doesn't know too much about; and a lot of things he is wrong on or puts it in a bad way. Like if he is talking about a person and makes him out a shit or something. So I just say to myself, "That's his opinion, and he's entitled to his opinions and the way he thinks about things even if I don't agree with them." I just accept it and think that everybody is entitled to his own opinions.

Therapist: Um hum; that's right. So you don't take him too seriously?

Joyce: No.

Therapist: Even if he attacks you as a person? What about that?

Joyce: Well, I listen to what he has to say; and maybe it's good and maybe it's not. But I don't necessarily agree with it. Because I think I'm old enough to discipline myself and take care of my own life; without him telling me how to do it. But I let him have his say-so. That's all right for some people, you know. But we're all different, and I don't have to agree with everything he says.

Therapist: Well, what else happened while you were home?

Joyce: Nothing much.

Therapist: Well, what in the nature of problems or difficulties do you feel that you still have to some extent—need to work through in order to be happier and enjoy life more?

Joyce: Well, some things I don't exactly like to accept; but I do. I just don't think I do entirely.

Therapist: For example?

Joyce: Well, things being my way. Certain situations I don't like. But I don't get disturbed about them now. I realize I can't have everything my way.

Therapist: Um hum.

Joyce: And I guess that's the main thing that bothers me sometimes, but not as bad as it used to—or at least I don't get too upset about it. It comes to my mind and I realize the situation. I want something I can't have; and so why worry about it?

Therapist: You're realizing that, while you may want it, it's not an absolute necessity that you have it right that moment; that you have no *need* for it; and that you are not going to die without it.

Joyce: Yeah.

Therapist: Huh?

Joyce: Yes.

Therapist: Well, let's take a recent experience in which you felt that way and use that as an illustration.

Joyce: Well, this is a little off the track; but it is similar in a way, too. It's something that bothered me a little bit. It was this friend of my mother calling all the time. In some way she found out that I was home and she would then call and want to know what was going on with me here at the hospital. She would say, "You know what I think? I think they're not doing anything for you and they're not going to do anything. They're going to leave you there." I could have told her off, but I figured that wasn't necessary—that it wouldn't have done any good and would have just made her believe more firmly that I was very sick or something. This is not just a matter of exactly having my way or not; but she gets me a little—oh, she agitates things all the time! It used to kinda make me mad, but I've kinda gotten used to it. And I now think to myself, "Well, she doesn't know any more about this hospital than a five-year-old child. So what can she say about it? She's not the one to judge how I've improved or how I haven't or anything like that. And she hasn't any influence on the hospital. So why should it bother me?" To heck with her and what she says! I really don't care whether she likes me or not. She's not the whole world, anyway.

Therapist: Um huh.

Joyce: I figure there's no love lost there. She's just another person.

Therapist: So you're saying you're not getting yourself upset any more by what she had to say?

Joyce: Yes. Where a few months ago, when she would call and say things like that, it kinda bothered me, now I realize that I shouldn't let her hurt me or upset me. I was upsetting myself to even let it worry me, because what she said didn't mean a damned thing. Because she didn't have any influence on what happened to me anyway.

Therapist: Except that you used to *let* her have this influence on you.

Joyce: In my own mind, I did. But I realize now that she's not right in what she says either. She doesn't have anything to do with me or the hospital; and I shouldn't let what she says disturb me or bother me because I know she hasn't anything to do with it; and if she did have anything to say, she would not be the only person involved, anyway.

Therapist: In other words, to hell with her ideas?

Joyce: Yes. Let them go! (laughs)

As can be seen from this excerpt, Joyce has apparently made considerable progress in coping with the difficulties of life, particularly in her relations with the same kind of people about whom she used to upset herself. Not content with this progress, the therapist looks for areas of her life in which she is still unduly bothering herself and tries to show her how to help herself in these respects. Thus, most of the rest of this session is taken up with her feelings of jealousy:

Therapist: Well, it sounds to me like you've been doing quite well in these areas. . . . What other things seem to bother you to some extent?

Joyce: Well, one of the problems I think that still exists, I haven't exactly been able to work on because I haven't come into any real contact with the problem recently. But it was previously a problem and I would say it still probably would be if I was to start going with someone and I didn't—if something came up in regard to getting along with men. If I'm going with them and they go out with someone else, I don't like it. I don't say I'm still that way; but I would say I could be.

Therapist: You're talking about feeling jealous.

Joyce: Yeah.

Therapist: What about it?

Joyce: Well, it's kinda a problem.

Therapist: How? In what way do you feel that it's a problem?

Joyce: Well, I don't really think that I should feel that way about it because it's——. That person, whoever it might be, would be free and should be able to make his own decisions and go with whoever he wants; and I don't have any business in thinking different.

Therapist: What do you mean? You shouldn't feel that way about it?

Joyce: Well, I don't say I shouldn't feel that way about it. But I shouldn't feel that way so strongly—saying that he's mine and you can't have him! I mean, I shouldn't have that kind of feeling or attitude in my mind toward him, toward the whole thing.

Therapist: Yes, but why shouldn't you feel that way? Even if you take it to the point of intense jealousy; why shouldn't you feel intensely jealous?

Joyce: Well, you can't have everything you want. And, uh, if I look at it this way: If it was him feeling that way instead of me, I wouldn't want to feel that someone's got a grip on me and is pulling me around on a chain. And I think that's what you make someone feel like when you act this jealous way.

Therapist: Well, I'm not sure that *you* make them feel that way, though they can certainly make that interpretation if you are very jealous. But aren't you trying to chain yourself to yourself in some respects? You're trying to throw the shackles on yourself.

Joyce: Yeah.

Therapist: The point I was trying to make was that there is nothing awful about your feeling jealous, even though it has inconveniences. What you really seem to mean is: "It would be best for me not to feel so jealous. I'd be a lot happier not feeling that way about this individual. I'd better more or less accept him even if he does go with other girls for the time being." But if you take the belief, "It would be better for me not to feel so jealous" and you translate it into "I've *got* to be less jealous; it's terrible when I'm jealous!" you then are saying that you *should* not be jealous instead of that it's *preferable* that you not be. That means you're blaming yourself for *having* the problem of jealousy to begin with, doesn't it?

Joyce: Yeah, in a roundabout way.

Therapist: So the first thing is to rid yourself of the attitude that you *shouldn't* have the problem of jealousy. You'd better recognize that you are a human being, that you do make mistakes, that being intensely jealous is nothing but one of these mistakes, and that you can calmly work at correcting this mistake. You'd better focus not on *how* you're doing—or, really, on how *badly* you're doing for being jealous—but on *what* you're doing to create the intense jealousy. Now how could you go about solving this problem?

Joyce: A good question.

Therapist: To answer it, I think the most important thing is to understand what you are doing to make yourself intensely jealous. Isn't that the main issue?

Joyce: Yes.

Therapist: All right, then: why do you feel jealous?

Joyce: I don't know.

Therapist: You really do—if you'll only look at exactly what you're telling yourself to *create* this feeling. In order to have the emotion of jealousy, you obviously must be telling yourself something about the situation you're in at the time you experience it. And what do you think you're telling yourself? Isn't it, first of all, the possibility of the fellow you're with going out with another girl?

Joyce: Well, it could be.

Therapist: Well, let's assume that he really is going out with another girl; that you see that he is; and that you feel very jealous. All right, now, in order for you to have this feeling you must be telling yourself something about the fact that here he is, out with another girl, and not with you. What do you think you are saying to yourself about this fact?

Joyce: He shouldn't be with her! He should be with me!

Therapist: Yes! But *why* shouldn't he be with her and *why* should he be with you?

Joyce: Because I think so!

Therapist: But who are *you?*

Joyce: Me (laughs)!

Therapist: So you're being kinda grandiose—demanding that he shouldn't be doing what he wants to do because *you* don't want him to do it.

Joyce: Um huh.

Therapist: You're saying, "The world should be the way I want it to be!" But isn't there something else involved here besides demanding that you get exactly what you want? *Why* would you be wanting him exclusively to yourself?

Joyce: Ummm. It could be that he's the person I think I can get along with and that I think's better than so-and-so; and that I don't think that someone else deserves him, but I do—that I'm better.

Therapist: In what way would you be better? What makes you think you're better than the other girl he might choose to go out with?

Joyce: I don't know.

Therapist: Well, how else are you really feeling if he's with this other girl? What else does your jealousy consist of besides your demand that he shouldn't be with her and should be with you? What else is there besides your feeling, your grandiosity, that you are better than she is and that therefore he should be with you? There's still something a little more basic—what is it?

Joyce: I don't know.

Therapist: Well, isn't it something along these lines: You're going with this guy and you're feeling kinda great in a sense; and when he goes out with another girl don't you kind of feel that he's rejecting you?

Joyce: Yeah.

Therapist: Don't you feel that you need this guy's love—otherwise you're just not much good? You feel also that it's a horrible thing that he is rejecting you, that this rejection means that he doesn't love you any more, and since he doesn't love you any more you return to being the kind of worthless shit that you think you really are.

Joyce: Indirectly, yes. I mean, I don't look at it that strongly; but in parts, I feel deserted.

Therapist: Deserted?

Joyce: Yeah.

Therapist: And what do you mean by feeling deserted?

Joyce: I don't know—just pushed back in somebody's past and forgotten.

Therapist: But so what if you really were pushed back in somebody's past and forgotten? How is this going to affect *you,* make *you* entirely rotten?

Joyce: I don't want to be forgotten.

Therapist: And why don't you want to be forgotten?

Joyce: I think that when I'm forgotten that I'm worthless, no good—that there's something wrong with me.

Therapist: Yes?

Joyce: That I'm goofy or something (laughs)!

Therapist: Well, now: How does your being rejected by a male, how does that make you worthless?

Joyce: I don't know.

Therapist: Neither do I—but you *believe* it!

Joyce: I *know* it. (laughs)

Therapist: You're defining your worth as a person in terms of extrinsic standards—in terms of what one fellow might think of you. That, of course, is nonsensical. If I were to say to you, "You're a red fire hydrant," would you believe me?

Joyce: No.

Therapist: Why not?

Joyce: Why should I?

Therapist: Well, prove to me that you aren't a red fire hydrant. Where's your evidence?

Joyce: Well, you haven't got any evidence that I am.

Therapist: Yes, but can you prove to me that you're not a fire hydrant?

Joyce: No.

Therapist: Well, don't you have *some* facts to prove that you're not a red fire hydrant?

Joyce: Yes, I guess so.

Therapist: Okay, what are they?

Joyce: Well, I look like a human being.

Therapist: All right, you don't look like a fire hydrant. What's another fact?

Joyce: A fire hydrant is motionless and I'm not.

Therapist: Right.

Joyce: And it doesn't talk and I do (laughs)!

Therapist: Right!

Joyce: And it doesn't consume food and I do.

Therapist: Okay. So there are at least four observable facts—and many more you could list. We have observable facts, scientific evidence that you are not a red fire hydrant. Right?

Joyce: Yes.

Therapist: Okay, so wouldn't it be kinda silly for you, in the face of that evidence, to believe that you *are* a red fire hydrant?

Joyce: Yeah.

Therapist: Okay, now. If somebody says to you, "You are worthless," does that *make* you worthless?

Joyce: No.

Therapist: But if you go along believing that you are worthless because someone says that you are, isn't that much the same thing as believing that you are a red fire hydrant because somebody tells you you're one?

Joyce: Yes, it is.

Therapist: And isn't that the problem—that you believe fundamental things about your total self just because some people, such as a man who deserts you for another girl, directly or indirectly indicates that they think you're not so hot in certain ways?

Joyce: Yes.

Therapist: Yes, that seems to be your assumption: that if my behavior is bad or poor, or someone merely thinks that it is, I as a total person am no good, a slob, a worthless individual. And you have the additional assumptions that, if you are deserted by a boyfriend, that proves, first, that he thinks you're worthless; and, second, that, if he believes this, it's true, you really *are* no good. This so-called "proof" that you're using is no proof at all, but only an arbitrary definition of yourself. It is a groundless statement for which you have no substantiating evidence. Actually, your worth as a person does not depend upon any external criterion. No matter what you do, you still have your own internal validity and you can be quite worthwhile to yourself just because you exist, because you're alive and capable of some kind of enjoyment. Even if no one else in the world likes you, that still does not make you worthless unless you *believe* that it does. You can still accept and enjoy yourself. Isn't it your dire need for love, then, which is the core of your intense jealousy? If you don't have this love that you think you absolutely need from the someone you have made the one significant person in your life, you convince yourself that you're a no-good slob. Isn't *that* the cause of the jealousy?

Joyce: Yes.

Therapist: And let's ask what's on the other side of the coin, too. It looks like, in order to try to compensate yourself for your basic feelings of worthlessness, when you have a special boyfriend you grandiosely tell yourself that you are better than other girls, and that therefore these girls have no right to go with him and that he *should* only go with you. Actually, however, why *are* you better than every other girl?

Joyce: I don't know.

Therapist: I don't either. Let's face it: that these others have just as much a right to a boy you like as you do. Not that you should not try to win him for yourself: because you *want* him and not because you *need* him or *have a unique right* to have him.

Joyce: Mmmm.

Therapist: So what can you do now to help yourself to become less intensely jealous?

Joyce: Refuse to believe that I'm no good and get myself to believe that I am good, in the sense of having a right to live and get what I want.

Therapist: That's right. To become less jealous you'd better question your basic assumption that, "If he dates other girls besides me, that makes me worthless; if he rejects me, it is a horrible thing." To question this assumption, you can keep asking yourself, "*How* does his going out with another girl make me no good? What is so *horrible* about being rejected?" And if you keep doing this kind of questioning and challenging, you will come to see that what he does cannot make you worthless to yourself (though you may be of little worth to him) and that it is not horrible to be rejected (though it may be terribly frustrating and inconvenient).

Joyce: It's just the things that I tell myself—the things I say I *should* have—that upset me, then, and make me jealous?

Therapist: Right. And you can replace these things with a more rational self-acceptance. Such as: "Okay, he's going out with this other girl in addition to me. Tough!—but he is. Now let me see what I can do to get him to be with me more, and be less with her or others." And then you can set about, in a reasonably calm manner, being nicer to him, being sexier, helping him with his problems, or otherwise giving him inducements to spend more time with you. If that's what you want, go after it—rather than bemoan the situation and denigrate yourself.

Two notable points are illustrated in this fairly typical segment of rational-emotive therapy: (1) Instead of the client spending much of the therapeutic time in talking at length about her past and present history and giving every possible nuance of her feelings, there is constant back and forth dialogue between her and the therapist. This is in contradistinction to her early psychoanalytic sessions, which largely consisted of her telling about the events of her past and present life. (2) Instead of reflecting the client's feelings and doing a considerable amount of passive listening to her, the therapist (a) instigates much of the dialogue; (b) continually asks probing questions; (c) doesn't allow an important topic to drop when the client seems willing to let it go; (d) does more talking than the client does; (e) does not hesitate to directly interpret, explain, exposit, and teach; (f) checks up from time to time to see whether the client is understanding the points he is making; (g) forces the client to repeat back to him, in her own words, the most usable parts of their discussion; (h) urges the client to perform some definite actions, or homework assignments, to back up the new ideas he is teaching her and to put them into actual practice.

For the next several sessions Joyce continued to show progress. She was offered a good job outside the hospital grounds but was not able to take it because it interfered with her hospital schedule; and she took this frustration with good grace. She also kept taking her parents' disappointment and criticism with more and more equanimity, though from time to time she relapsed into upsetting herself about their ways. When she did resent people in her family or at the hospital, she began to realize that she reacted toward them as she had always reacted toward her twin sisters: with jealousy and overcompetitiveness; and that she didn't *have* to react this way, didn't *have* to believe that she would always be favored. She admitted that her anger against others, including her anger at the child she killed and at her husband at the time she killed it, stemmed from her own nonacceptance of reality; and that she could effectively make herself much less angry by getting herself to accept this reality.

Although the main goal of the therapy was to get Joyce to accept herself fully and to live comfortably with the frustrations imposed on her by the world, she also reaped some side benefits from the basic changes in her attitudes. Where previously she had been prudish and condemnatory of herself and others in regard to premarital sex relations, she decided, in one of the last sessions of psychotherapy, that such relations were not necessarily wrong and that as long as she took proper precautions not to become pregnant, she could enjoyably have them. She noted, as her sex guilt decreased, that she could bring up problems in therapy that she previously could not talk about.

Joyce also successfully began to handle the problem of what people thought of her in her home borough. During the fifty-fourth therapy session, she indicated that she used to feel very hurt when she was home and passed old acquaintances on the street, because she knew they would remember her as a murderess and thought that they would despise her. She had recently stopped feeling that way; and, with insight, she remarked, "I don't think that these people have changed that much. It's me, I guess." She no longer was afraid to go out in public; she noted that when she did meet old acquaintances they usually told her that she didn't look anything like she looked a year ago (at the time she committed infanticide), but that she looked much more alive and happy.

She realized that at the time of the murder, she strongly felt that nobody, including her husband and her parents, understood her, and that it was a terrible thing not to be understood. Now, however, she thought that she didn't really need other people's understanding or approval, although she would like very much to have it. The therapist's notes at the end of the fifty-fourth session read: "She says she no longer views people and her home borough as bad and wanting to hurt her. She realizes that what she's done, she has done to herself; that it was her misperception of people and events, and not these people or events themselves, that caused her difficulty before and that led to her crime. With respect to her stepfather, she states that her feelings toward him have changed a lot and that she realizes he really is sick, where before she didn't want to accept this and just considered him something of an oddball."

At the close of the fifty-ninth session of psychotherapy Joyce's case was considered by the hospital staff and it was found that she had made considerable progress and improvement. Her basic problems had been extreme hostility and severe guilt, and she tended, at the time of her incarceration, to deny and to cover up the guilt by feeling angry and giving vent to violent behavior. What is more, not being able to face either her hostility or her guilt, she resorted to states of dissociation and confusion and at times literally did not know what she was doing. The murder of her child seems to have been committed when she was in one of these dissociational states.

The members of the hospital staff, including the therapist, felt that at the close of therapy Joyce's hostility and guilt both had been adequately uncovered and accepted by her and that she had been making concerted efforts to discover the philosophic sources of her negative feelings, to question and challenge these sources, and to change them. Her severe emotional difficulties largely seem to have been dissolved and her general progress was considered to be good. She was granted a complete discharge from the hospital.

Several years have passed since then. A recent checkup showed that about a year after returning home she married a boy of her own age whom she had known for some years and that a year after that she gave birth to another daughter. She was quite pleased with this new child and has been taking care of it more than adequately. She gets along well with her husband, even though he has his own problems, and is able to talk most of their difficulties out with him at the time they arise. She accepts her parents better than she ever did in the past and also, for the first time in her life, is getting along reasonably well with her twin sisters. As a result of an interview with her four years after her discharge, the social service department of the hospital concluded that she has largely resolved her presenting problems which were instrumental in leading her to murder her second daughter; that she shows no indication that she will ever again become homicidal; and that she probably will continue to lead a fulfilling life.

Chapter 11

Diagnostic and Therapeutic Interview with a Female Who Murdered Her Husband

This is an interview with a twenty-eight-year-old programmer, Clara, who in a fit of anger murdered her thirty-year-old husband. She was referred primarily for an emotional evaluation by the penal institution in which she was incarcerated. However, since the interviewer practiced rational-emotive psychotherapy, he felt that he might be able not only to diagnose this woman but that, even within the scope of a single interview, he might be able to help her. One of the main theories of rational-emotive therapy is that individuals can be helped in even a single session, and even more often within five to ten sessions: because little time is spent exhuming their background or analyzing their dreams and most of the therapeutic time is spent in showing them exactly what their major irrational premises are and what they can do to find these premises, to logically parse them, to question and challenge them, to do activity-oriented homework assignments that also challenge them, and finally to ameliorate or surrender them.

Knowing that he might not get anywhere with this interviewee, Clara, the therapist was nonetheless willing to take a chance that he might be able in part to reach her. Nothing is likely to be lost and much is to be gained in this process; since the basic philosophies of the interviewee which are sought out in a rational-emotive interview are indicative of what her fundamental personality patterns really are. Moreover, in noting how well the individual understands what the therapist is driving at, and how she reacts to his suggestions for helping herself, the therapist obtains a most important transactional picture of her. A good therapy interview, in other words, is likely to be an excellent diagnostic interview; and since an attempt at helping the individual is made at the same time, considerable professional effort is likely to be saved in the course of a rational-emotive session. The following is a transcript of the tape-recorded first interview:

Therapist: Now, Clara, can you give me some idea of why you're in prison? What happened?

Clara: Do you want the whole story?

Therapist: Yes, if you would.

Clara: Sure, if you've got enough tape.

Therapist: Oh, I've got plenty of tape.

Clara: Well, when I was about twenty, I'd fallen in love with a boy and I thought I was pregnant. And he didn't love me, apparently, so I tried to kill myself. And since then, I've tried it five more times. The last time was because of Dave. Dave—I met Dave through Dwight. I was going with Dwight, and Dave was engaged. And, uh, we double-dated a few times. Then Dwight went away to graduate school and Dave asked me out. And there was a strong attraction. And it was physical at first. I wanted to make love with him. And I said all right; so we went out. We went out more and more times. Then he started coming up to the office where I worked as a computer programmer and we would talk and laugh a great deal. He worked for the same firm in another department—as did Dwight, too. And then we started seeing each other every day. We'd both cut work every so often, and went off and spent the day together. We'd somehow manage to see a lot of each other almost every day, even though he had a regular girlfriend and, in fact, was engaged to her. And so by and by he left his girl; and he had to have a new place to live—since they had been living together—so he moved into an apartment near me. Then I moved in with him. It was an awful place. It was dirty, just filthy. The people that lived there just before were just, just animals. And so we fixed it up and made it rather nice. We suddenly decided to get married, although he was still sweet on his ex-girlfriend. We stayed in our cleaned-up place a couple of months; and then, just as suddenly as we got married, he decided to leave me and try to live with his girlfriend again. I couldn't believe it, because we were getting along all right and he was hardly seeing her at all. But he somehow decided to go back to her. And I told him, I said, "If you go back, I'll kill myself." It wasn't a threat, because I meant it. And so he left. I took a bottle of pills the night he was supposed to leave and I fell asleep. And he left and called my father and told him to come and get me. When I woke up, he was gone and father was there. He said he'd gone back to his girlfriend. So I went in the bathroom and took some more sleeping pills, as many as I could find. And I remember I was in the hospital, having my stomach pumped out, and they tried to find out whether I had any feeling and this and that. Then they drove me to another hospital to have a specialist look at me, operate on my windpipe, and do some more stomach pumping. I finally woke up, I was crying. I was all upset. And I wanted so bad to talk to Dave. There was a phone in my room; and dad finally said O.K., so I called him. And I told him, I asked him, I said, "Have you gone back to Josie?" He said, "Where are you, what's the matter?" I said, "I'm in the hospital. I had surgery. I took pills last night." He said, "Well, I've gone back to Josie. I'm going to send you some divorce papers. I want to marry her." And I ran out the exit of the ward I was in until I collapsed. And they gave me some sort of shot. I guess I was hysterical again. They had a man passing in a car and he helped take me back to the hospital. So I had the surgery. And dad didn't want Dave to come near me at all. He felt like it was his fault, which is how I wanted him to feel. And so Dave wanted to come see me. Dad said, "No, you leave her alone. She'll be all right if you leave her alone." But he smuggled a note in by Joe Slate, who is a good friend of dad's and a good friend of mine, as well as a good friend of Dave's. And he told me how much he still loved me and that he and Josie had parted again. They'd only been together for a few days. And so he said, "Call me and tell me when your father won't be there and I'll come up." I did, because I was just crazy about him. And so he came up, and he was crying and I was crying—you know, typical happy reunion. And so I was in the hospital a week and I had to wear high-necked dresses until the scar on my throat healed. Then we, we got back together; we were seeing each other. After I got out of the hospital, it was about a week later I moved back in with him. I wasn't with him, in our little apartment, but about two weeks. And I did all the washing and cleaning and ironing and that sort of thing. In fact, I just did too much and was too hard to get along with, I suppose. Ten days before we were to have a religious ceremony, to follow up on the civil wedding that we'd had, he decided to leave me and go back to Josie again. And so, I didn't want him to, but he decided to anyway. And he went back to her. And I was looking for another life. And he—they were back together a few days this time, too; and then he left her and he wanted me back. And then—I was put in prison Wednesday, and about a week before that we had had a fight. And he had another woman at our place, and to my knowledge this had been the first time he'd been with someone else but me and Josie. Of course I found out later that he had girls up to his apartment all the time when I wasn't living with him. The police had had complaints about it. But, anyway, I knocked at his door and he came outside and said, "I got company. Go home." I kicked out a window and then I ran. And I was running up the highway and a man wondered about this and picked me up. And he couldn't decide to take me to a motel or to let me stay with an alcoholic he knew.

Therapist: Or to what?

Clara: To take me to stay with an alcoholic woman he knew.

Therapist: Oh.

Clara: But he took me to see my own family physician, and he told me it would be best for me to see somebody, a psychologist or a psychiatrist. And I told him, "I just can't control myself. I used to be so level-headed. And I can't any more. I don't know what I'm going to do next." He said I needed help. I said, "I know that. I've known that a long time." So, anyway, the next morning I was supposed to take the car to work. I quit riding to work with Dave. See, we both worked at the same outfit. And up until about two days before I went to prison, we'd been riding together every morning and evening, which didn't make it any harder [Clara meant to say "easier"] to break up. So anyhow, I went to his apartment to make up again but I knew that if he didn't really want to make up still there was going to be something happen, because I had a cutting tool with a big razor blade in it with me. And

I had a blackjack with me. And so he didn't want to talk. He didn't want anything but for me to leave. He said, "Get out of here. I don't want anything to do with you." And so I said, "Well, you'll have to throw me out." And I locked the door while he was getting his shoes on getting ready to leave. And so he came to the door and he turned around to unlock it and I stabbed him in the back with the cutting tool. And he was furious [laughs]. He threw me outside, out the door and said, "Boy, you're going to jail!" He went downstairs and it scared me to death. I was screaming and crying. I didn't know how I could have done that to him. And so he went down to have someone call the police and I called an ambulance while he was downstairs. When they came he wasn't going to get in there, but I could see he was about ready to pass out. And they made him get into the ambulance and took him to the hospital, where he died. Then they took me to the D.A., and my doctor arranged an appointment with a psychiatrist that afternoon. By Monday evening I was in here, in prison.

Therapist: Why did you stab him?

Clara: Because I knew I'd either have to stab me or stab him. And I just wasn't up to stabbing me.

Therapist: Uh huh. What do you mean that you had to stab either him or you?

Clara: Because things just weren't worthwhile without him. I'd built my whole future, all my friends around him. We planned on quitting our jobs, going to graduate school together, and then moving to Canada, where he wanted to live and where I wanted to live. We'd work in the same place together. You know, we just wanted the same things at first. I think the biggest reason we got along was because he's the only man who could ever satisfy me sexually.

Therapist: Uh huh.

Clara: And I've always thought that was important in a marriage. Because so many marriages don't seem to succeed, because one or the other isn't satisfied.

Several important things can be seen from this opening dialogue:

1. Before killing her husband, she had tried suicide a half

dozen times. Apparently, whenever things went wrong for her in the world, and particularly when she thought that a boy in whom she was interested didn't love her, she convinced herself that life was intolerable, that she couldn't go on unloved, and that she had to kill herself.

2. This, of course, was exceptionally disturbed behavior, indicating that Clara had (a) a dire need to be loved and (b) an extremely low frustration tolerance. Her worth to herself mainly seemed to consist—as George Herbert Mead and Harry Stack Sullivan pointed out—of the reflected appraisals of others; and she dogmatically insisted that she could not accept herself and continue her existence unless she had a guarantee that a selected male would love her. As soon as she learned that her husband was going back to his old girlfriend, she ran and took a dose of sleeping pills; and, when she woke to find that he actually had gone, she took what would have been a fatal dose if she had not had her stomach pumped out quickly.

3. No matter how her husband treated her and how often he indicated that he really didn't care for her, Clara always insisted that she had to have him back; and, against her father's wishes, she kept going back to him. Even when they were separated, she continued to ride back and forth to work with him every day—obviously intent on getting him to return to her. As she reported to the therapist, she even let him know when her parents would not be around so that he could come to see her, because "I was just crazy about him." In her case, the word "crazy" was literally as well as figuratively true. She was obviously completely obsessed with getting his love; and she was consequently in a psychoticlike state throughout most of her association with her husband.

4. Clara, surprisingly like Joyce, the girl who killed her own child, was perfectionistic about the housework when she lived with Dave. Like Joyce, she noted, "In fact, I just did too much and was too hard to get along with, I suppose." This perfectionism was probably one of the main philosophic roots of her severe emotional disturbance: She irrationally believed that she *had* to do things perfectly and that she *had* to be approved for doing them. But even when her perfectionism led to poor results and served to antagonize others, including her husband, she compulsively clung

to it and refused to give it up—which indicates that she thoroughly believed that she *had* to act in a given way and that she *could not,* at all costs, change her ways. This dogmatic clinging to empirically unvalidatable beliefs, even when they are leading to undesired results, is one of the essences of psychotic thinking.

5. Clara obviously meant to kill her husband if he kept refusing her, since she brought along both a razor-bladed instrument and a blackjack. Quite possibly, however, she wanted to use these weapons to intimidate him and didn't really believe he would leave her. When he actually started to do so, and when he turned his back on her to open the door to get out of the apartment, she didn't hesitate to stab him. In other conditions, however, she might have only threatened him, hoping he would take her weapons away from her and would finally consent to stay with her. She mainly wanted—or thought she needed—to keep him with her; but she was prepared to do almost anything if her need was not fulfilled.

6. She is probably honest in saying that she only gave herself a choice between homicide and suicide. For, had her husband escaped from the apartment unscathed, she probably would have killed herself. The mere thought of living without him was so intolerable to her that she could think only of killing him (thereby getting her rejector out of the way) or killing herself (thereby being free of ever being rejected again). Because of the way things happened in the apartment, she killed him; but she could just as easily have killed herself. It is notable, in this respect, that the child killer, Joyce, and Clara convinced themselves to the *n*th degree that they could not stand a given set of circumstances—and therefore must either change it or change themselves in a drastic, sometimes death-dealing, manner.

7. Clara, like Joyce, had exceptionally low frustration tolerance. As soon as she saw she was not going to get her way about some important thing or person she desired, she set about some kind of violent action: whether it be having a hysterical fit, threatening suicide, attempting suicide, or committing murder. Stopping to think about possible solutions to her problems was not in her make-up. She had to have—or thought she had to have—a resolution *immediately;* and she would not for a second consider giving

up her desired object or making some kind of a compromise in regard to achieving it. Although she emphasized the importance of sexual satisfaction in marriage, and reported that her husband was the only man who ever satisfied her sexually, there is no reason to assume that it was only this kind of satisfaction that she craved and could not stand being deprived of. There is more reason to believe that she would have shown low frustration tolerance no matter *what* major desired thing was lacking in her life.

The interview with Clara continued:

Clara: That's one reason I don't believe in getting married without sex first. But as far as I know I kept him happy sexually. He kept me happy sexually, I know that. I never looked for anyone else when I was with him for several months. But I did something wrong.

Therapist: What do you mean did something wrong?

Clara: If we got along so well, we wouldn't have stopped getting along if I hadn't done something wrong. I think I pushed too hard, for one thing. But I knew he was changing and I kept trying to get him to say he wasn't. That things were still the same. But he has a peculiar honesty and he won't lie and say, "I love you," when he doesn't really love me. Rather, he'll avoid the question and it's just the same as saying, "I don't love you any more." And I know this because I know him fairly well.

Therapist: Uh huh. What did you mean before when you said you didn't think things were worthwhile any more?

Clara: Just the way I, I feel now. I mean, I've got a good job and a graduate education waiting for me if I get out of the charges that are against me. But what good is making a life for yourself without someone to share it with me? It's not. I *need* somebody to share things with. I don't like to be alone. And, I thought he was the right one. And I still think he would be but of course now he's dead. Naturally, I'll have to put on the same attitude because it's a matter of salvaging what's left of my pride. But it's going to be so hard.

Therapist: It still isn't entirely clear to me what you mean when you say that things aren't worthwhile any more, that you felt you either had to stab yourself or stab him.

Clara: Well, there's no question about which I'd rather have done. I'd rather have killed myself.

Therapist: Uh huh.

Clara: I don't—.

Therapist: Why was that?

Clara: I've always had a feeling, what people say, "Look at that—you're smart. You work as a computer programmer. You plan to go to graduate school. Look at that—you're pretty; you can get any boy you want." Now this isn't true. I'm too thin; I've got beady eyes. I've—I'm not smart. Some things come fairly easy, other things I can't get under any circumstances. I don't know why, I don't feel that I'm intelligent. I don't feel that I'm able to cope with things. But everybody else seems to think that I am, and can't understand why I find it so hard. As far as things being worthwhile, other people are all that make things worthwhile.

Therapist: How is that?

Clara: You can't live for yourself alone. It's just, it's no good. You've got to be there to make someone else happy, too.

Therapist: And if you're not making someone else happy, what does that mean?

Clara: That means you're wasting time or marking time until you find a person that you can make happy. I found him but he didn't want me.

Therapist: What kind of a person then do you think you are because you found this right guy and now he didn't want you?

Clara: I'm inadequate.

Therapist: Are there any other ways you could describe how you feel about yourself besides inadequate?

Clara: Well, I just feel that I've failed somewhere. And I feel like I'm not good enough. I've got some things going for me because I can finish my education. I can get into graduate school. I can qualify for it, I'm almost certain. But I don't see the point of doing all these things to make yourself a more intelligent and rounded person if you're not doing it for anyone but yourself. I want to be able to make a man happy.

Therapist: Why?

Clara: Because I want to love someone. And because I've never seen a happy marriage.

Therapist: Why do you want to love someone?

Clara: Because I'm lonely, all alone.

Therapist: And how do you feel when you're not loving someone? What kind of a person do you think you then are?

Clara: I'm just marking time. I always think it's better to be preparing yourself. But that's what I'm preparing for: to love someone and to make him happy. I thought it was Dave. I still think it would be Dave. But it's only my opinion. It's not his.

Therapist: And since Dave doesn't love you, and you love him, how do you feel about having failed in getting him to love you?

Clara: Well, a person can't help the way he feels. If he doesn't love me, there's something I don't have that he needs. I don't know what it was, because I gave him everything that I knew how.

Therapist: But you don't have what he needs. How do you feel about that?

Clara: Maybe some day I'll have what someone needs. I don't know. I doubt it.

Therapist: Why do you doubt it?

Clara: Well, because it seems like, whenever I care, the other person doesn't care. But when I don't care, I just wind up hurting someone. I guess that's just life. But it's an awfully poor way to run things.

Therapist: I'm still interested in seeing if I can get you to answer this other question, as to what kind of a person you think you are because you failed in getting Dave to love you.

Clara: What kind of a person?

Therapist: Uh huh.

Clara: Well, I'm a failure.

Therapist: You're a failure? A total failure?

Clara: No. I have some things I don't fail in. But with other people I don't succeed very well. I mean like in my job, I can work the computer and do well as a programmer. I can even talk to people usually fairly easily. But when it comes to a deep relationship, one that means something, I don't. I don't make it.

Therapist: Are you saying then that you feel that you're not a worthwhile person unless you're loving someone and someone's loving you back?

Clara: I think that's part of it. Unless you're doing some good. And I can think of no better good than loving someone and being loved in return. To me making someone happy is a worthwhile cause.

Therapist: I see. And when you're not making someone happy, then you're not worthwhile.

Clara: That's reducing it down pretty simply, but I guess that's about it.

In this section of the interview, the therapist drops his role of just being a diagnostician and tries to do some rational-emotive psychotherapy. He deliberately poses his questions in such a manner as to force Clara to see that she is severely disturbed because she has a self-defeating philosophy of life, and that she repeats specific irrational beliefs to herself which cause her to act suicidally and homicidally. He notes, from what she says to him, that she is quite perfectionistic. Actually, she is a beautiful girl, well developed physically and with lovely eyes. But she sees herself as being too thin and beady-eyed. She also does very well at her work and in school; but she sees herself as unintelligent. At times, of course, like most disturbed people, she *does* act rather stupidly: because that is what severe emotional disturbance tends to be—stupid behavior by a nonstupid person. But her real problem is her great perfectionism, which causes her to put herself down no matter what her assets are. The therapist notes this to himself and hypothesizes that Clara makes herself feel very inferior, by her perfectionistic demands, and that then, in order to make herself feel good or worthwhile, she believes that she must have the total approval of someone whom she loves and that she must devote herself to a worthy cause, such as "loving someone and being loved in return." The therapist hopes to get Clara to see clearly that this is her basic value system, and that it is this value system which directly and indirectly led her to murder her husband.

On her part, Clara at first clearly states, "I *need* somebody to share things with." Like nearly all highly disturbed individuals, she does not merely *want* to love and be loved; she desperately thinks she *needs* to be. And, if her need is not catered to, she has practically no choice but to feel hopelessly depressed and suicidal.

Clara states, again, "I don't see the point of doing all these things to make yourself a more intelligent and rounded person if you're not doing it for anyone but yourself." What she seems to mean is that she cannot really accept herself, as a person who *could* be independently happy if necessary, but can only conceive of gaining happiness through being symbiotically attached to some man. She says, "I want to be able to make a man happy," but she actually means that "I've *got* to be able to make a man happy if I am not to consider myself empty and worthless."

The theory and practice of rational-emotive therapy stresses that, although it is highly *desirable,* it is not *necessary* for people to be in a warm, loving relationship for them to accept themselves and to see value in living. The therapist tries to show Clara that she thinks it necessary, so that he can later demonstrate to her that this proposition is not valid.

Because of her perfectionistic demands on herself, Clara not only believes that she has to win her husband's or some other man's love, but that she probably never *can* do so. "Maybe," she states, "some day I'll have what someone needs. I don't know. I doubt it." It is her perfectionism-caused doubt that keeps making her depressed and suicidal.

Therapist: Now let's go back to something that you said much, much earlier. You said you weren't up to, you had to stab someone—either yourself or him—and you weren't up to stabbing yourself. What did you mean by that?

Clara: Well, blood frightens me and pain frightens me to death. I'm afraid of pain. And it didn't take courage. It just took desperation to take sleeping pills, because I didn't want to live; and I still don't.

Therapist: I see. And why didn't you want to live? And why still don't you want to live?

Clara: Because I don't have Dave.

Therapist: You don't have Dave. Why is that—why do you say that is a reason to no longer want to live?

Clara: Because I'm living and because it hurts to think I can't have him.

Therapist: How does it hurt?

Clara: Because someone else did things for him that I did. Someone else made him happy. And someone else is going to be hurt. I didn't know what he wants; I didn't understand him I guess. I thought he wanted me and I believed him when he said he did. But he changed his mind. You can't be blamed for that. And I shouldn't have hurt him because of it. But it just seems so unfair to lie all along. I told him in the beginning, I said, "I realize I want to make love to you, you want to make love to me. It's physical. You don't have to say 'I love you.' Because it's not necessary." I would react the same way if he didn't say that. "Don't say it and lie. It's not necessary." And later I told him, "If you're going to change your mind, change it now 'cause it's going to be too late later. I won't be able to get out." Because I knew what was happening. I knew how deeply involved I was getting. And I knew how hard it would be to get away from him once I loved him. And there was a time when I could have left. Could have gone away, put him out of my mind. But that time didn't last very long. Now it's awful hard to get him out of my mind. And it gets, it gets so I'm not thinking quite so much about him now. But you—the colors I wear are because he likes them. I sleep facing a certain direction because he faced that direction. He's just part of me. At least his memory is. He's not any more.

Therapist: You wanted initially to commit suicide, then, because you thought you were worthless if he didn't love you any more?

Clara: Because, well that's part of it; but mostly because life was worthless without him.

Therapist: Why did you think life was worthless without him?

Clara: Because he meant so much to me.

Therapist: And that therefore you couldn't go on living?

Clara: I guess that's it.

Therapist: "Since Dave isn't around any longer, I can't go on living. Life is a total bore. It's worthless without David."

Clara: I could go on living, but I don't want to.

Therapist: Yes. And why wouldn't you want to?

Clara: Well, I guess there's one way to say it. If they don't play the game the way I like it played, then I won't play the game.

Therapist: I think there's a little extra clause in there that you're saying that you may not be seeing: "If they don't play the game the way I want them to play it *and think therefore that they should play it,* there's no sense going on."

Clara: I have the choice of whether to live or whether to die. And if things don't go my way, and if things aren't the way I want them, if things don't make me happy, if I'm not happy, why be here?

Therapist: "If I don't have what I want which I feel I *should* have——."

Clara: Yes!

Therapist: "——then there's no sense going on living."

Clara: Yes.

Therapist: Now why should you——.

Clara: A very selfish attitude, which is one of the basic characteristics of my personality. I'm terribly selfish.

Therapist: Why do you think you should have what you want?

Clara: I don't want everything. I don't think I should have everything that I want. I think I should have Dave because he promised me himself.

Therapist: Why should you?

Clara: Because he promised.

Therapist: But that's your assumption. "Because he promised, I *should* have him." *It would be nice* if you had Dave; but why *should* you, just because it would be nice?

Clara: Oh, yes; it would be nice.

Therapist: Why should you have him just because he promised you?

Clara: Like I said before: He can't help it if he changed his mind. But I don't think he was fair to me. Because now I don't know how to get away from him.

Therapist: You mean you thought he was treating you unfairly and *shouldn't* be treating you unfairly?

Clara: When he went back and forth to his girlfriend after we were married and he said he'd stay away from her. Then shortly after that he changed his mind completely, after he was entirely separated from her. Don't you think that was a little bit unfair?

Therapist: Well, let's assume that you're correct that it was unfair. Why *shouldn't* he—or anyone else, for that matter—be unfair to you?

Clara: Well, why *should* he?

Therapist: Because that's the way he is!

Clara: I don't think he is.

Therapist: Well, obviously he is. That's reality; that's a fact. You can't erase what *is.* He was unfair to you. And your question is "Why should he be unfair?" My answer is: "That's the way he is—or was at that moment. In other words, that's the way the ball bounces, the cookie crumbles. This is the way people *are.*

The therapist first gets Clara to bring out the fact, in this portion of their interview, that she feels hurt because someone besides herself could make her husband happy. This she cannot tolerate—and clearly lowers herself, in her own eyes, because she could not exclusively win him and keep him. Her irrational idea here is: "I have to be everything to the one I love; else I am no good."

A second irrational idea is soon revealed: that once she is fully entangled with her husband, she won't be able to get out of the involvement; that her feeling for him, once it goes deep, cannot be controlled by her and has to master her. This unvalidatable notion, that one cannot change one's feelings and control one's destiny, is a common belief of highly disturbed individuals; and Clara holds it very firmly. Even when she has killed Dave, she still feels that, "It's awful hard to get him out of my mind," and she insists on wearing colors he liked and sleeping in the direction that he faced. She obviously keeps making herself follow well-knit pathways, to keep the thought of him alive; but she fools herself into believing that she has to continue this kind of behavior.

The next irrational idea Clara expresses is another one of her consistent definitional beliefs: that life is worthless without the man she loves. As long as she believes this, she will actualize her belief and feel worthless without her husband; but it is, of course, her belief in the horror of the loss of love, and not the actual loss itself, that makes her feel empty.

The therapist induces Clara to bring out a fourth irrational philosophy: that people must play any important life game her way, else she will not play it. This is a clearcut expression of her low frustration tolerance. Things *have* to be her way; else she believes she *can't stand* them; and she thinks she has to take desperate action to change them.

A fifth foolish assumption that Clara reveals is that if anyone, such as Dave, promises her something important, he *should* go through with this promise. The therapist tries to show her that this is only her definition. It would be nice if Dave fulfilled her promise to her; but that doesn't mean that he *has to* do what would be nice.

Clara then generalizes to a sixth irrational assumption: that Dave (and presumably other people) *should* be fair to her. Again the therapist tries to show her, in accordance with the principles of rational-emotive therapy, that conditions in life frequently *are* unfair; that that's too bad, but that's the way they *are.* He consistently confronts Clara with reality—especially the reality that people are fallible and that they do act unfairly at times. It is therefore highly unrealistic of her to demand that they not act unfairly and to claim that they *shouldn't.*

Clara: If that's the way people are, then I don't want to have anything to do with people.

Therapist: Because you believe that they should be treating you fairly, if that's what you mean?

Clara: They *should!*

Therapist: But why? Why should they?

Clara: Well, because I don't treat people unfairly if I can help it.

Therapist: All right, but now look at what you're saying: "Because I don't treat people unfairly, they shouldn't be treating me unfairly."

Clara: It's a give-and-take proposition.

Therapist: Is it really?

Clara: It should be.

Therapist: Well, why should people treat you exactly the same way you treat them?

Clara: Why shouldn't they? If I don't treat them—.

Therapist: Because they're different than you. That's the way they are.

Clara: Why should they want to hurt someone? That doesn't make sense.

Therapist: Well, maybe they don't realize at times that they're hurting people, for one thing.

Clara: You mean because I—when I took sleeping pills Dave didn't think I was hurt? He didn't think that it hurt me in my mind and in my heart?

Therapist: But you hurt yourself. He didn't hurt you.

Clara: No. He didn't hurt me physically, but his leaving me hurt me enough to make me try to take my life.

Therapist: No, it didn't. His leaving you did *not* hurt you. You hurt *yourself* over his leaving.

Clara: His leaving me hurt me inside.

Therapist: No.

Clara: He didn't hurt me?

Therapist: No, his leaving you did not hurt you inside. *You* hurt you inside because you took his leaving too seriously.

Clara: That's a hard distinction for me to grasp.

Therapist: Yes, it is. Because you've been believing this other nonsense all of your life. Because you go around telling yourself, "Whatever I want, I *should* have. If I treat other people nicely, they should treat me nicely." It's like the little boy in school who says, "How come Johnny didn't invite me to his party? I invited him to mine."

Clara: Well, I think that's fair. If I invited Johnny, why shouldn't Johnny invite me to his?

Therapist: Why *should* the little boy be invited to Johnny's party just because he invited Johnny to his party? How does that follow?

Clara: Well, that's not all that's the question here. Not why should he treat me fairly because I treated him fairly. But why should he try to hurt me? Why should he try to lie? Why should he time things so perfectly, just to get maximum damage done?

Therapist: For a number of reasons—assuming that you are right and he actually did try to hurt you and try to do the maximum damage to you. Either he's disturbed, or he's ignorant, or he's just plain stupid.

Clara: I don't think he's any of those things. He's intelligent. He's quick-tempered [she probably meant quick-witted].

Therapist: Well, that's not entirely true. Because if he weren't disturbed, ignorant, or stupid he probably wouldn't have treated you the way he did.

Clara: But it's not his fault if he changes his mind. It's my fault, because there's something I don't do to make it work.

Therapist: Well, how are you so sure you have that much to do with his decisions? Do you control whether he loves you or not?

Clara: If he loved me in the beginning and he changed his mind, then I did something and that's why he changed his mind. I did something to make him change his mind.

Therapist: Now why? Do you mean a person can't change his mind for his own reasons, that——.

Clara: Don't they? Isn't the reason they change it because of what someone else does?

Therapist: No, very often it is not that at all. And even if you did something wrong, he still would have his choice of staying or not staying with you. He wouldn't *have* to leave. In order for him to leave or change his mind, it's quite up to him. You have little to do with that decision. Do you have any real choice as to whether he loves you or not?

Clara: No. I just thought I was awfully lucky when he did.

Therapist: No. That's right: you have little choice in whether he loves you or not. And you're going around saying that, unless you push all the right magic buttons, he's not going to love you.

Clara: If I push the right magic buttons, shouldn't it work?

Therapist: No, it shouldn't necessarily work, for the simple reason——.

Clara: Well, how do you find someone to love you then?

Therapist: You go around and you look. And if they love you, they love you.

Clara: I've looked and I thought he loved me.

Therapist: But some people will and some people won't. You know, people do change. You know, today you may like toasted cheese sandwiches and ten years from now you may hate the damned things.

Clara: I've always liked toasted cheese.

Therapist: But maybe ten years from now you may not like them. The same is true of human relationships. This guy initially started out to love you but after a while he got to know you better and maybe he just discovered that you were not his cup of tea.

Clara: But there's something about me that makes him feel that way.

Therapist: No, it doesn't mean that there's necessarily anything rotten about you that makes him feel this way. Maybe it's just his taste. And doesn't he have a right to his taste?

Clara: Oh, he has a right to do what he darn well pleases.

Therapist: And you're saying: "He *must* take me, otherwise I'm no good."

Clara: Is that right? Am I saying that?

Therapist: Sure. Look at what you're saying to yourself. Think about it logically, for a moment.

Clara: That's where I have a lot of trouble, with logic. Did you know I made a "D" on my first logic test. How did I ever become a programmer?

Therapist: You have a lot of trouble because you've gotten yourself used to thinking unclearly in some areas of your life. Not in all, but in some.

Clara: I don't think I want to look any more. I don't think I want to be hurt any more.

Therapist: But *you're* the one who's hurting yourself by your attitude—by your belief.

Clara: Well, aren't you supposed to love someone?

Therapist: I don't see any reason why you're *supposed* to. It's nice if you love someone. But you're what we call other-directed. You have very little self-direction. The purpose of living is to have a ball on earth: to get as much of the things you like and as few of the things you dislike. But you're going around saying, "The only purpose of my living is to have somebody love me. When I'm not being loved, I'm worthless. I'm a total slob; I'm no good; I'm a piece of garbage unless someone I love loves me." And look where it's getting you, this crazy idea!

Clara: I think that's oversimplifying it a little bit. I don't know exactly how, but I don't think it's quite right.

Therapist: My view doesn't sound correct because you've taught yourself this other-directed belief all these years. That's why it doesn't sound quite right to you to live primarily for yourself; and you don't want to believe it. You want to believe that the purpose of your life is to be loving and be loved by someone else: to make someone else happy. And that's not the purpose of sane living. The purpose of living is for you to make *you* happy. You place yourself *first;* then you can legitimately love other people, too, and place them a reasonably close *second.*

Clara: That's the real reason for living?

Therapist: That's the sane reason.

Clara: But that's so selfish!

Therapist: Now what's wrong with being sanely selfish—getting what you want out of life, being true to yourself?

Clara: You know what I want out of life? I want to love someone and I want someone to love me.

Therapist: Ah, but you're saying two things: (1) the sane sentence, "I want someone to love and someone to love me," and then (2) the insane sentence, "therefore I *have* to love someone and that someone I love *must* love me. If I'm not loving them and they're not loving me, then I'm no damned good."

The therapist persists at trying to get Clara to see that there is no good reason why anyone she selects *should* love her, though it might be highly desirable that he did. He continues to emphasize the point that Clara can accept herself no matter how bad her behavior is and can tolerate others with their poor performances. Her main goal, he points out, would better be to put herself first and to put her desire to love and be loved in its proper place: as a strong desire and not a dire necessity. If she challenges her other-directedness, he contends, she will lose her depression and her anger, and be able to get along well in the world even when she is not loved in the manner she would very much like to be.

Clara: If you are here on this earth to get what you want—to look out for number one—then looking out for number one to me is being loved and loving; and that's what I *should* look for. Right?

Therapist: Yes, it would be well if you looked for it—if you tried to get something for yourself, such as loving and being loved. But remember that in a love relationship, the sane thing to do, usually, is to creatively, actively love the other person; and what love you get in return is important, but it doesn't mean *everything.* It's not necessarily even the greatest enjoyment that you get out of love; the greatest enjoyment usually comes from what you put into it—from your *own* feelings of loving.

Clara: But what could I have put in?

Therapist: You seem to be saying: "Because I put *in x* amount, I should be getting *x* amount *out.* And now I'm no longer getting *x* amount—he's no longer loving me. Therefore, I'm no good."

Clara: But don't you see that, when you put everything you know how to in a relationship, and then it doesn't do any good, that it's going to kind of make you feel just a little bit inadequate?

Therapist: No, it isn't going to make you feel inadequate at all—not if you think straight. *You* make yourself feel inadequate, by telling yourself, "How awful, how horrible it is that this person's not loving me! How can I go on any more? What a slob am I! If he doesn't love me, I can't love myself." You're doing the same thing that Romeo did when he acted so nutty with Juliet.

Clara: I always thought that was a beautiful story.

Therapist: Yes, people think it's so romantic! But it's really very nutty in many serious respects. For, thinking that he has lost Juliet, Romeo, instead of merely feeling quite sad for a while, and then eventually going out to find another Juliet to have a great romance with, convinces himself that he's no damned good and that he cannot possibly have *any* pleasure for the rest of his life without his beloved. So he crazily kills himself. What you could be more sanely saying to yourself is, "Well, Dave doesn't love me any more, but that's hardly the end of the world. Tough! Now let me see what I can do to go out and find someone else something like him who *will* love me. Maybe I won't make it today or tomorrow; but one of these days I will!"

Clara: How do I do that?

Therapist: By telling yourself what I just finished saying. "It's too bad that I lost Dave; it's terribly sad. But it's hardly the end of my life or the end of the world."

Clara: I've been doing that. And I've been doing it for the last two months.

Therapist: No, you haven't. You've been saying, "It's very sad that I'm losing Dave." But, in addition, you've been saying, "And it's *awful,* it's *terrible,* I *can't stand it!*" *That's* what you've been saying to yourself.

Clara: I'm saying I could stand it; but I don't want to if this is going to go on again.

Therapist: But that's a contradiction. If you really believe, "I could stand it," why *don't* you?

Clara: Because I don't want to. I don't want this to happen again.

Therapist: Because why?

Clara: I'm selfish.

Therapist: Because you think it's dreadful!

Clara: No, because I want to be happy. And if I'm not going to be happy, I don't want to be here.

Therapist: Because you think, "The *only* way I can be happy is when somebody else is loving me."

Clara: And when I'm loving someone else.

Therapist: Yes. Now is that *true?* Is that a true statement? Is that the *only* way you can possibly be happy? You mean that you can't ever go and be happy by yourself? That you can't ever like yourself?

Clara: I'm not much good.

Therapist: Why aren't you much good? Says who?

Clara: Well, if I were much good, then I would have friends and I would be loved.

Therapist: Why would you be?

Clara: Because people who are good are popular people.

Therapist: That's *your* belief. Is that a true statement?

Clara: Isn't it?

Therapist: No. I don't see that it's true. Since when does your worth as a person depend on somebody else loving you? And since when are all people with good traits completely loved by others?

Clara: Well, what does your worth as a person depend on?

Therapist: The fact that you're alive. You're a worthwhile person just because you exist—period. Because you are the only person in the world that you are fully and continually aware of, you are the most worthwhile person in your whole existence. You are worthwhile because you exist. No other reason. You're born worthwhile and you'll die worthwhile. You can never be worthless to yourself, except by your own definition.

Clara: Well, then, the murderer has the same worth as—.

Therapist: Exactly, exactly! Everybody in the world has the same worth, in that they're alive, they're able to enjoy themselves, and they can accept themselves just because they're alive and are capable of enjoying themselves. Even murderers can go on in life and enjoy themselves thereafter—if they don't falsely condemn themselves totally and thereby render themselves totally miserable.

Clara: That's not logical.

Therapist: But it is logical.

Clara: A person's worth is also dependent upon what he does with his life—not only on the fact that he has a life.

Therapist: No, it isn't. His worth as a person, his worth to himself, does not depend on what good deeds he performs, or on what the world thinks of him. Now, he may be more or less efficient than other people; and it is desirable, for several good reasons, that he be more, rather than less, efficient. But it doesn't make him worthless to himself if, unfortunately, he doesn't accomplish much or doesn't please others. If I called you a giraffe, would that make you a giraffe?

Clara: No; but I don't understand the parallel.

Therapist: Well, if I come to you and say that *I* think you're worthless, does that make you worthless?

Clara: You don't have to say I'm a giraffe.

Therapist: No, but, if I thought you were one, would that *make* you one; or in some way indicated that I thought you were one, would that *make* you one?

Clara: No, not really.

Therapist: All right. If I call you worthless, how does that make you worthless? How does my saying you're no good make you no good?

Clara: I'm afraid I missed the point.

Therapist: Well, just because I say I think you're a slob, just because I tell you I don't love you, does that mean you're a worthless person?

Clara: But you don't have to love me. You've got a wife.

Therapist: I'm just using myself as an example. Let's say I'm Dave. Does that make you worthless because Dave says he doesn't love you?

Clara: It doesn't make me worthless, but it makes me—.

Therapist: But that's what you believe: that Dave's not loving you does render you of no value.

Clara: Are you sure that's what I believe?

Therapist: Isn't it? You just said a moment ago quite clearly that, "I'm a person who's not much good unless I am loved."

Clara: Well, isn't that what you're here for—to make other people happy?

Therapist: No, you're here to make *yourself* happy. And *you* have no real life of your own; because you're going around trying to please everybody else.

Clara: I don't want a life of my own. I want one with someone. I want a life with two people, not just one person.

Therapist: Now, what are your chances of getting what you want, under the conditions you set up?

Clara: Right here?

Therapist: No, in general. Look what's happening to you. You tried to commit suicide several times because someone didn't love you. You were driven to try suicide, on the one hand, and to kill your husband, on the other hand. Now what are your chances, with your philosophy of life that compels you to perform this kind of self-defeating behavior, of getting what you want?

Clara: You think logically that I should change my philosophy because it isn't working too darn well?

Therapist: Isn't that true?

Clara: It's pretty valid. OK—you tell me your philosophy and I'll try yours a while.

Therapist: I just told you what mine is.

Clara: Tell me again.

The fact that Clara, who is a bright and educated girl, often fails to see what the therapist is getting at, and jumps from one illogical statement to another whenever he pins her down, tends to show how severely disturbed she is. She admits that she is not good at thinking logically; and she certainly isn't. Throughout the interview, she behaves more stupidly than one would expect from someone of her attainments—although she does cleverly think her way into rationalizing and untenable positions. She appears to have a true thinking disorder, in spite of her brightness; and in E. Bleuler's terms, she could therefore be diagnosed as basically schizophrenic. One advantage of rational-emotive therapy is that it forces the individual to confront several important issues of living and of moral values in a logical manner; and if she seems unable to do this, it is indicative of what Paul Meehl calls cognitive slippage. Even if Clara had never committed any crimes but considered herself worthless and responded to therapeutic intervention by stoutly insisting that she *was* no good as a person, the manner in which she maintains this conviction in her interview with the therapist might be enough to show her deep-seated psychological pathology.

Therapist: My philosophy is that I'm a worthwhile person—at least to myself—just because I'm alive and because, while I'm alive, it is possible for me to have more pleasure than pain. The purpose of my life is to have a ball and to avoid needless pain. I happen to have a set of likes and a set of dislikes—partly by inheritance and partly by my social training. Since this is so, let me see if I can get as many of the things I like and as few of the things I dislike. And if I fall in love with someone and she doesn't love me —tough! That's too bad; let me see what I can do to get her to love me. And if she still doesn't love me, then I'd better gracefully lump that fact. Too bad; so she doesn't love me! Does that really mean anything about me *as a person?* No. Her not loving me doesn't even necessarily mean that I have poor traits. But if I do have such traits, and she doesn't love me because of them, that still doesn't prove that I am totally no good. Her not loving me couldn't possibly make me worthless. Now let me see what I can do to go out and find other people who *will* love me, and whom I can love as well. That's *my* philosophy. But you, instead, are doing what most people do. You're confusing your internal value, or your worth to yourself, with your external value, or your worth to others. Let's suppose, for example, that I was the owner of a baseball team and I walked up to you and I said, "Clara, you're worthless to us as a baseball player." Would you feel very badly about that?

Clara: Oh, no. Not really.

Therapist: No, because I'm only saying that your worth to me, your external value as a baseball player, is low, since I'm only interested in you as a ball player. Now if I walk up to you and I say, "Clara, you're worthless to me as a wife." How would you feel?

Clara: You've got one wife. Why should you need two?

Therapist: No, let's assume that I'm Dave, and I'm still alive.

Clara: Oh.

Therapist: I walk up to you and I say, "Clara, you're worthless to me as a wife." Let's assume I'm single, too, and you like me and I could marry you.

Clara: If I really cared, I'd say, "How about a sex partner? Am I good enough to you as a sex partner?"

Therapist: "No, you're not good enough to me as a sex partner."

Clara: "Well, then, I suppose there's nothing else for us to do together."

Therapist: Let's say you really love me. How would you feel?

Clara: Hopeless.

Therapist: Yes, hopeless and worthless. Now, why? Because of this nutty idea that you're telling yourself—that if I don't like you as a wife or a sex partner, you're no good. Now what's the difference? Your worth to me as a sex partner or a wife is no different, really, than your worth to me as a baseball player. For they're both your external value. Your internal value is your value to yourself. You have your own internal validity. You're a worthwhile person to you—or at least can be—just because you're alive and kicking. You're walking around on the face of the earth. You see? You're saying, "If I'm not worthwhile to someone else, if my external value to him is low, I internally am worthless. I can't love myself. If he doesn't love me, I can't accept me. So onward to slobhood go I!" Is it true that just because I call you a piece of garbage that that *makes* you a piece of garbage?

Clara: You're saying that I'm not a piece of garbage just because I am alive, because I am here.

Therapist: That's right. I'm saying you're not a piece of garbage just because someone thinks that you are and refuses to give you value *to him.*

Clara: And that no matter what I do, I'm not anything less?

Therapist: That's right. As a person, as a human individual, you're not anything less.

Clara: It seems like a very revolutionary idea.

Therapist: It is a very revolutionary idea. That's why the world is so damned nutty today—because it resists this idea. Because most people believe what you believe in one degree or another—that their extrinsic value, or their worth to others, is the same as their intrinsic value, or their worth to themselves.

Clara: Then we're behind the times, huh?

Therapist: Yes.

Clara: How can you be so sure you're right?

Therapist: I can't be absolutely sure. But I have some evidence that I may be right. For one thing, I think that I can honestly say that I haven't had a truly miserable day for the last three years, since I read the principles of rational-emotive psychotherapy in Albert Ellis's book, *Reason and Emotion in Psychotherapy.* Before that, I used to have plenty of depressed days; but not since I began practicing what Dr. Ellis preaches. More to the point, since one case doesn't prove anything, we have thousands if not millions of cases like yours, where you have been miserable for many years, and all because you believe that you must win the love of some man whom you happen to love yourself. I myself, during the past three years, have seen many others like you. Most of them were just as depressed and felt just as inadequate as you do, even though they often had many assets and many possibilities of enjoying themselves in life. And in every case I found that they had philosophies similar to yours; and what is more, as soon as I induced them to begin giving up those views and changing them to more sensible ones, they became considerably less depressed and felt much less inadequate.

The philosophy that I now hold, incidentally, is time-tested, since it was first propounded by a famous philosopher, Epictetus, who lived about two thousand years ago. He said: "It's not things or events that happen to men that disturb them, but their views of these things or events." Shakespeare rephrased this many years later, in *Hamlet,* when he said, "There's nothing either good or bad but thinking makes it so." Agreeing as I do with Epictetus, Shakespeare, and Ellis, I now teach my clients that the only way you can hurt another human being is physically—as with a baseball bat. It's impossible for you to hurt someone emotionally, to hurt his feelings—unless he *makes* himself hurt by taking you too seriously. For the only way in which he can feel emotionally hurt is by telling himself some nonsense *about* what you are saying to him. For it's only words that you are telling him: and words cannot hurt unless he thinks they can. This is the way it invariably goes: At point A somebody calls you a nasty name, or refuses to love you madly; or at point A you make some kind of a mistake. Then, at point C, you feel terribly upset: grief stricken, depressed, anxious, or angry—not because of what happened at point A (though you may erroneously think this) but because at point *B* you're telling yourself two things—a sane and an insane belief. In the case of you and Dave, your sane belief is "Dave no longer loves me and I don't like that at all; in fact, I am terribly sorry about it." Your insane belief is "Because I don't like it, it's *terrible* that he doesn't love me. It's awful; it's dreadful; I can't stand it! If he doesn't love me, I can't like myself. What a worthless person I am!" Is that right?

Clara: Yes, that's what I'm saying. And it doesn't sound right when you talk about it; but it *feels* logical to me that if he didn't love me I was no good.

Therapist: Because—you feel that way because your feelings reflect your views, your ideas, your attitudes. And you're convincing yourself of this insane philosophy: "If I'm not loved or liked by other people, I'm a total slob. I'm no good. For a human being *must* be loved in order to be worthwhile." One of the nuttiest, most pernicious, beliefs ever invented!

Clara: Am I the only one that has it?

Therapist: No. Just about 99 per cent of the rest of the world also has this belief.

Clara: That makes me feel better.

Therapist: It's a very common belief.

Clara: Maybe I picked it up from someone who already believed it.

Therapist: Yes, you did. You picked it up from your parents, you picked it up from all the nutty movies you saw, from all the screwy magazines and novels and newspapers you read, and from all the people you went to school with. Because your whole damned society believes this!

Clara: What about the relationship between parents and children? Can they, the parents, enjoy freedom of action if their children displease them, if it makes them unhappy, the things that their children do? Should the parents just disregard these unpleasing things and go on and find something else to occupy their time?

Therapist: No, children do have to learn. Their reasoning capacity isn't as developed as is an adult's. There are differences between children and adults. And when children do the wrong things and act nastily, it's up to their parents to responsibly discipline the children. But they don't have to *condemn* them. They don't have to *depreciate* them as human beings—which is the sort of thing you're doing to yourself. You go around telling yourself all the time what a slob you are. And is that truly moral, truly right for you to do this? Because you're saying, "When I fail I'm no good. I must succeed; otherwise I'm worthless!"

Clara: And this is not right?

Therapist: Well, *is* it? What are your chances of always doing the right thing, of always having somebody love you? What are your chances?

Clara: Not very good.

Therapist: That's right. And you're not facing that fact. You're saying, "I must be on top all of the time." You want to be queen of the world. You're a perfectionist, in other words.

Clara: You know, my kindergarten teacher said that!

Therapist: Do you think that a human being has a right to be wrong?

Clara: Well, of course.

Therapist: That's what you say, but you don't really mean it. You don't really believe it. When you're wrong, as at times you are, you're saying, "When I'm wrong I'm no good. I *shouldn't* be doing this wrong thing. I *shouldn't* be failing. I should be doing exactly the right thing to get Dave. And if I'm not, if he's not loving me, that just proves what I originally believed: that I'm no good, that I'm worthless.

Clara: This is what I will think about before I go to bed—going over this conversation and digesting it.

Therapist: O.K., that's all the time we have now. Yes, you think about what I said!

For effective therapy with an individual like Clara to take place, it would be expected that many sessions would have to occur, over a considerable period, before she clearly got the message the therapist was trying to convey, and until she actually began to work on it in practice. Although prognosis does not appear to be exceptionally good in a case like hers, it is possible that a reasonably long period of rational-emotive therapy might be of distinct benefit to her and might help her to change her perfectionistic, self-condemning, and overtly hostile attitudes and actions.

In addition to the above interview, Clara was seen by the prison psychologist for psychological testing. Pertinent excerpts from his report follow:

"On examination, Clara was quite assertive and seductive, asking the examiner if he had any brothers, as she was 'looking for a man. . . .' Her thinking revealed rigidity, poor logic and inconsistency. Emotional tone was generally bland. She would narrate events of an emotional nature with a lack of emotion and a nonchalant depersonalized attitude. When she did show some emotion—for example, crying—it was shallow, ephemeral, and at times clearly inappropriate. The initial impression gained was that of a schizophrenic girl. . . .

"Psychological test data indicate that the patient is an acutely disturbed, somewhat intact psychotic who does not have adequate control to prevent herself from the overt expression of her disturbance. She is given to being worrisome, ruminative, anxious, and overideational. Her emotional turmoil is chronic with long-standing feelings of inadequacy and insecurity. Paramount is an almost complete lack of self-dependence or ability to stand on her own two feet."

Thus, the psychological testing bears out the findings of the therapist's interview with Clara. She is a classic example of a woman who has a chronic need of social acceptance and approval and who consequently is other-directed, with practically no life of her own. Even more importantly, she is convinced that she *must* live this way; and even in the face of the overwhelming self-defeat that accrues to her because of her demanding, self-denigrating philosophy, she refuses to modify her beliefs. It is the degree and the rigidity of her attitudes that make her behavior psychotic.

Instead of being self-assertive and self-interested in a healthy manner, Clara usually behaves compliantly and indecisively. She largely chooses to be inhibited, restrained, and overcautious. She handles relationships with others unrealistically; and while ignoring important problems, she daydreams incessantly. Her fantasies are rich and are frequently concerned with sex. She tends to view sex as a panacea and hence is prone to immediate relations with anyone she thinks she cares for.

At bottom, Clara is thoroughly perfectionistic. She demands infallibility in herself and in the people around her. She therefore castigates herself for her failings and is at times thoroughly hostile to others who do not meet her demands. Although she is above average in intelligence, she fails to accept the realities of her environment and has a clear-cut thinking disorder. She is often lacking in the ability to compare, criticize, reject inappropriate responses, and select a suitable response. She also is liable to the intrusion of strange thinking in the midst of otherwise accurate perception. She is quite unpredictable—which may be another characteristic of her schizophrenic kind of thinking.

Clara evidences considerable anxiety; and her emotional tone is explosive and largely at a primitive, infantile level. She shows some sensitivity to her environment, but is still unstable, immature, and egocentric. Her emotional stability frequently interferes with her judgment and she often appears to lack common sense in everyday matters. Moreover, she does not integrate what she has learned and does not profit from her own experience. In these respects, she is similar to Joyce, the mother who killed her child, who is discussed in the previous chapter of this book. Both women have a great need to be loved and approved, an incapacity to accept criticism, a strong tendency to condemn themselves, and exceptionally low frustration tolerance. These traits, and the crooked thinking which lies behind them, are the basic causes of their murderous impulses.

Chapter 12

Interview with a Bank Robber and Murderer

This is a typescript of a recorded interview with a twenty-one-year-old male who has led a most troublesome life and has frequently been in difficulties with legal authorities. He is unusually combative and dangerous. Shortly before the interview took place, he and two male companions attempted to rob a small bank. A gun battle ensued and one bank teller was wounded and another was killed, shot in the groin. The murderer, Ron, claimed that he wasn't trying to kill the teller but that he had only tried to shoot past him, in order to scare him. The following interview took place in prison, since Ron's lawyer wanted a psychological evaluation made. Although the purpose of the interview was entirely diagnostic, the interviewer tried to get in some therapeutic dialogue as well, as he was curious whether any therapy could be done with such a highly disturbed individual who was dogmatically set in hostile ways.

Therapist: Well, I'd like to get some idea from you as to how you got into trouble.

Ron: Well, I don't know. I just have urges to go out and do things. I'll be standing up a lot of times, just anywhere.

Therapist: Be what?

Ron: I'll be standing up, maybe shooting pool, and I'll get an urge to go out and start something or to get in a fight. Anything to just be doing something mean.

Therapist: Why?

Ron: I don't know why. I just do.

Therapist: Do the urges come at any particular time?

Ron: Just any time they hit me.

Therapist: What's it feel like?

Ron: I don't know. In a way, it's kind of like being a dope addict. And, it just hits me and I've got to let everything out. So I go out and do something.

Therapist: Yes. When you say "let everything out," what is it that you let out?

Ron: Well, I can't actually describe it. I don't know. It's just a feeling, you know, that after I do it, that I have inside of me, I'm content then. And after I go out and get into some meanness, then I'm content.

Therapist: Yes?

Ron: I sit around content. But other times, I mean, it don't hit me sometimes. I mean I can go a week, two weeks before this even hits me. But then, when it does, I go out and do something.

Therapist: How often does the urge come about?

Ron: Oh, it's—lately, it's being coming up just about every night. I've been wanting to go out and do something. Get in a fight, steal something.

Therapist: Can you control these urges?

Ron: I haven't tried. I haven't actually tried to control them. I get the urge and that's all I want to do. Just when the urge does come on me, then I want to go out and do something. Break into some place, steal something, or something.

Therapist: When did these urges start?

Ron: Oh, I've had these for quite some time—over a large amount of years.

Therapist: You remember when they first started at all?

Ron: No, I can't.

Therapist: Is there anything particular going on during the day that may set you off into getting one of these urges?

Ron: No. Same thing every day. Usually I sleep late. Go to the pool hall. That's what I do every day.

Therapist: Do you work?

Ron: No.

Therapist: Have you ever worked?

Ron: Yes.

Therapist: Where did you work?

Ron: I worked at a gas station. I worked at a laundry. I worked on an assembly line.

Therapist: What did you do at these places?

Ron: Nothing special. I sold gas at the gas station.

Therapist: When was that?

Ron: Three months ago.

Therapist: And what happened to that job?

Ron: I quit.

Therapist: How come you quit?

Ron: The work didn't interest me. I didn't care for it.

Therapist: Then what'd you do after that?

Ron: Skipped town for a while. The cops were after me.

Therapist: For what?

Ron: Assaulting someone.

Therapist: And how did that come about?

Ron: I was having a drink in one of the local bars that I hang out at. I seen this boy. I had been having trouble with him, quarreling over our views on different things. So the urge just hit me to beat him up. So I just started fighting with him. I felt better afterwards. I was content. They wanted to pick me up and charge me with assault, but I skipped town.

Therapist: How'd you feel then?

Ron: Well, it didn't bother me, actually. I figured that I would be in trouble after I did do it. I was just content for beating him up.

Therapist: How'd you feel after they were out looking for you and you had to skip town?

Ron: Well, I didn't want to be in the town I was hiding in, with an old friend of mine. I felt, I felt like killing the guy I beat up for calling the police. I felt just like going back to this town and killing him. But when I finally decided to go back to town, since it then seemed to be safe enough, I was picked up by the police on another rap they had against me—a boss I had worked for and who I had been bothering after he let me go. While I was still out on bond from that rap, I was picked up for robbery. I broke into the gas station where I used to work and got caught. Got put in jail this time; and because of all the things against me, I got sent away for nine months.

Therapist: Where were you sent then?

Ron: To the county court house.

Therapist: And you got out of there when?

Ron: I was released on July 21.

Therapist: So you did a full nine months in there?

Ron: Yes, eight months and twelve days.

Therapist: What was it like in prison?

Ron: It wasn't bad—a lot of fighting and stuff. You know, you have to hold your own ground.

Therapist: Did you get in any fights?

Ron: Yes.

Therapist: How did they come about?

Ron: Just argued, started fighting. Lot of times I would hunt them.

Therapist: Lot of times you would hunt them. These urges would come on?

Ron: I would hunt a fight, yeah.

Therapist: Why would you hunt a fight?

Ron: Just to have something to do; the urge hit me. It's the only way to do anything. So I thought I'd start a fight with somebody.

Therapist: Can you remember the last time you were in a fight?

Ron: It was last month, if I'm not mistaken.

Therapist: And where was this at?

Ron: It was at my friend's house.

Therapist: Tell me what happened.

Ron: Well, I went to my friend's house and they told me that this other fellow I knew asked someone if I'd banged up his bicycle. And when he did pull in, the urge just hit me to go out and beat him up. So I went out and started fighting with him.

Therapist: This was the guy that—?

Ron: My pal, an old friend of mine.

Therapist: One of the two fellows who is charged with you for this latest offense?

Ron: No, this was another friend of mine.

Therapist: Now wait a minute. Just before he pulled up in the driveway, your other friend said what now?

Ron: My other friend had told me that this one accused me of banging up his bicycle. And I just had one of those urges anyway. I was trying to find him 'cause I wanted to go out and steal something. When he came up, he got out of the car and I walked out on the front porch. The only thing he said was "Hi!" and I started hitting him.

Therapist: Then what happened?

Ron: Well, then after the fight was over he came in the house and he set down and we talked. And then we went out. Me and him, we rode around. Content. Didn't want to do anything then.

Therapist: What were his feelings when you started to attack him?

Ron: He didn't actually know what was going on. And after the fight I explained to him why I jumped him. And, uh, he didn't know how to take it, really. But I just have urges like that.

Therapist: Now you say you had this urge before your other friend said anything to you?

Ron: Yeah. I had had the urge, been just about the whole day I had the urge.

Therapist: What part of the day did the urge start to come on you?

Ron: I was up in the barber shop, playing poker. Was in the afternoon that the urge started to come on.

Therapist: What was going on just before the urge started?

Ron: I was playing poker.

Therapist: And?

Ron: I don't know. I lost a couple of games, and I just wanted to go out and tear something up.

Therapist: Ah!

Ron: I was mad, depressed.

Therapist: Yeah. So before your urges come, something is going on?

Ron: Yes, I guess.

Therapist: And this was when you started getting depressed. And what do you mean by depressed?

Ron: Well, I was losing money.

Therapist: Yes, and how'd you feel about this?

Ron: I didn't like it too well.

Therapist: "What a goddamned shit I am for losing!"

Ron: Yeah.

Therapist: "And these bastards are not going to like me any more if I keep losing like this. They'll think I'm a real slob!"

Ron: I felt like knocking them in the head, taking my money back.

Therapist: 'Cause you felt they were unfair?

Ron: Yes, I thought that I should be winning instead of them.

It is fairly evident, from the way the interview progressed up to this time, that Ron is an exceptionally disturbed individual. It is difficult to see his act of murder as a sort of accident, as he claimed when he was arrested, since he obviously has been looking for fights, and finding them, most of his life. He is in the habit, according to his own story, of suddenly getting an urge to go out and get into a fight; of fighting even with his closest friends; and of engaging in armed robberies and other adventures that are very likely to lead to violence.

Ron believes, moreover, that he really cannot control his combative urges; and he makes no attempt to control them. On the contrary, when he feels upset about anything and thinks that he has an urge to fight coming on, he almost goes out of his way *not* to control it, and practically makes certain that it will lead to an actual brawl.

The therapist, on the basis of the theory of rational-emotive psychotherapy, assumes that Ron is being compelled to violence by his own value system, and he tries to get him to reveal what this value system is. He soon ascertains that Ron tends to get depressed when he loses at a game like poker; that he considers himself rather worthless for losing; that he also feels that he should be winning and that it is unfair if his opponents win. His main values, therefore, include: (1) "I can't stand losing, especially when I am playing a game that I am good at." (2) "If I do lose, it likely is my fault; and if so, I am pretty worthless for having such a fault." (3) "If they are winning from me, when I am a better player than they are, then they are unfair and should not be allowed to win." With these kinds of values—which are not dissimilar from the values of Joyce, the infant-killer, and Clara, the husband-killer, that we have previously examined in this book—it would be difficult, if not impossible, for Ron to control his anger and avoid violent altercations.

Therapist: You felt what?

Ron: I felt that I should be winning instead of them.

Therapist: Now, why did you feel you should have been winning?

Ron: Oh, I just knew I was better than they were.

Therapist: O.K., let's assume that you could really play poker better than they could. Why does that mean you *should* win?

Ron: I just *should.*

Therapist: Why?

Ron: 'Cause I'm a better player.

Therapist: But how does that prove that you should win?

Ron: Well, it really doesn't. It's just that, I don't know. It's just something inside me.

Therapist: Yes—that's the thing that's inside you. That's the idea that makes you get these feelings. You couldn't possibly get these feelings that you *should* win and that the people you're playing with are unfair and no good for winning instead—you couldn't get them from nowhere, out of a clear blue sky. That's almost impossible for a human being to do. Feelings like yours just don't come from nowhere. In order to *feel* anything, you have to *tell yourself* something. And frequently we tell ourselves ideas, thoughts, attitudes, beliefs, philosophies, values—whatever you want to call them—and in a split second we get an emotion or feeling from them. Usually, we don't even realize that we've even told ourselves anything to create the emotion, because it comes so fast. We tend to think in shorthand. Let me give you an example. Let's suppose you're walking down the street and somebody kicks you in the shins. Aside from feeling hurt physically, what emotion do you usually experience?

Ron: Well, my emotion would be to turn and fire on him, to hit him.

Therapist: Right! That's exactly the way most people would react. Now, as you turn around to face him and you're about to strike him and you've got your fist six inches from his mouth, you happen to notice that he's blind. Now what happens to your emotion?

Ron: I'd still hit him.

Therapist: Would you still hit him?

Ron: Yes.

Therapist: You might. But what do you think other people would do in this same situation? Would they hit a blind man?

Ron: No.

Therapist: Now, what do you think would happen to those people who wouldn't hit him?

Ron: Probably just go on about their business.

Therapist: Well, what do you think would happen to their anger?

Ron: Probably go away slowly.

Therapist: Yes; or it might even go away quite fast. What would happen to most people is that their anger would go away immediately. They would see that this guy is blind; and they would tend to feel sorry for him and say to themselves, "Isn't it too bad that this poor guy is blind? No wonder he accidentally kicked me in the shins." Or they might even get angry at themselves for almost hitting him back. Now, of course, if you're in the habit of making yourself angry, then you can do like you said you'd do: you can easily go all the way and hit the guy, in spite of the fact that you notice he's blind, because of your lack of control. This lack of control is something you learn. Over the years, through many experiences, you've taught yourself—whether you realize it or not—to have no control, to just explode, to just cut loose. Do you see what I mean?

Ron: Yeah.

The therapist, seeing by this time that Ron is exceptionally upsettable and is not in touch with reality, knows that he will not be able to go far in teaching him why he is combative and what he can do about changing. But he figures that he has nothing to lose, and wants to see how far he can get with Ron, so he continues his rational course of therapy, just as if Ron were more amenable to logical reasoning. He also, diagnostically, wants to see just where Ron's crooked thinking lies; so he keeps trying to see how much logic he can follow.

Therapist: So it means that you have to force yourself to stop and think for a moment what you're saying to yourself to create these feelings that you have. Have you ever been on any kind of medication? Any pills or tranquilizing medications?

Ron: I had convulsions when I was young, my mother told me, and they gave me phenobarbital and a lot of other drugs.

Therapist: Well, it's quite possible that you may have some physical problem and that some mechanism in your head may trigger off some of this compulsive fighting you get into. But then it's also possible that it's not physical, which is frequently the case. You may be upsetting yourself psychologically, emotionally. You get depressed, as you said a moment ago. And then your feeling of depression can trigger some chemical reaction in your brain—in which case your compulsion to strike out at others gets going. Lots of times, if this is so, you won't be able to control yourself, until your rage has run its gamut. Then, as you say, the urge is all over with and then you feel content. A third possibility is that your compulsion to get into fights has no physical or organic basis at all, that it's entirely emotional or psychological. But it doesn't make any difference which one of these three possibilities is true. Whether it's purely psychological, mainly physical, or a combination of both, you still can train yourself to control these urges much more than you have managed to control them up to now. It requires work to do so, lots of effort. I'm not saying that it would be easy. In fact, if you try to do so, it's going to be goddamned hard to achieve it, especially at the beginning. But, like anything else, like learning how to play the piano and do other activities, you could, with practice, learn how to control your strong urges to fight. You did learn how to drive a car, didn't you?

Ron: Yeah.

Therapist: And that takes time. You have to think about what you're doing here, and how to shift the gear there, in first, second, third, and reverse, and so forth. If you drive a truck, you have four gears, maybe five—a dual low and maybe two kinds of reverses, or something like that; and you have to learn how to do all that kind of business. So that when you first start driving, you have to keep thinking all the time about what to do next. Well, once you start to drive the car for a while, it becomes second nature, and you hardly think about it at all. Do you see what I mean?

Ron: Yes.

Therapist: So that it would certainly be hard for you at first to learn to control your emotional reactions; but you can do it. Anything you learn, you can unlearn, can't you?

Ron: Yes.

Therapist: How much education have you had?

Ron: Half of my freshman year in college.

Therapist: What happened that you didn't finish? You had to quit?

Ron: I got kicked out. I was skipping, tearing up the place.

Therapist: Yes. Now do you ever have any blackout spells or anything like that?

Ron: I have dizzy spells.

Therapist: Yes?

Ron: And blackouts when I get up real fast. Kind of blackout.

Therapist: Yes. Now when do the dizzy spells come?

Ron: They just come on now and then. I mean, I don't know. Just whenever it comes, it comes. I mean, I'd be working or anything, and it'd come.

Therapist: Are they like the urges? Are they connected with the urges in any way?

Ron: I don't believe they are, because I just get up and I'll have a blackout. In a few seconds, I'll be all right and just go on about my business, what I was doing.

Therapist: Have you had dizzy spells today?

Ron: No.

Therapist: You said you have a girlfriend?

Ron: Yes.

Therapist: And how old is she?

Ron: Sixteen.

Therapist: Does she go to school?

Ron: No.

Therapist: How long have you been going with her?

Ron: Several months.

Therapist: Was she in with you on this last deal?

Ron: No.

Therapist: Do the girls have anything to do with your stealing?

Ron: No. Just do it to be doing it.

Therapist: What do you mean?

Ron: Well, we'll be riding around. Maybe the girl will be low on money. She'll say, "Why don't you steal some money or something?" And I go out and steal some money. I've done it several times. One of my girlfriends was with us a year ago when I was picked up for breaking into a store.

Therapist: So when she says, "Steal some money," why do you do it?

Ron: Just steal it to be stealing it. Not for myself, but for her.

Therapist: But why do you steal for her?

Ron: I don't know.

Therapist: Yes, you do.

Ron: She wants money, so I steal the money for her.

Therapist: But if I tell you to commit suicide, would you do it?

Ron: No.

Therapist: Why not?

Ron: I don't want to die.

Therapist: Do you want to steal money?

Ron: No, not really.

Therapist: Then why do you do it when she asks you to do it?

Ron: I don't know. I guess to make her think I'm big or something.

Therapist: Yes. So you *do* know. Now, why do you have to make her think you're big?

Ron: I don't know.

Therapist: Because you think she'd think you're a slob if you didn't do this? She'd think you a square?

Ron: Yes.

Therapist: Well, what difference does that make? Let's say, now, she really thought you were a slob. Why would that make such a terrible difference?

Ron: I don't know.

Therapist: But it does, doesn't it?

Ron: Yeah.

Therapist: Well, why?

Ron: Well, you don't want to be a square if there's a bunch of guys around.

Therapist: Why not?

Ron: Everybody else looks down on you.

Therapist: So?

Ron: For being a square.

Therapist: Let's say they look down on you for being a square. What difference does that make?

Ron: You don't like to be looked down on.

Therapist: That's true; you don't like to. But you also seem to be saying, "I must not be looked down on as a square. It's awful, terrible if I am!" Is that what you mean?

Ron: Uh huh. Yeah.

Therapist: What's *really* so awful about somebody looking down on you as a square?

Ron: I don't know.

Therapist: I don't know either. Look where it's getting you, this belief. As long as you have it, what are your chances of not getting into trouble?

Ron: Probably slimmer than what they are without it.

Therapist: That's right! In other words, when you have the belief that you must not be looked down upon as a square, and whenever anybody becomes intimate with you—somebody like this gal—and says, "Ron, why don't you steal something?" or, "Ron, why don't you start a fight?" you're always going to be getting into trouble, aren't you?

Ron: Probably.

Therapist: Is that what you want?

Ron: No.

Therapist: Well, how do you think you can stop this kind of behavior which keeps getting you into trouble?

Ron: Stay away from the type of people who keep urging me to do that kind of thing.

Therapist: That's one way. But how can you do it another

way—even if you stay intimate with people like this girl who keeps urging you to steal?

Ron: Just keep refusing. Stay with it.

Therapist: Yes, stay with your own views. And what would you have to tell yourself differently, in order to do so, from what you're now telling yourself?

Ron: That I'm not a square if I don't do what they ask me to do.

Therapist: That you're not a square?

Ron: Yes.

Therapist: Do you think you could convince yourself of that?

Ron: Probably could.

Therapist: How would you do this?

Ron: Have enough gumption to.

Therapist: Well, who is really running your life? You or other people?

Ron: Well, I feel that I am.

Therapist: You really feel you are?

Ron: Yes.

Therapist: I feel that you're running your life only about one per cent of the time. I think that 99 per cent of the time you're not in the saddle seat. You're letting other people run your life with this crazy idea that, "If they look on me and think I'm a square, then that makes me a no-good square, a no-goodnik!" And that's running your life by their standards, not by yours. You see what I mean? So you're kissing their asses—that's what it amounts to—in order to get them to like you. Now if I walked up to you and said I think you're a goddamned camel, would that make you a camel?

Ron: No.

Therapist: Why not?

Ron: It just wouldn't.

Therapist: That's right. Now if I walk up to you and say, "I think you're a goddamned square," does that make you a square?

Ron: No.

Therapist: But that's what I don't think you fully believe. If you really believe that you weren't a square, that you were cool, then when this gal or somebody else would say to you, "Look, why don't you steal money? Look, if you're such a big guy, why don't you do this?" Or "Let's see you fight this guy! You claim to be a bigger and better guy than he is, so let's see you beat him at poker, or let's see you beat the shit out of him!"—when they said these things to you, and if you really didn't believe that you were a shit when they called you one, you know what you'd say to yourself? You'd say, "Just because they say that I'm not a cool guy or I'm square, that doesn't make me a square. Sticks and stones will break my bones but names will never hurt me!" No matter *what* anybody calls you, that can't make you out to be a square unless you *believe* it—unless you go around agreeing with the people who called you one. If they think badly of you, the only way in which you can be upset is if you *agree* with their evaluation. You're saying to yourself, "If they don't like me, I can't like myself. And since I need them to like me, I guess I'd better do what they want me to do—to steal, to beat somebody up, beat some guy in a poker game, and so forth." You see what I mean? You have a low opinion of yourself. You don't value yourself very much. And, like most people, you're confusing external worth, or your value to other people, with your internal worth, or your value to yourself. Suppose, for example, the coach of a basketball team on which you wanted to play came up to you and said, "Look, Ron, I think that you're worthless to us as a player." Do you think you'd feel very bad?

Ron: No.

Therapist: Why not?

Ron: 'Cause I know his team consists of better players than I am.

Therapist: Yes. They're better basketball players. They may be more efficient than you at that particular game. But if I walked up to you and said, "Look, Ron, if you don't steal, I think you are a louse," then I bet you would feel bad and that you'd try to please me by stealing, as you tried to please this gal. You see what I mean?

Ron: Yeah.

Therapist: That's because you're exaggerating the significance of your external value, or your worth to me or to other people, and you're confusing it with your internal worth: the value that you have to yourself. You're telling yourself, "If I am worthless to somebody else, because he or she doesn't approve of my ability to play cards, to hit a baseball, to make love, or to do something else, then I'm valueless to myself. Actually, of course, you as a person, as a total human being, are not crummy just because someone thinks that some of your traits are. As a person, you're worthwhile—or at least worthwhile to yourself just because you're alive, kicking, walking around and can do certain things to please yourself. But, instead of accepting yourself because you're alive and potentially able to enjoy yourself, you're demanding that you've got to be the best—be King of the May—and insisting that you're the lowest dog if you're not. "I've got to be the best poker player those guys have ever seen! I've got to be the best bully on the block!"—or something like that. See what I mean? And you don't realize that you can fully accept yourself just because you're alive and kicking. And even if you are a better poker player than all the guys you know at the barber shop, that doesn't make you a better *person.* You don't gain greater worth, greater personhood, by being better than somebody at something. By your definition, you would have to think that I was a better person than you and you were lower than me just because I'm a professional and I'm educated, wouldn't you? Which is horseshit of the worst sort! I'm *not* better than you; and you're *not* better than me. And even if you and I go down to the barber shop and play poker—which I haven't actually played in years—and if I beat the hell out of you at the game, that still won't make me a better individual than you. And it wouldn't make you a better person than me if you beat me. You see what I mean? You may be more efficient than others; and if you and another guy are dating a girl and she chooses you as a better love-maker than he, that shows she thinks you are more efficient in that respect. But that doesn't make you a better person; nor would it make him one if he were more efficient as a love-maker than you. It certainly makes neither of you a louse just because the other is more proficient in a certain trait, such as love-making. Moreover, the fact that a girl chooses him as a better lover than you may not even mean that he is; it may only mean that she has peculiar taste. And her taste doesn't necessarily mean anything about you; it's merely *her* preference. She's got a right to have her taste, doesn't she?

Ron: Yes.

Therapist: You like cookies and I don't like cookies. Does that make me no good? That's your taste and my taste. And we all have different tastes, don't we? And the same goes for any friends that you may have. Because someone likes you, that's his preference, his taste; and because he doesn't like you, that's also his taste. As a matter of fact, I probably have more people who dislike me than you have. 'Cause I see more people than you do. But I don't tell myself what a louse I am because I make these mistakes or because those people don't like me. I don't get upset. When people hate my guts, I merely tell myself, "Maybe they're right about what they think is wrong with me. In that case, I'd better do something to try to change it. But maybe they're wrong, and dislike me for the wrong reasons. In that case, they have problems. They're unnecessarily critical. Isn't that sad for them?" So I don't get upset. Now if I could really get you to believe this, that you can accept yourself fully even when others dislike you, you wouldn't be getting upset and would be much less angry. What it sounds to me like you're doing is, first of all, making yourself feel guilty, depressed, worthless, blue, because you take others' criticism too seriously. And then, in order not to feel so blue and so worthless, you externalize your feelings. You take them outside yourself. And you say something like, "Those sons-of-bitches out there have no right to treat me this way! They're unfair to me. They should be losing the game, especially if I'm a better poker player than they are. They're no damned good!" You see what I mean? This is your kind of way of defending yourself. "Boy, what a no-good person I must be if I can't beat these guys at poker!" And so I think this is why you're getting angry lots of times. Because of your tendency to view yourself as such a low person in life. Now if you would do less of that, I'd be willing to bet you wouldn't have your hostile urges most of the time. Making any sense to you?

Ron: Uh huh.

Therapist: But let me tell you that, if you want to change yourself, and not make yourself so underlyingly depressed and then very angry, you're going to have to do a little work. As I said earlier, it's not going to come easy. You have to first admit that it's you who is angering or upsetting yourself. It's not other people who are doing it. It's you. The only way that one human being can hurt another human being is by hitting him physically. If you get upset in any other way—any emotional way—if you get depressed or angry, it's the result of what you say to yourself and not of what others do or say to you. You get upset by first telling yourself a sane and then an insane sentence. It all starts out with A-B-C. A is something that happens to you—like this gal saying to you, "Look, why don't you steal some money?" A is a fact, something that happens in the outside world. She tells you to steal. After A occurs, you start feeling something at point C—you usually feel bad, upset, depressed, angry. Now you may think that your feeling at point C stems from what happens to you at point A; but this is not true. At point B you're telling yourself what I said before: one sane and one insane sentence. The sane sentence may be something like, "Wouldn't it be nice if I had some money to give her? Isn't it disappointing that I don't have it and that she's going to be displeased with my not having it to give her?" This sane sentence, as I say, is at point B-1. Then, at point B-2, you're adding an insane set of beliefs: "Isn't it awful that I don't have any money to give her? If I don't get her some money, she'll think badly of me; and that would be terrible! I couldn't stand it. If I don't do what she says right away—steal some money for her—I'll be a sissy!" It's these B-2 crazy beliefs that get you into difficulty. It's not the girl that's upsetting you, making you depressed. It's not this guy calling you names or thinking you're a lousy poker player that's upsetting you. It's your nutty beliefs, that you can't stand the girl's criticism or the guy's calling you names. I've had all kinds of people call me all kinds of names during my life. But I refuse to get upset about these names. I say to myself, about the people who blame me, "That's their problem. If they have to be children and call me names and egg me on to fight, let them. I'm not going to fall for this nonsense. If they think me a chicken, that doesn't *make* me a chicken." As a matter of fact, it takes a really mature person to refuse to fight, to say to himself, "I can accept myself, whether they think I'm good or not. And I don't have to fight them if they try to insult me or think poorly of me." So I don't get into fights—because I don't think that I have to. Well, we're getting close to the end of this interview. If you'd like me to see you again for some counseling, I think I may be able to be of help to you. However, this will have to be your decision. What do you think? Do you think you need or want some help?

Ron: No.

Therapist: But you can't go through life with the thoughts that you have and be happy and keep out of trouble. What do you think will happen to you if you keep going on like this?

Ron: I don't know.

Therapist: So you're not interested in any kind of counseling then?

Ron: No. I don't think nothing's wrong with me.

While there seems to be a single hope left, the therapist persists. He realizes that there is very little chance of his making an important impact upon Ron; but he feels that, as long as there is any chance whatever, he has nothing to lose. Moreover—as we pointed out previously—Ron's resistance itself is good grist for his diagnostic mill: It shows the therapist exactly where he stands and what the chances are of his benefiting by future therapy. In a purely diagnostic interview, it can only be guessed with a fair degree of accuracy how well the individual is going to respond to later therapy. In a diagnostic-therapeutic interview, such as this one with Ron is, it can be guessed with a much higher degree of accuracy what the chances are of his being therapeutically helped. According to the findings of this interview, prognosis is obviously poor.

Therapist: You mean you get into all this difficulty and you don't think there's anything wrong with you for getting into that amount of trouble? You mean you think all the things you do are all right?

Ron: Yeah.

Therapist: Well, why do you think all that's all right?

Ron: 'Cause I do it, I guess.

Therapist: You mean you don't think there's anything wrong in anything you've done?

Ron: No.

Therapist: In the stealing and killing?

Ron: No.

Therapist: You think that's all right? Why do you think so?

Ron: I just think that it is.

Therapist: Well, why?

Ron: I don't know. I just do.

Therapist: Well, would you like everybody else in the world to be like you?

Ron: No, not really.

Therapist: Well, what makes it right for you, then?

Ron: I don't know.

Therapist: Maybe you're just afraid to admit to yourself that you've got problems.

Ron: I know I'm not crazy.

Therapist: I didn't say you were crazy. You think you have to be crazy to see someone for counseling?

Ron: I don't know.

Therapist: I see a lot of fairly normal people for counseling. People who don't get into any kind of trouble, in fact. I think you're going to have to face the fact that, unless you start controlling some of these urges, there's a damned good probability that you're going to continue to get yourself into difficulty. And the consequences may be that you're going to be thrown in jail time and time again. You may even spend the greater part of your life there—unless you get the death penalty first. Now is that what you want?

Ron: No.

Therapist: If you really don't want that, then you're going to have to do something to stop yourself from getting into difficulty. How are you going to do that?

Ron: Just have to try to control myself.

Therapist: Yes, you are right. But the only real control that you're likely to get is to think more clearly along the lines that I've been suggesting to you. Did you ever, by the way, hear voices or anything like that?

Ron: Yes.

Therapist: When nobody's around?

Ron: Yes. People talking to me.

Therapist: Which people?

Ron: I don't know. I can't see them. Hear, though.

Therapist: What do they say?

Ron: They tell me to do things.

Therapist: Such as.

Ron: To steal, to go out and beat the hell out of somebody. I had an urge like that when I was home last time. Just standing on the corner.

Therapist: Are they male or female voices?

Ron: Male.

Therapist: And do you recognize any of them?

Ron: I recognize one.

Therapist: Young or old?

Ron: They sound old.

Therapist: Yes?

Ron: I don't know—just like a ringing voice, ringing voice.

Therapist: When did these start?

Ron: Oh, I've had them over a period of time, years. Just be standing around somewhere. Just like somebody's there. They say something and I go do it. Standing downtown one night by myself. Heard this voice. Then I seen this boy riding around, voice said to bust his head open. I pulled him in. Went out and punched him and busted his head open. Then I was content.

Therapist: Now doesn't this sound strange to you?

Ron: No.

Therapist: You think that most people experience what you experience?

Ron: Yes.

Therapist: You do? That most people hear voices like that?

Ron: Yes.

Therapist: Well, I can tell you that they don't. I don't.

Ron: Fifty per cent of them do.

Therapist: Where do you get your statistics? What makes you think fifty per cent of them do?

Ron: I make my own.

Therapist: Yes. Over 90 per cent of people don't hear voices like you do. But even if everybody did, that still wouldn't make it healthy, would it?

Ron: Not really.

Therapist: But you think that it does. It might be normal statistically but that doesn't make it normal in a healthy sense. I believe that the main reason you're hearing these voices is the reason I talked about a while ago. You first make yourself feel guilty, depressed, upset. And then you get angry to cover it up. And lots of times the anger comes to the surface, when you hear these voices and think they tell you to do something violent. That's all that it really is. You keep making yourself terribly upset. Aren't you the kind of person who tends to hold your anger inside of yourself a long time before you let it out?

Ron: Yes. And when I let it out, it all goes!

Therapist: Yes. Well, I don't know what more I can say or do for you, except that I'll tell you frankly you could use counseling.

Ron: I feel that I don't.

Therapist: You're entitled to feel that way.

Toward the end of the session, when there is really not time to explore much further, Ron admits that he actually hears voices and that some of his violence is related to the voices telling him to get into fights with others. As if this were not strange enough, Ron even more strangely insists that it is not unusual for him to hear such voices, and he maintains that most people hear them. Obviously, he is not only psychotic in this respect, but has no insight whatever into his condition. On the whole, his lack of insight is perhaps his most outstanding aberration. For he is not really stupid (although at times he appears to be) and he is able to relate to others to some extent and to hold down jobs when he wants to do so. But he is clearly driven to prove himself, especially his masculinity, to others; and he becomes exceptionally hostile when he is thwarted or feels that his ego has been downed. He then invents voices and other forces that compel him to get into a vicious fight, and thereby temporarily to blow off some of the steam that he himself has generated by his grim insistence on proving himself. And he fails completely to see what is going on in his head, and even to admit that anything of the sort is transpiring when the therapist objectively brings some of his underlying thought processes to his attention.

We could justifiably conclude, therefore, that Ron (and probably many other thugs and murderers like him) really *want* to remain ignorant of their underlying motivations to violence and *want* to retain their defensive-offensive ways. It is apparently much easier for them to build up an enormous feeling of hostility and then to do something aggressive to temporarily appease this feeling than it is for them to question the motives for their behavior and to do something to change these motives and control their violence. Self-discipline is too much of a hassle for them, even psychotherapy appears to be much too hard and valueless. By remaining the way they are, they get the rewards of (1) defensively feeling greater and more manly than others; (2) exerting themselves violently and pleasurably from time to time; (3) avoiding the difficulties of self-control; and (4) enjoying the fact that they keep getting away with things and are thereby, again, "better" or "cleverer" than are others. They are classic short-range hedonists; and they have little or no intention of growing up and ordering their lives along the lines of longer-range hedonistic principles. Most of the time, their childish brand of hedonism does not really work, so that they are self-defeating. But they maintain the illusion that sooner or later it will work; thus they rigorously refuse to accept reality.

Chapter 13

The Treatment of Murderers and Assassins

Until the beginning of the twentieth century, there were few authorities who believed in any kind of treatment of serious criminals, and particularly of murderers, other than long imprisonment or death. Even today, the vast majority of police officials, judges, legislators, and other individuals concerned with the making and keeping of our laws think in somewhat similar terms—except that in recent years the view has been increasingly promulgated that capital punishment, the death sentence, is too harsh and inhumane, and that therefore life imprisonment should be meted out to murderers instead.

The concept remains, though it is being increasingly attacked, that we should let the punishment fit the crime, and that the only fair and sensible way to deal with criminals is to penalize or punish them in some definite manner, in order to deter them and others from committing further offenses. This concept of punishment is, of course, of ancient origin, originating among the earliest civilizations. On purely logical grounds, it would seem to be correct: since if we exact an eye for an eye and a tooth for a tooth, we presumably "pay back" the criminal's victim for the wrong that has been done him and we teach the criminal a lesson that he and others who might think of stealing, assaulting, or murdering will not easily forget.

Unfortunately (or fortunately), man does not operate in the simplistic manner that the proponents of the theory of punishing criminals assume that he does. He is a much more complex, and in many ways more irrational, animal than the punishment hypothesis implies that he is. Very frequently, he is not deterred by being heavily punished; nor does he necessarily learn from this grim experience. In fact, he may become so angry and otherwise upset by being punished, that he may engage in more antisocial behavior in the future.

As A. V. Huffman, state criminologist of Illinois, notes: "David Glaser, in his outstanding and scholarly report entitled *The Effectiveness of a Prison and Parole System,* reports as one of his principal findings—one supported by extensive data—the conclusion that in the first two to five years after their release, about a third of all the men released from an entire prison system are returned to prison. Other studies have reported substantially higher return to crime, indicating that further research in this area is needed. In brief, we have come to know that too substantial a percentage of offenders are not likely to be salvaged by any method we have thus far developed."

Moreover, as C. H. Rolph points out, "Any law which punishes without seeking to redeem is based upon hate. I wish to advance the proposition, though I be the millionth man to do it, that punishment without love is an unmitigated evil. . . . Everyone recognizes that, in the very last resort, the offender who resists every other kind of effort to make him conform to minimal standards of social decency will have to be locked up. But such a man (unless he is mentally disordered) is a confirmed hater; and though we may be little to blame for it, we have made him into a hater by punishing him. . . . 'Our criminal system,' as Bernard Shaw said, 'is an organized attempt to produce white by two blacks.' "

Moreover, criminals by no means have full control over their performing or not performing an immoral act. They are frequently neurotically or psychotically compulsive, basically driven to do what they do out of motives that they do not themselves comprehend or explain. They are something like little children, who impulsively and compulsively often do what they know is incorrect, but who cannot easily keep themselves from so doing. They are also, of course, like millions of "normal" adults, who compulsively overeat, smoke, overdrink, and do various other acts which they know are undesirable or "wrong," but which they nonetheless keep repeating. It is not that it is utterly *impossible* for these "normal" individuals to refrain from overeating or from smoking, but they find it so *easy* to continue these practices and so *hard* to discontinue them, that they very frequently remain addicted for their entire lives. Similarly, it is not impossible for most criminals to stop stealing, cheating, and assaulting; but, again, they have an inborn tendency *easily* to take the "easy" way out, to go for immediate satisfactions rather than long-term gains, and to rationalize away the disadvantages of their criminal behavior.

Noting this underlying tendency of criminals to be more or less driven to their unethical deeds, W. N. Thayer in the 1920's stated that criminal law far too much stressed the idea of punishment for crime and gave practically no consideration to its underlying psychological and sociological *causes.* J. Drever, C. Kellogg and his collaborators and G. Tului tended to agree with Thayer and, like him, to stress that attention be given to the personality of offenders and to the possibility of treating instead of punishing them.

Thayer advanced the "Naponoch Plan," which called for the scientific study of all convicted criminals by a board which would make recommendations to the court about what kind of facility they should be committed to. In order to safeguard the public from further depredation by convicted criminals, the Naponoch Plan called for indefinite sentences for confirmed offenders and recommended that a minimum length of incarceration should be suggested for them. Similarly, Tului advocated that prisons be converted into re-educational systems and that punishment per se be minimized or eliminated.

A couple of years after Thayer's pioneering article on the humane and psychological treatment of criminals, A. Vollmer came out with somewhat similar views but advocated much more comprehensive treatment guidelines. Vollmer's plan included: (1) intensive study of the offender prior to sentencing; (2) giving the offender psychological and medical treatment congruent with his mental and physical state, rather than punishment for his act; (3) segregating prisoners within the prison population, on the basis of diagnostic and sociological criteria; (4) handing out indeterminate sentences to many criminals; (5) giving appropriate types of education to incarcerated offenders; and (6) making provision for adequate post-discharge supervision of prisoners.

Since these early thinkers on the subject of prison reform promulgated their views, there has been considerable further discussion of this important problem; and a good many reforms in prison philosophy and treatment have been instituted. Nonetheless, as N. Cantor pointed out some years ago, penal theory in the United States appears to have two conflicting aims, which have resulted in considerable confusion. On the one hand, its goals are retribution or punishment; and on the other hand, reformation or prevention. He maintained that the protection of society is best achieved through a sane and rational theory of treatment—by "curing" and reforming the improvable prisoners and by permanently segregating from them the unimprovable ones. Punishment as such, he held, should no longer be utilized because it is ineffective in preventing offenders from committing further crimes.

Our own theory of treating prisoners is derived from the theory and practice of rational-emotive psychotherapy. We distinguish between *penalization* and *punishment* and feel that, although the former is often legitimate in human affairs, the latter practically never is. To penalize an individual means, in our terminology, to assess his deeds as wrong or antisocial and to calmly and unangrily show him that if he continues to do certain of these deeds in the future, he will be deprived of certain benefits or will suffer certain unfortunate consequences. Thus, a child may objectively be taught that if he eats forbidden food, or runs across the street without seeing whether it is safe to do so, or destroys his parents' furniture in a needless manner, he will (1) probably suffer certain intrinsic poor consequences (such as becoming ill from the food, getting hit by an automobile, or getting splinters in his hand from the broken furniture); and will (2) quite definitely suffer certain imposed consequences (such as his parents depriving him of his allowance or insisting that he rebuild or pay for some of the broken furniture). If the child observes that these intrinsic and extrinsic penalizations normally follow from his self-defeating or antisocial behavior, he will usually learn to inhibit this behavior or to behave differently.

To punish an individual, however, means not only to penalize him but *also* to denigrate him as a human being, to communicate to him that he is no damned good, and to retaliate against him in order to humiliate him. Thus, a child may punitively be taught that if he eats forbidden food, or runs across the street without seeing whether it is safe to do so, or destroys his parents' furniture in a needless manner, he will (1) probably suffer certain intrinsic and extrinsic penalties (such as those listed in the previous paragraph) *and* that (2) he will be hated by his parents and others long after his specific misdeeds have been forgotten. He will be enthusiastically encouraged to hate himself (for a while or forever), and he will be made to believe that he *deserves* all possible penalties because he is just utterly *rotten.* This does not mean, of course, that every time a child is deliberately punished instead of penalized for his wrongdoings he will be literally cast into hell and made to feel miserable for the rest of his life; but it does mean that at least for some period of time, short or long, he will be encouraged to feel like a slob, a failure, or a villain. And it means that his punisher, of course, takes the risk that he *always* and *utterly* will castigate himself for the particular misdeed or series of wrongs that he has committed.

Penalization, in other words, refers to the disadvantages, inconveniences, and frustrations which ensue when an individual makes an error or commits a crime; while punishment, in our usage, refers to the negative attitudes toward his person, by others as well as by himself, which accrue in addition to the other kinds of disadvantage, inconvenience, and frustration that will probably come his way. In rational-emotive therapy, therefore, we hold that penalization is often (though not always) legitimate when an individual acts badly or antisocially; but that punishment is practically never legitimate (although, like certain other forms of unfair, impractical, and illegitimate actions, it may sometimes accidentally bring about fairly good results).

The main reasons that an individual would better not be punished for his misdeeds, even when he commits serious crimes like murder, are as follows:

1. Wrongdoers, and particularly serious criminals, are often so badly emotionally or mentally disturbed that they are not even

truly responsible for their acts. As we have seen consistently throughout this book, murderers are usually in the psychotic or borderline psychotic range; and even though they may fully "know," at the time they commit homicide, what they are doing and know the consequences of their acts, they still can often hardly stop themselves from doing them. Therefore, it is hardly fair or just to hold them fully accountable under the famous M'Naughten rule. This rule usually states: "An act done by a person who is an idiot, imbecile, lunatic or insane is not a crime. A person cannot be tried, sentenced to any punishment or punished for a crime while he is in a state of idiocy, imbecility, lunacy or insanity so as to be incapable of understanding the proceeding or making his defense. A person is not excused from criminal liability as an idiot, imbecile, lunatic, or insane person, except upon proof that, at the time of committing the alleged criminal act, he was laboring under such defect of reason as: (a) not to know the nature and quality of the act he was doing; or (b) not to know that the act was wrong."

Unfortunately, this rule does not realistically acknowledge the fact that many (probably most) psychotic and borderline psychotic individuals do, at the time they commit murder, know the nature and quality of the acts they are doing and do know that the act is wrong. Nonetheless, they convince themselves, at this time, that they *must* murder, that the Lord told them to do so, that they cannot stop themselves, that their victims *deserve* to die, that they are acting in self-defense, etc. For this is the way that temporary and permanent psychotics frequently think; and it is foolish to contend that they "know what they do" when they are deluded by these kinds of powerful rationalizations.

2. Psychotic and borderline psychotic individuals, therefore, are indubitably wrong about many of their deeds, but there seems to be no good reason that they should suffer anything but the intrinsic penalties that often accompany these misdeeds. Thus, if they get into a murderous rage and kill someone, they may easily be killed, in turn, themselves; and that is the risk they of course must take. If, however, they are captured after committing murder, there is no reason that the law *should* electrocute them or jail them for life in order to make them feel pain somewhat equal to

that of their victim and his loved ones. There is no law of the universe that says that people *deserve to* or *ought to* suffer because they have caused someone else to suffer. This is only a man-made law; and, like most other man-made laws, is fair if it is applied to so-called "normal" individuals, who may be deterred by penalties if they are realistically imposed, but is hardly fair if it is applied to mentally abnormal individuals, who only formally "know" what they do and are therefore truly unaccountable.

3. The theory of penalization is that normal humans (and lower animals) usually learn from penalizing experiences and therefore change their behavior in the future. This hardly applies to emotionally aberrated individuals, who are very unlikely to learn, in many instances, from the usual kind of penalties. For many of them were unable to learn, in the first place, that it was unwise to commit assaultive or murderous deeds, even though, in one sense, they "knew" that it was. Many of them were even certain that they would be penalized for their crimes; and that knowledge did not deter them. C. R. Tittle studied the crime rates for the states of the United States and their relationship to certainty and severity of punishment for various crimes. He found that, although for several offenses there was consistently a positive though low correlation between severity of punishment and several crime rates (such as sex offenses, assault, larceny, and burglary), there was actually a negative association between severity of punishment and homicide rate. J. P. Gibbs and T. D. Chiricos and G. P. Waldo largely confirmed Tittle's findings. Why, then, should the condemning and executing of murderers be expected to teach a lesson to individuals who, at least to a large degree, seem to be incapable of learning by this kind of deterrent?

More and more authorities are coming around to the view that punishing, in the sense of condemning, an individual for his offenses against others is of dubious value. The psychiatrist, Karl Menninger, the lawyers, Lon Fuller, Herbert L. Packer, and John A. Robertson, and the social scientist and cybernetician, Norbert Wiener, have all spoken out against it. Robertson, reviewing Packer's *The Limits of Criminal Sanction,* notes that "the book begins with the unsurprising fact that the criminal sanction exists to prevent antisocial behavior by punishing offenses called crimes. In spite of its inevitability (there is simply nothing else to do the job), punishment is logically as well as morally ambiguous: We have no proof that it really works, and we cannot be sure that it does not cloak barbaric impulses of vengeance. Therefore, we must use it sparingly."

E. Bergler contends that the reason punishment is invalid and produces such poor results in preventing further criminal behavior is that criminals unconsciously desire to be punished: "Criminotics, in contrast to neurotics, act under the influence of pre-oedipal rather than oedipal conflict. The deepest and dynamically most effective core in the unconscious conflict of the criminotic is the compensatory, concealed helplessness, expressed originally toward the mother and only later shifted toward society."

This Freudian-inspired view is probably mainly mistaken; since it is most doubtful whether pre-oedipal or oedipal conflicts have much to do with the need for punishment. For one reason or another, however, some criminals *do* seem to want to be punished—probably because they think they will ultimately be purified, and even get to some kind of heaven, that way. Such criminals, of course, will not be deterred by the kinds of sentences that we now hand out to them. Moreover, many other criminals, although not exactly looking for punishment, think crookedly in various other ways. Because they *are* criminals, they tend to be highly disturbed; and because they are disturbed, they are prone to believe in all kinds of irrational ideas. Or, otherwise stated, confirmed criminals are the kinds of individuals who dogmatically hold to illogical and irrational hypotheses, thereby make themselves upset, and consequently keep committing punishable crimes. Since they think sloppily in *several* different ways, it is likely that they are not going to be deterred from committing future crimes by punishment: which is aimed at *logically* making criminal behavior too costly for them.

4. This does not mean that putting a murderer in jail for life or electrocuting him does no good whatever: obviously, it deters him from committing any other murderous acts while he is in jail or when he is dead. Deterrence of this kind clearly has some social value; and it is wise, in many instances, for us to put hardened criminals in protective custody, to make sure that they will not

commit future crimes. But it would better be clearly understood, if this is done, that our motive is not to punish the individual, especially if he is so disturbed that he is not logically to be held responsible for his acts. Our motive, instead, is merely to keep him from harming others; and, preferably, to treat him psychologically while he is in protective custody so that the day may come when he is able to resume his regular life in the community again, without any considerable chance that he will revert to criminal behavior.

5. If the individual is not seriously disturbed and can therefore be held accountable for his criminal deed, it may or may not be sensible to penalize him, depending on the kind of person he is and the circumstances of his act. If, for example, an individual with low frustration tolerance becomes enraged because his wife spends all their hard-earned money on silly luxuries while serving him and their children the cheapest kind of food, and if in a fit of rage he actually kills his wife, it is questionable whether any special penalty that is meted out to him for this murder will prevent him from killing his next wife or will enable him to have higher frustration tolerance. The chances are that his very act of murdering his wife will have such a dramatic and sobering effect on him that it will be most unlikely that he will ever kill anyone again; while depriving him of his freedom (and his children of a father) for the next five or ten years will probably teach him nothing that is very useful and may actually help him to become so embittered that he turns into a worse rather than a better citizen. Penalizing an individual for his crime may work in many cases—but may not work in many others. Such penalization, when employed, should probably be used at the discretion of a psychological board which examines every convicted offender, rather than merely leaving it up to the routine or accidental behavior of some judge or jury.

6. Punishment, as distinct from penalization, is unjustified in practically all cases of human error, because it rests on assumptions that are unprovable and theological. It assumes that just because an individual's *act* or *performance* is wrong or antisocial, *he,* as an entire *person,* is bad or worthless. His act, however, is obviously just a *part* of his being; and how fair is it to condemn this whole being for the part that is wrong? To condemn a person for

his poor deeds is, moreover, an arrant overgeneralization. It is to jump from the perfectly sane statement, which can often be empirically validated—namely, "He committed this deed, by which he needlessly and definitely harmed himself or some other human being"—to the foolishly overgeneralized set of statements: (a) "Therefore, this proves that he *as a whole* is worthless"; (b) "therefore, he was probably born no good"; (c) "therefore, he never will be any good"; (d) "therefore, he deserves to be denigrated as a human being for his harmful deed"; (e) "therefore, he ultimately deserves to roast in some kind of hell for being the way he is." All these statements from (a) to (e) are illogical deductions from the original empirical statement; are derived from a value system ("original sin") that has no empirical referent but is essentially theological in nature; can never really be proved or disproved; and tend to lead to highly unfortunate, inhumane results.

7. Man obviously, because of his heredity and his environment, is a fallible creature and therefore has to make innumerable mistakes and commit countless misdeeds. To expect him *not* to do so and to condemn him for being the way he is makes one patently unrealistic and perfectionistic. As noted in *Reason and Emotion in Psychotherapy*: "The sentence, 'He made a serious blunder; I hope he does better next time,' is perfectly sane. But the sentence, 'He made a serious blunder; he *should* not have made it and *should* do better next time,' is perfectly nonsensical. For it really means: 'I unrealistically expected him to be an angel instead of a human and not to make any mistakes; and now that he has proven that he is fallibly human, I even more unrealistically demand that he start being a perfect angel in the future.' "

8. The theory of blaming and punishing individuals for their "sins" is rooted in the assumption that blame and punishment will usually encourage a man to stop his wrongdoing and to behave much better. But almost the entire history of crime and punishment shows just the opposite: namely, that people who are hatefully punished for their misdeeds frequently do not change for the better but actually often become worse. Psychologists commonly penalize rats, guinea pigs, and college students in a calm, objective manner when they make mistakes on mazes or other problems, and thereby help them make fewer mistakes. But no psychologist

that we know of yells at his subjects, humiliates them, or angrily calls them vermin when they go into the wrong passageway or fail to solve the experimental problem.

There is considerable clinical, experimental, and anecdotal evidence that shows that when human beings are punished in a hating, deprecating manner for their errors, they tend to make even more mistakes than they otherwise would do. In many instances, in fact, as the individual internalizes the condemnation of others, and convinces himself that he really *is* no good because he has failed at certain projects, he gets the concomitant notion that he *has* to keep failing, and he consequently becomes a *compulsive* failure. This has probably been true of numerous criminals over the years; and even some multiple murderers may compulsively keep killing new victims, because they are convinced that they are no damned good and that they therefore *cannot* stop killing.

9. People tend to commit serious crimes for three main reasons: (a) They are relatively stupid and cannot easily tell right from wrong; (b) they are terribly ignorant and therefore do not realize how wrong their acts are; and (c) they are emotionally disturbed, and feel that they must act in a manner that they know is wrong. In none of these instances is condemning and punishing the criminal (instead of objectively reeducating him) likely to do any good; and in all of them it may do considerable harm. For blaming a stupid individual will not make him more intelligent; condemning an ignorant person will not make him more knowledgeable; castigating an emotionally disturbed criminal will only tend to help him be still more disturbed. Condemnatory punishment may certainly in some instances help some persons be more careful and law-abiding in the future. But most of the time the condemnation is likely to do far more harm than good, while only the penalization is likely to have (on occasion) a fortuitous effect.

10. In the final analysis, blame, condemnation, hostility, anger, and similar emotions are probably the most important core of human disturbance. When we blame ourselves, we tend to become anxious, guilty, and depressed; when we excoriate others, we tend to become hostile, bigoted, grandiose and violent; and when we blame the difficulties of the world and the things in it, we tend to become unduly frustrated and self-pitying. Moreover,

when we blame other people, and they accept our condemnation of them, they become just as upset as we would become if we were self-flagellating. Since—as we have seen in the course of this book—severe emotional disturbance is one of the main reasons for violent and murderous behavior, and since emotional disturbance is itself so closely connected with damning, it should be fairly obvious that blame and punishment, in the long if not the short run, will tend to result in more rather than less criminality, and that they therefore foment exactly what they are designed to cure.

For the foregoing reasons—as well as several others which can be brought forth—we, as rational-emotive therapists, object strenuously to the concept of blaming and punishing criminals for their behavior. We would much rather see them sanely and objectively penalized at times, in order to help them learn more efficient behavior; and at other times, we would rather see them not even penalized, but intensively treated, often while being kept in protective custody, until it has been reasonably ascertained that they will no longer be a community menace.

This means, of course, that we are entirely opposed to capital punishment. We believe that a human being has a right to live, even though he has taken away someone else's right to live. We can, in this connection, not do much better than to quote the arguments of Clarence Darrow, who in a famous debate with Judge Alfred J. Talley of New York City at the Manhattan Opera House on September 23, 1924 (a short time after he obtained a life sentence rather than a death sentence for Nathan Leopold and Richard Loeb), opposed capital punishment with these words:

"I might just observe, in passing, that in all of these states where the mortality by homicide is great, they have capital punishment and always have had it. A logical man, when he found out the death rate increased under capital punishment, would suggest some other way of dealing with it. . . .

"We teach people to kill, and the State is the one that teaches them. If the State wishes that its citizens respect human life, then the State should stop killing. It can be done in no other way. There are infinite reasons for killing. There are infinite circumstances under which there are more or less deaths. It never did depend and never can depend upon the severity of the punishment. . . .

"There isn't, I submit, a single admissible argument in favor of capital punishment. Nature loves life. We believe that life should be protected and preserved. The thing that keeps one from killing is the emotion they have against it; and the greater the sanctity that the State pays to life, the greater the feeling of sanctity the individual has for life. . . ."

While Darrow's arguments tended to be a bit extreme, we think that basically they are good ones; and we think that the recent removal of the death penalty in many of our states was originally sparked by Darrow's forthright views. Although, along with Darrow, we must admit that most murderers are definitely wrong, if we do not give an antisocial wrongdoer the inalienable right to be wrong, we are really depriving him of his humanity; and by the very act of his being born (which, of course, he did not ask to be), he normally deserves to be alive and to be human—which means to be incredibly fallible. Once we deprive a person of his right to live, on almost any conceivable ground, we are verging dangerously close to a fascist or Nazi philosophy: The typical fascist or Nazi condemns an individual to annihilation because some of his important traits (such as his non-Aryanism or his antifascist beliefs) are held to be wrong and heinous. Not only are these traits damned (as presumably the fascist or Nazi, with his own peculiar value system, has a right to damn them) but *he,* the whole person, is consigned to oblivion for possessing such "reprehensible" characteristics.

If, therefore, we (1) rate an individual's traits, such as his tendency toward violence or murder, and find them seriously wanting, and (2) take away his right to live and to have *any* traits whatever because of those that we happen to find heinous, how are we essentially different from the fascist or Nazi? If *any* human characteristic or performance is deemed so wicked as to justify the expunging from life of the whole person himself, who among us will ever be safe? And who is to judge *which* traits the performer must possess in order to be legitimately liable to capital punishment?

The other side of the case, the one in favor of killing killers, of course, has its advantages. If we electrocute or otherwise dispose of murderers, we save the state a great deal of expense, we rid the world of many individuals who could probably not be helped with any amount of treatment, we mercifully cut short the miserable lives of many killers who would otherwise spend a half century or more in prison, we give cathartic release to some of the angry emotions of the relatives or close friends of slain individuals, we perhaps deter some persons from committing murder who might otherwise do so, etc. C. S. Lewis and several other Protestant ministers, quoted in R. Ingram's *Essays on the Death Penalty*, forcefully uphold this penalty as the most just disposition of murderers. Says Lewis: "The humanitarian theory wants simply to abolish justice and substitute mercy for it. . . . Mercy detached from justice grows unmerciful."

The case for capital punishment is dramatically presented in a letter to *Playboy Magazine,* which appeared in August, 1968. It reads as follows:

"Though I had read your rather asinine views on capital punishment, I had not taken any particular stand on the subject until November 1, 1967, when my father was struck down. He was not hit merely for the sake of being robbed, but was brutally beaten with a piece of iron pipe to make sure that he could not be a witness against the criminals. He died the following morning, but not before he was able to give the police information that helped in the capture and the conviction of the killers.

"My father, though not a saint, hardly deserved this fate. Throughout his life, he gave money, food and clothing to many of his so-called friends. It was three of these friends who murdered him. Since then one has been convicted and sentenced to die in the gas chamber. The two others are up for trial soon.

"You, in your grand manner and disconnected slop, would want me to say that his killers should be given a jail term during which they should be rehabilitated so they can return to society. It's easy (as I remember) to say noble things about capital punishment while on the outside looking in, since you have never been touched personally by the horror. I wonder what your views would be if murder really came close to you. I have noticed that you have never interviewed families of the murder victims and asked what they would want done. It might be interesting to see how the other side feels. Instead of just listening to the so-called experts, listen to the real experts: Talk to the families who have had to view the mutilated bodies of their loved ones and who have had to watch them die slowly, very slowly. Ask what hit them hardest and what lasting effect it has had on their lives. Print these so that people can see what the other side is like. (Signed) Herbert Kay, San Diego, California."

This is a highly emotional letter, and it says something that is very true: that murder is a terrible crime, that it cruelly snuffs out the lives of its victims and tortures some of them in the process, and that it leaves countless relatives and friends of the slain individual who may be grimly and lastingly affected by the results of the gory deed. All this cannot be gainsaid. But the fact remains that any person who would brutally beat to death another person who had befriended and helped him is a sadly disturbed individual; and it is a sorry commentary on human affairs that a "friend" will sometimes steal from another and bludgeon him to death so that he cannot be a witness against this "friend." But that's the way some—fortunately not too many—humans are: thieving, inconsiderate, brutal, murderous; and it is difficult to see how they or anyone will be truly helped to become more humane by impassionedly damning them and sending them to the gas chamber.

What the writer of this pitiful letter has also failed to note is that not every close relative of a savagely murdered person feels the way he does about his father's death. A fine example was set in 1959 in the City of Philadelphia, when a three-and-one-half-year-old girl was sexually attacked and killed by a young man who was taken into custody soon after. Thousands of Philadelphians were literally screaming murder and yelling for this young man's blood when her father, Professor Anatol Hold of the University of Pennsylvania, wrote a remarkable letter to the *Philadelphia Bulletin,* in which he asked that the murderer be brought to justice, psychologically treated, and not be made to suffer the death penalty. For as much as he missed and grieved over his dead child, this father wrote, he could not help acknowledge that the slayer was an exceptionally disturbed individual who had been driven to his deed by his terrible feelings of inadequacy and worthlessness; and he could not, in all conscience, desire the death of such an emotionally aberrated person. The closing sentences of Professor Hold's letter are most notable: "My final word has to do with the operation of the machinery of justice. Had I caught the boy in the act, I would have wished to kill him. Now that there is no undoing of what has been done, I only wish to help him. Let no feelings of caveman vengeance influence us. Let us rather help him who did so human a thing."

Man, alas, is not always as enlightened, especially in the hour of his deepest sorrow, as this bereaved father. When he becomes so, there is every reason to believe that capital punishment, for almost any crime one can conceive, will be eliminated from our statute books. Meanwhile, there are some promising signs in this direction. During the closing days of 1969, the death penalty was permanently abolished in Britain, in spite of the fact that public opinion polls in that country showed a preponderant majority in favor of bringing back the hangman after capital punishment had been temporarily discontinued. In the debate that raged, before Parliament acted decisively against the death penalty, it was pointed out that this kind of ultimate punishment hardly deters murderers. Thus, in the preceding year when it was without hanging, Britain had five reported murders per million of population, while the United States, with capital punishment in most states, had seventy per million. It was also shown that a great many murders are the result of family tensions and psychological explosions, to which the deterrent of the criminal law is irrelevant. Thus, one of the largest categories of murder in England for many years has been killing followed by suicide.

Other modern nations have similarly restricted or abolished capital punishment in recent years. All western European countries except France have abolished the death penalty; and the French guillotine has been used only rarely. Even where the law has not been formally abolished, Rupert Townshend-Rose tells us, "it has largely fallen into disuse. In Belgium there has been no execution for murder since 1863, and none in Luxemburg since 1822. In the last ten years there have been only two executions in

Northern Ireland, and none in Eire. In France, during the same period, there have been less than two executions a year. Eleven of the fifty states in the United States have outlawed capital punishment. In three others it is sanctioned only for such special cases as the murder of a prison guard or a prison official. There is still a move on foot to have the United States Supreme Court abolish all capital punishment on the grounds that it is 'cruel and unusual' punishment, which is prohibited by the Constitution. Most Latin-American countries have abolished the death penalty for all but military cases."

Both capital punishment and severe physical treatment of prisoners—especially flogging—have been for many years advocated as deterrents to crimes of violence. But, as briefly noted before, no empirical evidence has been brought forth to prove that these types of punitive treatment actually do deter criminal acts; and there are several important indications that they do not. In fact, H. Staub argued against the use of capital punishment because, he hypothesized, a killer's desire for vengeance often stems from the punitive drives of the group in which he resides. Consequently, the more punitive the group is, the more violent crime there will tend to be. E. R. Calvert similarly held that capital punishment is actually self-defeating and that consequently modern nations will abolish it; and to some extent his predictions have now come true.

Rolph points out that many countries and regions of countries that once utilized capital punishment have abolished it or let it fall into abeyance; but "their murder rate seems to have been unaffected." Among the countries he includes are Austria, Belgium, Denmark, Finland, Western Germany, Holland, Iceland, Israel, Italy, Luxembourg, Nepal, Norway, Portugal, Sweden, Switzerland, several states of the United States, and several Central and South American nations.

Rolph additionally notes that in 1893, after the city of Liverpool, England, had punished robbery with violence by flogging for ten years, this crime "was more frequent than it had been at the beginning." At the same time, in 1948 all forms of corporal punishment were abolished in England by the Criminal Justice Act; and this time robbery with violence decreased. E. Lewis-Faning also reports on flogging in England: "From a statistical examination of the published records of the volume of crime and robbery with violence, and of the number of persons sentenced to be flogged for this crime during the period 1863–1936, there is no evidence that the infliction of corporal punishment has in any way acted as a deterrent to prevent others from committing such crimes. Rather, does it appear that there is no relation at all between the number of floggings and the amount of crime in the same year."

E. H. Johnson observes that not enough attention has been given to the finding that the effects of capital punishment differ according to the type of offender and crime: "The deterrent and eugenic arguments in support of capital punishment rest on a consistent and certain application of the penalty according to carefully formulated principles. It would appear that consistency, certainty, and principles are lacking."

Does what we have said about the treatment of ordinary murderers apply to the treatment of assassins, assuming that they are apprehended and convicted? Yes, we do not see why it does not. Assassins, in our estimation, would better be placed in protective custody, often for the rest of their lives, and while incarcerated treated with psychotherapy and other available methods, just as we recommend for other killers. There are several special reasons why we recommend this kind of treatment for convicted assassins:

1. The vast majority of them seem to be seriously disturbed and are more or less driven or compelled to follow their murderous bents. It is highly academic to assume that they could have acted otherwise if they really wanted to do so. They are therefore not exactly responsible for their deeds in most instances.

2. Even when an assassin is not forced, by his own disordered ruminations, to kill one of his political opponents, and even when he is sufficiently integrated to plot and scheme his crime with due malice aforethought, there is obviously something radically wrong with his thinking which leads him to believe that his kind of violence will do considerable good or that it is the only logical way out of the dilemma that he thinks his victim has foisted upon the community. Hence, again, he is seriously emotionally aberrated.

3. The assassin, like other murderers, is highly disturbed and murderous because of his biological inheritance and his social upbringing. But obviously he did not rear himself or contribute to his own genes; therefore he is not entirely responsible for his deranged condition and would better not be denigrated and punished for it.

4. Assassins (like murderers) are to some degree influenced by the social environment and the atmosphere of violence that exists in their countries. Our nation, for example, is a land where rage and violence *are* specifically encouraged. Witness our ubiquitous cowboy and gangster films and television shows, where *verbal* assassination of political figures *is* commonplace. Witness the editorials and speeches of both right- and left-wingers where moralism *is* rife. Witness the absolutistic *shoulds, oughts,* and *musts* of our religions, our schools, and our courts, where all of us *are* urged to condemn the sinner as well as his sins and to despise the writer or speaker as well as his views. It is only to be expected that in this kind of atmosphere we will breed rabidly hating and murderously vengeful people even among our nonpsychotics, and it is to be expected further that we will push our severely disturbed individuals into committing fairly frequent mayhem. The blame and the guilt for assassinations, therefore, if any is validly to be levied, would perhaps better be laid at society's rather than the assassin's door.

Lest we seem too harsh on the social structure, let us note that, as an aftermath of the assassinations of Robert F. Kennedy and Martin Luther King, several leading American citizens pointed out the same thing that we are emphasizing. Dr. David Abrahamsen, a governor of the Lemberg Center for the Study of Violence at Brandeis University, said Americans not only condone violence, "We love it. We love to fight. The frontier days made the gun manly. In France they can riot for three weeks and only two people get killed. Can you imagine how many would have been killed here?" Dr. Herbert A. Otto, a well-known psychologist, commented: "America accepts violent acts as commonplace." Arthur Schlesinger, Jr., the Pulitzer Prize-winning historian who was an aide to President John F. Kennedy, called the American people "the most frightening on this planet." Dr. John Spiegel, director of Brandeis University's Lemberg Center, thought that the assassination of Senator Kennedy resulted from the nation's "gun fetish" and said there is an emotional addiction to use guns "as strong as any other addiction, such as drugs." His colleague at the center, Dr. Ralph W. Conant, pointed out that, since the assassination of Lincoln in 1865, one-fifth of America's presidents have been murdered and one-third have had attempts made on their lives.

In spite of the evidence that assassins tend to be severely disturbed emotionally and that there are many influences in our social structure which encourage and help them to give in to their murderous urges, we still irrationally sentence assassins to death. Thus, in the case of Sirhan B. Sirhan, Robert F. Kennedy's slayer, twelve solemn-faced jurors who had previously found him to be guilty condemned him to the gas chamber. In spite of a plea for compassion from Senator Edward M. Kennedy, brother of the victim, Judge Herbert V. Walker rejected a motion for a reduction of the death penalty to life imprisonment. "My brother," the Massachusetts senator wrote the court, "would not have wanted his death to be a cause for the taking of another life."

United States Attorney General Ramsey Clark concurred, to no avail, with Edward Kennedy's plea. When asked whether, had Lee Harvey Oswald lived, he would have wanted to spare his life, Clark (according to T. Wicker) replied: "Yes. In opposing the death penalty, I do so knowing that all murder is ghastly, that some may wound an entire country, that someday I or a member of my family may be the victim. The death penalty lowers the state to the level of the killer by attempting to redress a private execution with a public execution. Either human life—*all* human life—is sacred or it is not. I think it is. In his appeal for mercy in the sentencing of Sirhan Sirhan last May, Senator Edward Kennedy—who might be expected to feel the desire for revenge as deeply as any man—also acknowledged the sacredness of what he called 'God's gift of life itself.' "

Once an individual is arrested for a misdemeanor or a felony, one might think that he would be treated at least kindly and humanely, and preferably with psychological methods. For there are presumably reasons why humans commit crimes, and two of the main reasons are (1) he is emotionally disturbed and therefore cannot tell right from wrong or else compulsively does wrong even though he knows what is right, and (2) he significantly differs with the Establishment's laws and does not agree that its rules and laws are valid. In either of these eventualities, a prisoner would normally be expected to be benefited or "rehabilitated" by proper reeducation when he has been convicted and jailed for an offense. Actually, however, only a small degree of psychological treatment is usually available to him under our present system of incarceration.

Thus, B. Jackson notes that "fewer than seven per cent of all correctional employees (psychologists, social workers, vocational and academic teachers, and chaplains) are qualified to treat inmates. Half the states have no educational requirements at all for custodial officers; in 28 percent of the prisons, according to the report done for the President's crime commission, 'One can be a "professional worker" without having graduated from high school. In at least one [prison system] the mail clerk is called a social worker.' "

Karl Menninger concurs: "The legal and political structure handicaps a jail warden when he tries to provide decent treatment for his prisoners. I'll give you an example. Until just a few months ago, the warden of the Cook County [Illinois] jail was forced to feed his prisoners on fourteen cents a day per man. . . . The whole business is brutal and cruel. I worked as a cowhand when I was young and we were far gentler when we ran steers than the police are when they run their prisoners. There have been improvements in the *prisons,* yes. But nobody tries to do rehabilitation in the *jails.*"

M. T. Kaufman points out that jail crowding in New York City has reached enormous proportions. The various detention centers tend to be 60 percent over their capacity: "About 60 percent of those arrested are granted bail and raise it. The rest will be sorted and routed into other vans headed for remand facilities, where men sleep two and three to a cell and where solitary confinement is sometimes regarded as a pleasure, the only place an inmate can be alone. For some of those arrested the shock of confinement ends in suicide. Observation and surveillance are stretched thin by the demands of moving masses of prisoners."

After Kaufman made this report, several notable riots took place in New York City jails as prisoners protested their conditions.

McGarry and Bendt point out that many offenders, especially those guilty of crimes of murder and violence, are actually psychotic; and that if these psychotic criminals are given a pretrial commitment as criminals they do not do as well psychotherapeutically as do equally disturbed individuals who are given civil commitment. Penn and his associates also review the kinds of judicial review and decision-making processes applied to individuals who are psychiatrically committed as being "criminal" or "mentally ill." They find that the former are usually discriminated against in various ways and that this kind of discrimination often mitigates their being properly treated and rehabilitated.

A large-scale study made by the Census Bureau for the Law Enforcement Assistance Administration, an arm of the United States Department of Justice, was released in 1971 showing that city and county jails in the country had 52 per cent of their inmates who had not been convicted of a crime and included many inmates, whether convicted or not, who endured "less-than-human conditions." The report of the Bureau indicated that four jails still in daily use were built before George Washington's Administration, and that a quarter of the 97,500 local jail cells in the country are more than fifty years old.

Former United States Attorney General Ramsey Clark, in *Crime in America,* points out that "long delays in trials dissipate any deterrent effect that might possibly result from convictions." He also points out that "we practice no theory of penology in America today. We do what we do. And what we do has almost no relationship to what we say we do. Essentially, we use penology to confine as inexpensively as possible and thus separate from society people who have committed crime." Our penological treatment of murderers, Clark insists, is even more irrational: "Some crimes are acts of momentary irrationality by people who will never commit another serious crime. Murder is often such an act. Occurring most often within families and between friends and neighbors, it is sometimes the result of an uncontrollable impulse, of sudden overwhelming anger—spontaneous, unpredictable, and nonrecurrent. Placing the tormented people who have committed such a crime among men who lead lives of crime can be cruel and senseless."

At the same time, Henry Raymont reports that Dr. Joseph E. Goldstein, who helped draft the Durham Rule in 1954, which allowed many more murderers and other criminals to plead insanity than were allowed to plead it under the old M'Naughten Rule, now feels that the new rule often results in injustice: "Though the Durham Rule expanded the courts' use of expert witnesses and inspired other liberalizations, the record of its application shows that if a defendant is acquitted because of mental 'defect' or 'disease,' he is automatically committed to an institution for the criminal insane, sometimes receiving longer confinement than if he had pleaded guilty. . . . Inadequate clinical attention in state mental institutions combined with society's continued ambivalence about mental illness, Dr. Goldstein added, sometimes makes imprisonment more desirable because the chances for parole are often better than the possibility of release from a mental institution for an individual stigmatized as criminally insane."

Dale Wittner excoriates American criminal "justice" by contending that in New York, anyone who commits a serious crime has odds of 200 to 1 that he will never go to prison on that charge; and in Washington the average delay between a felony arrest and trial is ten months. He further notes: "The criminal courts of troubled urban America are failing. Like once-fearsome scarecrows put out to keep away birds of lawlessness, they are tattered by neglect, familiar and even accommodating to professional hoodlums and incorrigible terrorists of society who walk free for months and years, waiting for trials that never come. To the innocent, the poor, the uneducated, to the victims of crime and witnesses to it, and to honest policemen, many big-city courts are already a sham and a broken promise. So strained, so clogged with humanity have they become that substantial justice is only an occasional, almost accidental, product. A system drafted nearly two centuries ago to protect four million people does not work for 200 million. . . . Prosecutions are haphazard. Justice is the subject of bargaining. The possibility of punishment diminishes—and with it, respect for the law."

Ronald L. Goldfarb welcomes the fact that America's new

breed of political prisoners—such as Civil Rights movement leaders, war and draft resisters, and college rebels—are making more clear than ever to us our court and prison inadequacies. "They have not been complaining simply about the food or making grumbling recriminations about their lot; their indictments go to fundamental flaws in the system—bail practices, trial delays, gross physical conditions. The shock waves are reaching main street. The word is getting out about the inept and evil American prisons." John P. Frank, in his book, *American Law: The Case for Radical Reform,* heartily concurs: "If a fundamental social value of the rule of law is to permit people to settle their disputes in an orderly and efficient way, then the system itself is failing. . . . The gloom is unadulterated by a ray of hope."

From objective reporters, such as David Burnham and Nat Hentoff—who revealed almost unspeakable conditions in New York City's famous jail, the Tombs—to subjective first-hand reports by inmates H. Jack Grisold, Mike Misenheimer, Art Powers, and Ed Tromanhauser—who revealed equally unspeakable conditions at the Indiana State Prison—the observations that we keep receiving on conditions in our city, county, and federal jails are almost uniform. Burnham tells us that "a world of fear, violence, filth and degradation has been described by many of the prisoners who answered an uncensored questionnaire about their living conditions while awaiting trial in the Tombs, the Manhattan House of Detention for men. . . . More than four out of ten prisoners said they had seen a guard assault an inmate. Fewer than one out of ten said they had a mattress and blanket during their first few days in the Tombs." The Indiana State Prison inmates insist that a deputy warden sold jobs, cells, punks, and even freedom to any con who had the cash; that many "penitentiary punks" (effeminate homosexuals) purr like a kitten for the right "jocker" (masculine prisoners), who for sex favors will see that they are well taken care of; and that violence and degradation prevail in their prison system.

Even more objective first-hand reports on prison conditions are also available. At a congressional hearing on the abuse of prisoners, reported by *Newsweek* Magazine, we learn " 'Sexual assaults are epidemic,' concurred District Attorney Arlen Spector of

Philadelphia in testimony about his city's prison system. 'Almost every slightly built young man is sexually approached within an hour after his admission to prison. Many of these young men are beaten and repeatedly raped by gang aggressors.' Spector cited a report on sexual assaults in the city's prisons that traces the awful fate of such victims. 'After a young man's body has been defiled, his manhood degraded and his will broken,' says the report, 'he is marked as a sexual victim for the duration of his confinement. This mark follows him from institution to institution. He eventually returns to the community ashamed, confused and filled with hatred.' And another subcommittee witness, Milton Luger, director of the New York State Division for Youth, added a logical conclusion to the illogic of such a 'correctional' system. 'It would probably be better for all concerned,' he said, 'if young delinquents were not detected, apprehended or institutionalized. Too many of them get worse in our care.' "

A still more gruesome report comes from Tom Murton, who was appointed superintendent of Cummins Prison in Arkansas by Governor Winthrop Rockefeller, to investigate and correct some of the flagrant abuses there. Before he was subsequently fired for literally digging up *too* much evidence—including the bodies of several prisoners who presumably had been secretly and brutally murdered by guards or inmates under previous prison administrations—Murton discovered and reported incredible conditions at this and other Arkansas prisons. He found, for example, that the inmates at Cummins were much better armed than the guards and troopers assigned to control them; that "for offenses as trivial as failure to pick an established quota of cotton, men were forced to lie naked while a warden struck them as many as 60 times with a five-foot-long, wooden-handled leather strap"; that some men were disciplined by having electrodes "attached to their big toe and penis and wired to an old-fashioned rural telephone. When the handle was cranked, six volts of electricity discharged into his body. . . . Some men were rendered permanently sterile; others went insane"; that some men "were beaten with pipes, clubs or rifle butts"; that "most 'short hairs,' as new inmates are called, got a spoonful of rice a day, plus some soybeans, corn bread and water. They ate meat once a *year,* usually pigs'-knuckles soup. The food was rancid and often contaminated with weevils." Homosexuality, often of a forced nature, was rife. "We had serious situations develop, where kids were raped, and one even had his eye knocked out of his head." At the Women's Reformatory at Cummins, the inmates, especially those who were black, were miserably housed and fed, and "worse than that, they were beaten; they had the hide laid on them. They were put without clothing into the hole—a concrete-block structure with no heat and no water, no bedding—and they would have to defecate in a number-ten can. One of my predecessors as superintendent had a buzzer installed beside his bed and he'd just punch it and some gal would have to come trotting over from the reformatory to perform sex acts on him. If it matters, this guy was married. The women were transported to the prison in the back of a van with male convicts—no separation, no supervision. Consequently, they were all raped before they got to the prison." Finally, said Superintendent Murton, "At the last convention of the American Correctional Association, I introduced a resolution condemning acts of murder in the Arkansas prison system and urging that state to take action against such crimes by holding a thorough investigation to see that justice is done and the guilty parties punished. It was voted down 36 to 70. One hundred members of the association didn't even vote. Couldn't decide which way to stand on the issue of murder."

Although it is impossible here to detail completely police brutality against supposed perpetrators of violence—since that subject would require many volumes—we may briefly note that police and national guard maimings and killings of "riot" participants and of innocent bystanders have taken place quite frequently in recent years. Blacks, for example, have been killed in Augusta, Georgia; Jackson, Mississippi; Des Moines, Iowa; Memphis, Tennessee; and New Bedford, Massachusetts. University students have been seriously mussed up and shot at Columbia, Berkeley, Wisconsin, San Francisco State, and, most notably, Mississippi and Kent State.

In nonpolitical cases, convicted prisoners have often been mistreated and sometimes even killed by guards—notably at Arkansas and Indiana penitentiaries. Mistreatment of prisoners has helped to start riots in recent years at a large number of prisons, including several jails in New York City and New York State which have been, until recently, known for their relatively fair treatment of convicted criminals. In other countries of the world there have also been many instances of prisoners being treated cruelly and inhumanely, as especially noted in the books depicting the barbarous treatment of convicted criminals on Devil's Island by R. Belbenoit, H. Charriere, and C. Rickards.

Reports such as those just cited do not prove that prisoners are uniformly dealt with in an arbitrary, unjust, and cruel manner that sabotages rather than helps their rehabilitation. On the contrary, various treatment and reeducational programs for those who have perpetrated crimes of violence (and other kinds of offenses) have been in effect for over a century, and new methods of treating offenders are continually being tried. For example, Zinberg and Fellman show how enraged and violent individuals can be treated by a therapist helping them "to become genuinely aware of what they really felt." Schumacher and Molnar indicate how adjudicated juvenile delinquents can be improved by a non-giving therapist's deliberately frustrating their infantile dependent needs, arousing hostility and anxiety in them, and then getting them to understand and talk out their hurt and their hatred. W. A. McClain reports an experiment in which the almost impossibly aggressive, acting-out behavior of a ten-year-old impulsive boy was brought under good control by the use of a combination of operant conditioning (a form of behavior therapy) and relationship therapy that achieved the extinction of surplus conditioned responses and the building up of missing stimulus connections. He believes that similar reconditioning methods could be effectively employed with other overly impulsive, hostile individuals. B. R. Brooks presents a method, mainly consisting of conceptual interpretations of aggression, that is useful with medical patients who are verbally hostile and who exhibit disruptive behavior.

A. Ellis reports the successful treatment of convicted psychopaths in *Reason and Emotion in Psychotherapy*. P. L. Gallway shows how an analytic approach can be used in the rehabilitation of violent prisoners. The Massachusetts State Department of Corrections and Mental Health gives data on a psychotherapy program at the Massachusetts Correctional Institution in Walpole which has helped to lower recidivism significantly. Melitta Schmideberg notes that psychotherapy can be helpful with criminals but that emphasis on the here and now rather than on childhood factors that supposedly led to the offense is likely to be effective. S. W. Engel discusses various types of criminal behavior and examines seven different kinds of therapeutic measures: (1) improving the prison atmosphere, (2) mitigating initial reactions, (3) helping the offender to come to terms with the offense and the penalties enacted against him, (4) preparation for release from prison, (5) pedagogic approaches, (6) individual therapy, and (7) group therapy.

Bostow and Bailey used behavior therapy techniques to control the aggressive and disruptive behavior of two institutionalized patients. Following the leads of Wolf, Risley, and Mees; Hamilton, Stephens, and Allen; and Tyler and Brown—all of whom had success in reducing the angry and violent actions of different types of disturbed individuals—Bostow and Bailey took two exceptionally hard to control patients and, by simple methods of reinforcement and penalization, induced them to be much more tractable. As they note, "this demonstration that brief, 'non-painful,' and easily administered consequences can prove to be extremely effective in reducing severe and even violent behaviors, may provide an attractive alternative to the use of electric shock for such purposes."

A. W. Rachman developed a method of group therapy for adolescent delinquents who showed marked patterns of aggressive and hostile behavior and was successful, with this therapy, at preventing a gang war. Kuehn and Burton described a therapeutic approach to college students with homicidal impulses and were able to forestall violent action by some hostile and paranoid individuals by using this plan. B. Wedge outlined a method of training psychiatrists so they would better understand international problems and be available for the possible solution of combative behavior by national groups.

Kuehn and Burton, working with highly disturbed college students who were suffering from the "Whitman syndrome"—that is, were exceptionally hostile, tended to be good marksmen, and could possibly have killed close associates or innocent bystanders

—developed a treatment method including recognition, consultation, hospitalization, the use of drugs, and brief psychotherapy, which seems to be effective in calming down such individuals and at least temporarily eliminating their murderous impulses.

Harjit S. Sandhu worked with violent psychopaths in an Indian prison community and, with the help of a well-planned therapeutic milieu, succeeded in resocializing thirteen out of eighteen of these very difficult individuals.

H. M. Feinstein and his associates developed an effective form of group therapy for outpatients with elements of violent behavior, including mothers with infanticidal impulses. Scheidlinger and Holden used group methods with women with severe character disorders, including tendencies toward violence. Lion and Bach-y-Rita employed group therapy to good effect with violent male outpatients who referred themselves to the Psychiatric Division of the Massachusetts General Hospital in Boston.

How would we better treat individuals who are arrested and convicted for crimes of violence in general and of murder in particular? The information that we have examined throughout this book shows that there is much to be desired in this regard. Especially as far as arrest is concerned, individuals who have violently resisted the laws of the Establishment would better be much more carefully apprehended than had hitherto been true. Not that they should not expect to accept some of the consequences of their violent behavior: For any Establishment which foolishly allows its laws to be broken or which is easily blackmailed by the threat of violence is not likely to remain established very long! And any revolutionaries who are not prepared to encounter some kind of police or military intervention are hardly worth their salt and would better go back to purely verbal attacks on the powers that be.

But it is one thing for the authorities to arrest the key protesters in a violent rebellion, and quite another thing for them to corral any spectator who happens to be around at the time. It is also, perhaps, legitimate for guards to bodily haul a building-occupying rebel off a besieged premise, but hardly equally legitimate for them to pull him cruelly by the hair. We would hope that, if the Establishment is to stay in power and legislate and act against crimes of violence, it would do so within the limits of due process of law and not itself appreciably and needlessly contribute to the violence which it is trying to prevent.

Once individuals are convicted of violent depredations, and especially of murder and assassination, we would like to see a treatment program set up for them that would use some of the psychological and psychotherapeutic knowledge that is now accumulating and that could appreciably grow in the course of instituting and experimenting with this plan. Such a program might include the following:

1. All murderers (and preferably all criminals) would be psychologically examined before trial, to see whether they were responsible for the commission of their alleged crime or whether they were so emotionally disturbed that they could hardly be held responsible for it. If they were held to be nonresponsible, they would not be charged with any crime, but would be remanded for treatment, either in a psychiatric facility or in the community. If they insisted on being brought to trial, this would be done; but if they voluntarily agreed to a pretrial psychological examination and to being sent for treatment if they were found to be seriously disturbed, trial would then be waived.

2. Once an individual was put on trial for a serious crime, such as homicide, and was convicted, he would be sent for psychological examination (if none had already taken place) with or without his consent. He would not be sentenced before such an examination took place, and the results of his examination would always be available to the judge or judges who were to determine his sentence. Partly on the basis of these results, they would send him to some kind of treatment facility, such as a psychiatric hospital, which might or might not be a maximum security hospital; or they would place him on probation and arrange for his treatment in his community. Placement or referral of serious criminals would usually be on an indeterminate basis: that is to say, the convicted individual would be placed in a psychological facility or put on probation for an indefinite period of time, until his therapists or other collaborators felt that he was no longer a menace to society.

3. Lesser offenders could be given specific terms of incarcera-

tion in psychological facilities or specific terms of psychological treatment in their community. At the end of these terms, they would normally be under no further obligation to stay in protective custody or to be treated locally. But if their psychological supervisors found that they were really seriously disturbed and could constitute a menace to members of their community, they could be recommitted in much the same manner that psychotic individuals are now sometimes committed to mental institutions, and would only be released from incarceration or from treatment in the community when it was shown that there was little chance of their committing further crimes.

4. While incarcerated for treatment purposes, criminals would not be looked upon as blackguards, villains, or knaves, but as exceptionally human individuals who have thus far been a little more fallible than most people are, and who can nonetheless be accepted with their liabilities and handicaps. Those who care for them and treat them would always accept the fact that their very aliveness, as human beings, gives them personal "worth" or "value"—by which is simply meant the right to continue to exist in the world, and the right to seek out maximum happiness and minimum pain and misery. Although their deeds would be seen as distinctly wrong or mistaken, *they* would not be damned as total persons, but would be given the same kind of respect we commonly give to a child who behaves stupidly, nastily, or even criminally. We often negatively assess the child's deeds—but not the child himself: We realize he very easily and naturally can do the wrong thing, but that he is not a louse for having done it, and if we resist the temptation to denigrate him for doing it, there is a good chance we can help him act better in the future.

A convicted criminal, in other words, like most other human beings, almost always has a potential for acting better than he has behaved to date. He is also a process rather than a product: an ongoing, ever-changing person rather than a static thing. Consequently, there is no legitimate way of assessing *him,* in toto, though there may be legitimate ways of measuring most of his performances. Because he lives and changes, his performances can usually be modified or bettered; by calm practice and determination, they frequently are. Because he has in his repertoire, during his lifetime, literally millions of possible performances, there is no real way, no accurate mathematical method, of weighting them all, adding or multiplying them, and giving him one precise and for-all-time mark or report card.

Even if it were somehow possible to add a person's entire assets and subtract his entire liabilities and to come out with a final score, and even if his score were far below that of "excellent" or "average" individuals, there would be no justification for condemning him. For if he really *is,* let us say, a 10 per cent goodnik and a 90 per cent no-goodnik, then that is sad and regrettable—but it is obviously the way he is. And why should he be excoriated for being the way he is?

5. When murderers or other criminals are incarcerated, and especially when they are incarcerated for long periods of time, they would best not be deprived of normal and accustomed sexual outlets; for whether the court intended so or not, this kind of deprivation is usually taken as a form of punishment by the prisoners. Thus, Robert Neese (1959), a prisoner at Iowa State Prison who wrote a book called *Prison Exposures,* notes that "to make certain there is no contact with the opposite sex, even the visiting room has double thicknesses of screen wire plus a guard. Man and wife are not permitted to touch hands. While officials claim the screens are used to prevent smuggling, we know better. We know searches could easily be made of prisoners after visits. We resent fiercely what we believe is extra punishment imposed by the prison itself, and not by law."

I. D. Levine notes that the Spanish penal system allows prisoners to copulate with their wives or girlfriends; and, in fact, Leon Trotsky's assassin, Mercader, was permitted to have a girlfriend with whom he copulated in his cell. A. V. Huffman points out the hazards of sexual deprivation in prison, including the encouragement of fixed homosexuality: "Homosexuality in prison is frequent; we cannot tell how frequent because we lack reliable statistics. It is, we think, so frequent that we may call it an 'occupational hazard' to being an inmate. . . . Deprivation of conventional sexual outlet in a one-sexed person can be a harmful experience. An inmate who serves a prolonged prison term may become confused about his sexual role and may not carry over into the free community a normal sexual concept. Consequently, it is not unusual for us in the Diagnostic Depot to find before us as a classificant a recidivist who previously had shown himself to be without gross personality deviation as well as a conforming prisoner who had gone along uneventfully conduct-wise. Now, however, he is back before us for having sought out children or adolescents as sexual objects. It is only on the new reexamination that we really uncover what was there all along: his immaturity and inadequacy." What Huffman is referring to here is the phenomenon that has previously been noted in regard to fixed homosexuality. Although it is true that the *average* or "normal" male does not become a confirmed deviant if he is seduced into some homosexual activity, it is also true that a certain number of individuals are so generally and psychosexually immature that if *they* are induced to engage in homosexual relations, particularly during their adolescence, they easily give up on later heterosexual affairs and become fixed deviants. Since murderers and criminals are so often in the immature category, it is highly likely that a fair proportion of them, when they are forced to engage in homosexual activity because nothing else of an interhuman nature is available, will become psychologically fixated on homosexuality and will, in a sense, become addicted to it.

It is interesting to note, in this connection, that Cormier and Williams found that long-term imprisonment, with its consequent excessive deprivation of liberty, is frequently "accompanied by emotional regression, the extent of which is predetermined by the personality of the offender." It may lead to suicide, homicide, psychotic withdrawal, or incessant rage.

Some moralists, such as the absolutistic and dogmatic followers of Ayn Rand, would contend that, if the individual has some degree of potentiality and free will, and if he *volitionally* chooses to think irrationally and to commit antisocial deeds (when he presumably could choose to do otherwise), he clearly *is* a villain and consequently *deserves* to be verbally castigated and physically punished. But this (as A. Ellis shows in *Is Objectivism a Religion?*) is specious thinking because (1) it is almost impossible to prove that a wrongdoer entirely *volitionally* chooses to do wrong, since he usually believes (though for bad reasons) that his acts are right when he commits them, and even when he knows he is wrong he feels compulsively driven to make his errors; (2) if an individual volitionally does choose to do wrong when he knows perfectly well that he is wrong and that he is likely to be heavily penalized or punished for his mistakes, he is obviously not entirely sane—and, once again, we must question how "volitional" his wrongdoing actually is; and (3) even if it is possible for a person volitionally to do wrong when he is perfectly aware that he is acting badly, and for him not to be disturbed at the time he does his misdeeds (as, for example, when he deliberately steals in order to gain money, even though he knows full well that he is unfairly harming his victim and that, in the long run, stealing is socially harmful and therefore against his own interests), he still is only committing a mistaken, erroneous, or foolish act, which as a fallible human being we can only expect that he will at times commit, and (unless we posit a blaming, sadistic god) there is no law of the universe which says that he *should* not be wrong and that he *ought* to be condemned and punished for being humanly mistaken.

We are often gratified by finding that many of our theories and practices of rational-emotive psychotherapy, which we have largely derived from our work with disturbed individuals rather than from reading books on the theory of psychotherapy, are independently arrived at by other practitioners in the field, many of whom have a much different orientation than we do. Similarly, we were gratified to find that, as we were working on this book, Dr. Karl Menninger, the famous Freudian-oriented psychiatrist who has an outlook that is often quite different from ours, published a book, *The Crime of Punishment,* in which he agrees with much of what we say.

"It is a well-known fact," Menninger states, "that relatively few offenders are caught. But society makes a fetish of wreaking 'punishment' on an occasional captured and convicted one. This is supposed to 'control crime' by deterrence. The more valid and obvious conclusion—that getting caught is thus made the unthinkable thing—is overlooked by all but the offenders." He goes on to note that vengeance mainly brutalizes prisoners and confirms them in their criminal way of life; that few people should be put into prison and that those that are should normally be there for indeterminate terms; and that psychiatric or psychological services should be offered to criminals after conviction but before sentencing. Menninger clearly sees that it is not the crime but the reasons for doing it which would better be intensively studied, and that criminals are really *persons who* commit crimes and not merely *criminal persons.*

For reasons such as these, we'd better accept people with their misdemeanors and crimes and try to help them by showing them how to think straighter, how to work more effectively in the noncriminal world, and (by giving up their condemnation of themselves and others) how to lead highly satisfactory lives without resorting to criminal acts. Preferably, we could teach them this mode of thinking and behaving in the course of their regular schooling and family upbringing; but, if we fail to do this, or if they prove to be essentially unteachable, then we'd better have an alternative plan of teaching them socialized conduct in some kind of educational or rehabilitative facility after they get into difficulties—or, as we noted previously, keeping them in protective custody in a nonpunitive manner indefinitely until it can be ascertained that they are teachable.

We do not feel that our plan for the rehabilitation or treatment of criminals will act as a panacea that will eventually do away with all crime or even insure that criminals will never repeat their antisocial deeds; for as long as humans are anywhere like the way they presently are, this is most improbable. We do feel, however, that it might well reduce recidivism; that it would protect the public in ways that are better than our present penal system protects them; that it would largely put a halt to prisoners' learning how to be *more* disturbed and more antisocial while they are incarcerated; and that it would be a much fairer and more humane system of treating mistake-making people than the one which has been in effect in most civilizations for many centuries. Best of all, perhaps, it has built into it some important aspects of the general prevention, as well as the after-the-fact solution, of crime. For, if society itself takes the nonpunitive attitude toward offenders that we recommend, we believe that it will create a climate of opinion that will encourage individuals to accept themselves and others with their wrongdoings, to focus on how to become less wrong rather than on how to punish themselves and others for already committed errors, and thereby to truly solve the problem (as well as human beings can ever solve it) of minimizing antisocial behavior.

Bibliography

Altman, J., and Ziporyn, M. *Born to Raise Hell: The Untold Story of Richard Speck*. New York: Grove, 1967.

Ancona, L., and Fontanes, M. *La dinamica della aggresivita* [The dynamics of aggression]. *Quaderni di Criminologia Clinica,* 1965, 1–28.

Ansbacher, H., Ansbacher, R., Shiverick, D., and Shiverick, K. Lee Harvey Oswald: An Adlerian interpretation. *Psychoanalytic Review,* 1966, 53, 55–68.

Arendt, H. *Eichmann in Jerusalem*. New York: Viking, 1964.

Atkins, S. D. Susan Atkins details her diary. *Philadelphia Inquirer,* December 14, 1969, Section 1, 20–23.

Bach, G. R. (ed.). Constructive aspects of aggression. *Proceedings of the Annual Conference of the Group Psychotherapy Association of Southern California,* 1962.

Bach, G. R. *Intimate violence, understanding and prevention.* Beverly Hills: Institute of Group Psychotherapy, 1967. Mimeographed.

Baker, J. C. Indians, alcohol, and homicide. *Journal of Social Therapy,* 1959, 5, 270–75.

Ball, J., and Butes, W. M. Migration and residential mobility of narcotic drug addicts. *Social Problems,* 1966, 14, 56–69.

Banay, R. S. Study of a murder for revenge. *Journal of Criminal Psychopathology,* 1941, 3, 1–10.

Barnes P. "An outcry": Thoughts on being tear gassed. *Newsweek,* June 2, 1969, 37.

Bartholomew, A. A. The extra Y chromosome and criminal behavior. *Australian and New Zealand Journal of Psychiatry,* 1968, 2, 1.

Batt, J. L. Homicidal incidence in the depressive psychoses. *Journal of Mental Science,* 1948, 94, 782–92.

Belbenoit, R. *Dry Guillotine*. New York: Dutton, 1938.

Belberg, J. Psychoanalysis and crime. *Journal of Criminal Psychopathology,* 1943, 4, 729–50.

Bergler, E. Crime and punishment: Why punishment fails to prevent crime. *Psychiatric Quarterly Supplement,* 1947, 21.

Bigart, H. Portrait of a killer. *New York Times,* October 25, 1967, 26.

Bishop, G. *Executions.* Los Angeles: Sherbourne, 1965.

Black, J. The "speed" that kills or worse. *New York Times Magazine,* June 21, 1970, 14–26.

Blackburn, R. Personality in relation to extreme aggression in psychiatric offenders. *British Journal of Psychiatry,* 1968, 114, 821–28.

Blackman, N., Weiss, J. M., and Lamberti, J. W. The sudden murderer. *Archives of General Psychiatry,* 1963, 8(3), 289–94.

Bonaparte, M. *Der Fall Lefebure, sur psychoanalyse einer morderin* [The Lefebure case: psychoanalysis of a murderess]. *Imago,* 1929, 15, 15–62.

Bostow, D. E., and Bailey, J. B. Modification of severe disruptive and aggressive use of brief timeout and reinforcement procedures. *Journal of Applied Behavior Analysis,* 1969, 2, 31–37.

Botwin, C. Violence and the city child. *New York Times Magazine,* January 11, 1970, 73–78.

Brill, H. Drugs and aggression. *Mental Health Digest,* 1970, 2(1), 11–13.

Brody, J. E. In the mind of the assassin. *New York Times,* June 9, 1968a.

Brody, J. E. Rate of crime-linked genetic flaw is devised. *New York Times,* August 7, 1968b, 34.

Bromberg, W. *The World of Murder: A Psychiatric Study of Homicide.* New York: Grune & Stratton, 1962.

Brooks, B. R. Aggression. *American Journal of Nursing,* 1967, 67, 2514–22.

Brophy, J. *The Meaning of Murder.* New York: Crowell, 1967.

Buckley, T. Central Park killer was moody and untrusting. *New York Times,* July 8, 1968.

Buckley, W. F., Jr. The politics of assassination. *Esquire,* October, 1968, 163–65, 228–36.

Bunker, H. A. Mother-murder in myth and legend: A psychoanalytic note. *Psychoanalytic Quarterly,* 1944, 13, 198–207.

Burnham, D. Psychologist says pressures of big-city life are transforming Americans into potential assassins. *New York Times,* April 20, 1969a, 49.

Burnham, D. The tombs called "dungeon of fear." *New York Times,* April 8, 1970, 45.

Butter, J. R., Spruill, V. J., and Frye, R. L. The generality of deviant perception. *Corrective Psychiatry and Journal of Social Therapy,* 1966, 12, 263–66.

Bychowski, G. *Przestepca w seietle psychoanalyizy* [The criminal from the psychoanalytic point of view]. *Rocznik Psychjat.* 1935, 24, 30–52.

Bychowski, G. *Evil in Man.* New York: Grune & Stratton, 1968.

Calder, N. (ed.). *Unless Peace Comes: A Scientific Forecast of New Weapons.* New York: Viking, 1968.

Caldwell, E. Youth testifies Manson urged him to murder sheriff. *New York Times,* October 28, 1970, 53.

Caldwell, E. State rests in Tate murder case; Manson bid denied. *New York Times,* November 17, 1970, 32.

Caldwell, E. Manson co-defendants allowed to testify after defense rests. *New York Times,* November 20, 1970, 22.

Caldwell, E. "Robot theory" cited in defense of Manson's three co-defendants. *New York Times,* January 13, 1971, 36.

Caldwell, E. Girl's letters reread to Manson Jury. *New York Times,* January 20, 1971, 39.

Caldwell, E. Manson, three guilty; prosecution to ask death. *New York Times,* January 26, 1971, 1, 14.

Caldwell, R. G. *James A. Garfield: Party Chieftain.* New York: Dodd, Mead, 1931.

Calvert, E. R. Murder and the death penalty. *Nation,* 1929, 129, 405–7.

Cantor, N. Conflicts in penal theory and practice. *Journal of Criminal Law and Criminology,* 1935, 20, 330–50.

Capote, T. *In Cold Blood.* New York: New American Library, 1965.

Casey, M. D., Segall, L. J., Street, D. R. K., Blank, C. E., McDougall, J. H., McGrath, P. J., and Skinnert, J. L. YY chromosomes and antisocial behavior. *Lancet,* 1966, 2, 859.

Casey, M. D., and others. Patients with sex chromatin abnormality in two state hospitals. *Annals of Human Genetics,* 1968, 32, 53–63.

Catlin, G. *In the Path of Mahatma Gandhi.* Chicago: Regnery, 1950.

Champion, D. L. *The Sexual Psychopath.* New York: Lancer, 1967.

Charriere, H. *Papillon.* New York: Morrow, 1970.

Cher, M. *Charlotte Corday and Certain Men of the Revolutionary Torment.* New York: Appleton, 1929.

Chiricos, T. G., and Waldo, G. P. Punishment and crime: An examination of some empirical evidence. *Social Problems,* 1970, 18, 200–17.

Clark, R. *Crime in America.* New York: Simon and Schuster, 1970.

Cleckley, H. *The Mask of Sanity*. St. Louis: Mosby, 1950.

Clemens, L. S. Presidential killings fall into one pattern. *Illinois State Journal,* November 21, 1968.

Clemens, L. S. Failure common among presidential assassins. *Illinois State Journal,* November 22, 1968, 17.

Cloward, R. A., and Ohlin, E. E. *Delinquency and Opportunity*. Glencoe, Illinois: The Free Press, 1961.

Cole, K. E., Fisher, G., and Cole, S. S. Women who kill: A socio-psychological study. *Archives of General Psychiatry,* 1968, 19, 1–18.

Condon, R. " 'Manchurian Candidate' in Dallas," *The Nation,* December 28, 1963, 449–51.

Cormier, B. M. Psychoanalysis of homicide committed in a marital relationship. *Corrective Psychiatry and Journal of Social Therapy,* 1962, 8, 187–94.

Cormier, B. M., and Williams, P. J. Excessive deprivation of liberty. *Canadian Psychiatric Association Journal,* 1966, 11, 470–84.

Cousins, N. The conquest of violence. *Saturday Review,* June 22, 1968, 20.

Darrow, C. *Attorney for the Damned*. New York: Simon and Schuster, 1957.

Dawnay, P. Conspiracy. *Los Angeles Free Press,* June 13, 1969, 6.

DeFord, M. A. *Murderers, Sane and Mad*. New York: Abelard-Schuman, 1965.

DeFord, M. A. *The Real Bonnie and Clyde*. New York: Ace Books, 1968.

Donaldson, F. J. On the physiological interpretation of anger. *Central African Medical Journal,* 1969, 15, 79–82.

Donovan, R. J. *The Assassins*. New York: Harper and Brothers, 1952.

Dumas, F. R. *Madness in Power*. Philadelphia: Chilton, 1969.

Edwards, A. E., Bloom, M. H., and Cohen, S. The psychedelics: Love or hostility potion? *Psychological Reports,* 1969, 24, 843–46.

Ellis, A. A young woman convicted of manslaughter. *Case Reports in Clinical Psychology,* 1951, 2(1), 9–34.

Ellis, A. *How to Live with a Neurotic*. New York: Crown, 1957.

Ellis, A. *Reason and Emotion in Psychotherapy*. New York: Lyle Stuart, 1962a.

Ellis, A. *Homosexuality: Its Causes and Cure*. New York: Lyle Stuart, 1965a.

Ellis, A. *Suppressed: Seven Key Essays Publishers Dared Not Print*. Chicago: New Classics House, 1965b.

Ellis, A., with Wolfe, J., and Moseley, S. *How to Prevent Your Child from Becoming a Neurotic Adult.* New York: Crown, 1966.

Ellis, A. *Is Objectivism a Religion?* New York: Lyle Stuart, 1968a.

Ellis, A., and Harper, R. A. *A Guide to Rational Living.* Englewood Cliffs, N.J.: Prentice-Hall, 1961; Hollywood: Wilshire, 1967.

Ellis, A., and Harper, R. A. *Creative Marriage.* New York: Lyle Stuart, 1961. Reprinted as *A Guide to Successful Marriage.* Hollywood: Wilshire, 1968.

El-Rawy, M. *Okadato Oedipus waatharoha fel egrami* [Oedipus complex and criminality]. *Egyptian Journal of Psychology,* 1947, 3, 97–106.

El-Rawy, M. *Alkatlo'l syasy* [Political murder]. *Egyptian Journal of Psychology,* 1947, 3, 207–14.

Engel, S. W. Offender therapy in prison and on the outside. *International Journal of Offender Therapy,* 1967, 11, 43–50.

Ewart, A. *The World's Wickedest Men.* New York: Taplinger, 1965.

Eysenck, H. J. *Crime and Personality.* Boston: Houghton Mifflin, 1964a.

Eysenck, H. J. Biological factors in neurosis and crime. *Abhand ungen der deutschen Academie der Wissenschaften zu Berlin,* 1966, 2, 169–75.

Feinstein, H. M., *et al.* Group therapy for mothers with infanticidal impulses. *American Journal of Psychiatry,* 1964, 120, 882–86.

Ferri, E. A character study and life history of Violet Gibson, who attempted the life of Benito Mussolini. *Journal of Criminal Law and Criminology,* 1928, 19(2).

Flugel, J. C. *The Psychoanalytic Study of the Family.* London: Hogarth Press, 1950.

Foreman, P. Against conspiracy. *Look,* April 15, 1969, 112.

Fosburgh, L. Sirhan: The only issue is how much punishment. *New York Times,* March 2, 1969a, Sect. E, 6.

Fosburgh, L. The strange portrait of a mysterious assassin. *New York Times,* March 9, 1969b.

Fosburgh, L. Sirhan tells court why he wanted to kill Kennedy. *New York Times,* March 5, 1969c, 24.

Frank, G. *The Boston Strangler.* New York: New American Library, 1966.

Frank, J. P. *American Law: The Case for Radical Reform.* New York: Macmillan, 1970.

Frankel, C. The meaning of political murder. *Saturday Review,* June 22, 1968, 17–18.

Franklin, C. *Woman in the Case*. New York: Taplinger, 1968.

Franklin, C. *The World's Worst Murderers*. New York: Taplinger, 1965.

Freedland, N. Charlie Manson's greatest hits. *Other Scenes,* October, 1970, 4(8), no paging.

Freud, S. *New Introductory Lectures on Psycho-Analysis.* New York: Norton, 1933.

Freud, S. *The Problem of Anxiety*. New York: Norton, 1962.

Freud, S. *Collected papers*. New York: Collier, 1963.

Freud, S., and Breuer, J. *Studies in Hysteria.* New York: Basic Books, 1957.

Gallagher, J., and Felcher, B. Mother, grandma victims. *Chicago Daily News,* October 22, 1969, 1.

Gallwey, P. L. The rehabilitation of the violent prisoner: A synopsis. *Psychotherapy and Psychosomatics,* 1967, 15, 24.

Garber, C. M. Eskimo infanticide. *Scientific Monthly,* New York, 1947, 64, 98–102.

Garrison, L. French murder jury rejects chromosome defect as defense. *New York Times,* October 15, 1968, 5.

Giannell, A. S. Giannell's criminosynthesis theory applied to female homosexuality. *Journal of Psychology,* 1966, 64, 213–22.

Gibbens, T. C. N. Sane and insane homicide. *Journal of Criminal Law and Criminology,* 1958, 49, 110–15.

Gibbs, J. P. Crime, punishment, and deterrence. *Southwest Social Science Quarterly,* 1968, 48, 515–30.

Gibson, W. B. (ed.). *The Fine Art of Murder*. New York: Grosset and Dunlap, 1965.

Gillier, H. Murder in the west of Scotland. *British Journal of Psychiatry,* 1965, 111, 1087–94.

Gillin, J. L. Murder as a sociological phenomenon. *Annals of the American Academy of Political and Social Science,* 1952, no. 284, 20–25.

Glueck, S. Theory and fact in criminology: A criticism of differential association. *British Journal of Delinquency,* 1966, 7, 92–98.

Glueck, S., and Glueck, E. *Unraveling Juvenile Delinquency*. New York: Commonwealth Fund, 1950.

Glueck, S., and Glueck, E. *Family Environment and Delinquency*. Boston: Houghton Mifflin, 1962.

Goldfarb, R. L. The horror of the prisons. *New York Times,* October 28, 1970, 47.

Goodwin, F. K., Brodie, M. H., and Murphy, D. L. Report on sustained high doses of L-DOPA with depressed patients. *Health, Education and Welfare News,* May 15, 1970, 1–2.

Graff, H. F. Review of C. E. Rosenberg, *The trial of the assassin Guiteau. New York Times Book Review,* September 8, 1968, 46.

Graham, H. D., and Gurr, T. R. (eds.). *Violence in America.* New York: New American Library, 1969.

Greenberg, D. S. Review of Nigel Calder's *Unless peace comes. New York Times Book Review,* July 7, 1968, 6.

Gribble, L. *Such Women Are Deadly.* New York: Arco, 1969.

Griswold, H. J., Misenheimer, M., Powers, A., and Tromanhauser, E. *An Eye for an Eye: Four Inmates on the Crime of American Prisons Today.* New York: Holt, Rinehart and Winston, 1970.

Gurr, T. R. *Why Men Rebel.* Princeton: Princeton University Press, 1970.

Guttmacher, M. *The Mind of the Murderer.* New York: Grove, 1962.

Gwertzman, B. Soviet finds '69 Kremlin gunman is insane. *New York Times,* March 21, 1970, 3.

Hamilton, J., Stephens, L., and Allen, P. Controlling aggressive and destructive behavior in severely retarded institutionalized residents. *American Journal of Mental Deficiency,* 1967, 7, 852–56.

Harris, T. G. Sirhan B. Sirhan: A conversation with Bernard L. Diamond. *Psychology Today,* September, 1969, 3(4), 48–56.

Hartogs, R., and Freeman, L. *The Two Assassins.* New York: Crowell, 1965.

Haskell, M. R., and Yablonsky, L. *Crime and Delinquency.* Chicago: Rand, McNally, 1970.

Hauck, P. *The Rational Management of Children.* New York: Libra, 1967.

Hausner, G. Eichmann and his trial. *Saturday Evening Post,* November 3, 1962, 10, 17.

Helfer, R. E., and Kempe, C. H. (eds.). *The Battered Child.* Chicago: University of Chicago Press, 1968.

Hellwig, A. *Kritiken des Gattenmordes* [Critical notes on uxoricide]. *Krim. Montash.* 1930, 4, 62–63.

Henry, A. F., and Short, J. F. *Suicide and Homicide.* New York: Free Press, 1964.

Hentoff, N. Prisoners: Men or animals. *Evergreen Review,* 1971, 86, 57–59.

Hinsie, L. E., and Campbell, R. J. *Psychiatric Dictionary.* New York: Oxford University Press, 1960.

Hooten, E. A. *Up from the Ape.* New York: Macmillan, 1946.

Horton, D. The functions of school in primitive societies. *Quarterly Journal for Studies in Alcoholism,* 1943, 4, 199–320.

Huffman, A. V. The behavior pattern of criminals. *Journal of Social Therapy,* 1962, 8, 15–33.

Huie, W. B. *He Slew the Dreamer.* New York: Delacorte, 1970.

Hurley, J. R. (chairman). Symposium: Murder within the family. *American Psychologist,* July, 1967, 22, 502.

Ingram, T. R. (ed.). *Essays on the Death Penalty.* Houston: St. Thomas Press, 1963.

Jackson, B. Our prisons are criminal. *New York Times Magazine,* September 22, 1968, 44–66.

Johnson, Elmer H. Selective factors in capital punishment. *Social Forces,* 1957, 36, 165–69.

Johnson, T. A. Expert deplores year in solitary. *New York Times,* October 21, 1969d, 46.

Jones, E. *Hamlet and Oedipus.* New York: Anchor Books, 1954.

Jones, E. *The Last Two to Hang.* New York: Stein and Day, 1966.

Kaiser, R. B. Conversations in jail with Sirhan, a name meaning wolf. *Life,* January 17, 1969, 66(2), 21–25.

Kaiser, R. B. *"R.F.K. Must Die!"* New York: Dutton, 1970.

Karpman, B. A psychoanalytic study of a case of murder. *Psychoanalytic Review,* 1951, 38, 139–57.

Kaufman, M. T. Talks scheduled on jail crowding. *New York Times,* January 12, 1970a, 11.

Kaufman, M. T. In street, store and subway, rudeness infects the life of the city. *New York Times,* March 2, 1970c, 31.

Kellogg, C., and others. New plan of criminal procedure presented by the Committee of the Los Angeles Bar Association. *Journal of Delinquency,* 1927, 11, 309–18.

Khrushchev, N. *Khrushchev Remembers.* New York: Little, Brown, 1970.

Klein, M. *Contributions to Psychoanalysis.* New York: McGraw-Hill, 1963.

Kneeland, D. E. Manson testifies on "harassment." *New York Times,* August 2, 1970, 21.

Kneeland, D. E. Tearful Manson witness unyielding when shown death photos. *New York Times,* August 8, 1970, 47.

Kneeland, D. E. Manson witness given immunity. *New York Times,* August 11, 1970, 17.

Kneeland, D. E. Tate witness tells murder jury of thinking she was a witch. *New York Times,* August 12, 1970, 3.

Kneeland, D. E. Witness says Manson gives off "vibrations" in the courtroom. *New York Times,* August 14, 1970, 16.

Kneeland, D. E. Witness calls Manson the Devil and says she is God's emissary. *New York Times,* August 18, 1970, 26.

Kneeland, D. E. Five slain on coast and left in pool. *New York Times,* October 21, 1970, 1, 95.

Kuehn, J. L., and Burton, J. Management of the college student with homicidal impulses—the "Whitman syndrome." *American Journal of Psychiatry,* 1969, 125, 1594–99.

Lachman, J. H., and Cravens, J. M. The murderers—before and after. *Psychiatric Quarterly,* 1969, 43, 1–11.

Laing, R. D. *The Divided Self.* Baltimore: Penguin, 1965.

Lalli, M., and Turner, S. H. Suicide and homicide: A comparative analysis by race and occupation levels. *Journal of Criminal Law, Criminology and Police Science,* 1968, 59, 191–220.

Lamberti, J. W., Blackman, N., and Weiss, J. The sudden murderer: A preliminary report. *Journal of Social Therapy,* 1958, 2–15.

Lando, B. It's a gas! *New Republic,* June 28, 1969, 17–18.

Langford, G. *The Murder of Stanford White.* Indianapolis: Bobbs-Merrill, 1962.

Lehrman, P. R. *Über einige unbewusste komponenten geim mord* [Some unconscious components in murder]. *Int. Z. Psychoanal.,* 1937, 23, 527–35.

Leon, C. A. Unusual patterns of crime during *La Violencia* in Colombia. *American Journal of Psychiatry,* 1969, 125, 1564–75.

Lester, D. Suicide, homicide, and the effects of socialization. *Journal of Personality and Social Psychology,* 1967a, 5, 466–68.

Lester, D. The relation between discipline experience and the expression of aggression. *American Anthropologist,* 1967b, 69, 734–37.

Levine, I. D. *The Mind of an Assassin.* New York: Farrar, Straus and Cudahy, 1959.

Lion, J. R., and Bach-y-Rita, G. Group psychotherapy with violent outpatients. *International Journal of Group Psychotherapy,* 1970, 20, 185–91.

Lion, J. R., *et al.* The self-referred violent patient. *Journal of the American Medical Association,* 1968, 205, 503–5.

Lipset, S. M. The political thrust motivating campus turmoil. *Saturday Review,* March 1, 1969, 22–25, 47.

Littenun, Y., and Gaier, E. L. Social control and social integration. *International Journal of Social Psychiatry,* 1967, 9, 165–73.

Lombroso, C., and Ferrero, W. *The Female Offender.* New York: Wisdom Library, 1961.

Mackenzie, F. A. *Landru.* London: Geoffrey Bles, 1928.

Malnic, E. Tate murder suspect had a plan to foment a race war, hippies say. *Chicago Sun-Times,* December 8, 1969, 18.

Manchester, W. *The Death of a President.* New York: Harper and Row, 1967.

Maria, G. M. *Malattie Mentali crimingenetiche* [Criminal-genetic mental disease]. *Difesa Sociale,* 1962, 41, 113–20.

Mark, V. H., and Ervin, F. R. Is there a need to evaluate the individuals producing human violence? *Psychiatric Opinion,* 1968, 5(3), 32–34.

Martin, J. B. The criminal mentality. *Playboy,* December, 1967, 165, 249–56.

Masters, R. E. L., and Lea, E. *Sex Crimes in History.* New York: Julian, 1963.

McGarry, A. L., and Bendt, R. H. Criminal vs. civil commitment of psychotic offenders: A seven-year follow-up. *American Journal of Psychiatry,* 1969, 125, 1387–94.

McKnight, C. K., Mohr, J. W., Quincy, R. E., and Erockko, J. Matricide and mental illness. *Canadian Psychiatric Association Journal,* 1966a, 11, 99–106.

McKnight, C. K., Mohr, J. W., Quincy, R. E., and Erockko, J. Mental illness and homicide. *Canadian Psychiatric Association Journal,* 1966b, 11, 91–98.

McLoughlin, E. *An Inquiry into the Assassination of Abraham Lincoln.* New York: Lyle Stuart, 1963.

McMillan, P. The real Lee Harvey Oswald. *New York Times,* November 20, 1970, 41.

McWhirter, W. A. The story of the accused killer of Dr. King. *Life,* May 3, 1968, 64, 20–29.

Mead, G. H. *Selected Writings.* Indianapolis: Liberal Arts Press, 1965.

Meehl, P. Schizotaxia, schizotype, and schizophrenia. *American Psychologist,* 1962, 17, 827–38.

Meltzer, R. Charles Manson was my bunkmate. *Realist,* May–June, 1970, 87, 1, 9–11.

Menninger, K. *Man Against Himself.* New York: Harcourt, Brace, 1938.

Menninger, K. *The Crime of Punishment.* New York: Viking, 1968.

Merton, R. K. Social structure and anomie. *American Sociological Review,* 1938, 13, 672–82.

Mills, C. A. Suicides and homicides in their relations to weather changes. *American Journal of Psychiatry,* 1934, 91, 669–77.

Mosse, H. L. Individual and collective violence. *Journal of Psychoanalysis in Groups,* 1969, in press.

Mowat, R. R. *Morbid Jealousy and Murder*. London: Tavistock, 1966.

Murton, T., and Hyams, J. *Accomplices to the Crime*. New York: Grove Press, 1970.

Nash, M. Machine age Maya. *American Anthropologist,* April, 1958, Memoir 87.

National Commission on the Causes and Prevention of Violence. Report on assassinations. *New York Times,* November 3, 1969e, 41.

National Commission on the Causes and Prevention of Violence. *Violent Crime—Homicide, Assault, Rape, Robbery: The Report of the Commission*. New York: Braziller, 1970.

National Institute for Mental Health. *Report on the XYY Chromosomal Abnormality*. Washington: U.S. Government Printing Office, 1970.

Newman, A. H. *The Assassination of John F. Kennedy*. New York: Clarkson Potter, 1970.

Norman, G. Playboy interview: Tom Murton. *Playboy,* February, 1971, 59–78.

Novitski, J. Ex-student after Rio arrest. *New York Times,* December 3, 1969d.

O'Connor, R. *Courtroom Warrior*. Boston: Little, Brown, 1963.

Oelsner, L. Many kept in jail by lack of aides. *New York Times,* February 21, 1970, 1, 19.

O'Neil, P. Clarence the Ripper? *Life,* November 13, 1970, 85–88.

O'Neil, P. The wreck of a monstrous "family." *Life,* December 12, 1969, 20–31.

O'Neil, P. Ray, Sirhan—what possessed them? *Life,* June 21, 1968, 24.

Opotowsky, S. *The Longs of Louisiana*. New York: Dutton, 1960.

Oswald, R. L., with Land, M., and Land, B. *Lee: A Portrait of Lee Harvey Oswald by His Brother*. New York: Coward-McCann, 1967.

Packer, H. L. *The Limits of the Criminal Sanction*. Stanford: Stanford University Press, 1968.

Palmer, S. Murder and suicide in forty non-literate societies. *Journal of Criminal Law, Criminology and Police Science,* 1965, 56, 320–24.

Parker, S. The Wiitiko psychosis in the context of Ojibwa personality and culture. *American Anthropologist,* 1960, 62, 603–23.

Penn, N. E., Stover, D., Giebink, V., and Sindberg, R. Some considerations for future mental health legislation. *Mental Hygiene,* 1969, 53, 10–13.

Penrose, L. S. Genetics and the criminal. *British Journal of Delinquency,* 1955, 6, 15.

Perlmutter, E. Chief Justice Burger scores panel system for rating punishment over rehabilitation. *New York Times,* February 18, 1970b, 16.

Piaget, J. *The Language and Thought of the Child.* New York: Humanities Press, 1952.

Pippin, L. L. *The Roman Era.* Stanford, Calif.: Stanford University Press, 1964.

Pittman, D. J., and Handy, W. Patterns in criminal aggravated assault. *Journal of Criminal Law, Criminology and Police Science,* 1964, 55, 462–70.

Podolsky, E. The diseased brain and homicide. *Journal of Nervous and Mental Disease,* 1956, 124, 621–24.

Podolsky, E. Organic brain conditions and homicide. *Corrective Psychiatry and Journal of Social Therapy,* 1965, 11, 91–94.

Pokorny, A. D., and Mefford, R. B., Jr. Geomagnetic fluctuations and disturbed behavior. *Journal of Nervous and Mental Disease,* 1966, 143, 140–51.

Porter, B. The many faces of murder. *Playboy,* October, 1970, 97–98, 209–20.

Porterfield, A. L. Ecological correlates of alcoholism. *Social Problems,* 1958, 5, 326–38.

Quinney, R. Suicide, homicide and economic development. *Social Force,* 1965, 43, 401–6.

Rachman, A. W. Taking it out rather than fighting it out: Prevention of a delinquent gang war by group therapy intervention. *International Journal of Group Psychotherapy,* 1969, 19, 518–21.

Rand, A. *Atlas Shrugged.* New York: Random House, 1957.

Rand, A. *For the New Intellectual.* New York: New American Library, 1961.

Raymond, H. Modern legal test on insanity attacked by one of its drafters. *New York Times,* August 30, 1970, 55.

Redston, G., and Crossen, K. F. *The Conspiracy of Death.* Indianapolis: Bobbs, Merrill, 1965.

Reinhardt, J. M. *The Psychology of Strange Killers.* Springfield: Charles C Thomas, 1962.

Renaud, H., and Estes, F. Life history with 100 normal American males: Pathogenicity of childhood. *American Journal of Orthopsychiatry,* 1961, 31, 786–802.

Rickards, C. *The Man from Devil's Island.* New York: Stein and Day, 1968.

Ritter, J. P. Nightmare for the innocent in a California town. *Life,* August 15, 1969, 49–54.

Rivera Silva, M. *Lapena y el psicoanalisis* [Crime and psychoanalysis]. *Revista Mexicana Neuro-Psiqiatria,* 1938, 5, 15–24.

Robertson, J. A. Review of H. L. Packer, *The limits of the criminal sanction. Psychiatry and Social Science Review,* 1970, 3(12), 3–10.

Robinson, D. Psychiatrist says Sirhan saw himself as a "savior." *New York Times,* March 21, 1969.

Robinson, D. Psychologist, testifying for the defense, says tests indicate Sirhan has paranoid tendencies. *New York Times,* March 11, 1969.

Robinson, D. Defense attacks doctor's view that Sirhan was not legally ill. *New York Times,* April 3, 1969.

Robinson, D. Psychiatrist concedes Sirhan has "substantial mental illness." *New York Times,* April 4, 1969.

Robinson, D. Psychiatrist tells Sirhan trial killing was not psychotic's act. *New York Times,* March 3, 1969.

Robinson, D. Sirhan plea to die is denied by court. *New York Times,* March 1, 1969, 1, 16.

Robinson, D. Manson called a megalomaniac by prosecutor as trial begins. *New York Times,* July 25, 1970, 47.

Robinson, D. Manson family member testifies on Tate killings. *New York Times,* July 29, 1970, 27.

Robinson, D. Witness says Manson led second murder expedition. *New York Times,* July 30, 1970, 20.

Robinson, D. Third murder plan is laid to Manson. *New York Times,* July 31, 1970, 19.

Robinson, D. Key witness says that she once regarded Manson as a "Messiah." *New York Times,* August 1, 1970, 21.

Rolph, C. H. *Common Sense About Crime and Punishment.* New York: Macmillan, 1961.

Romano, C., and Paolella, A. First results from an inquiry into the personality of imprisoned murderers. *Di Fesa Sociale,* 1958, 37, 41–47.

Rose, G. J. Screen memories in homicidal acting out. *Psychoanalytic Quarterly,* 1960, 29, 328–43.

Rosen, J. N. *Direct Analysis.* New York: Grune and Stratton, 1953.

Rosenberg, C. E. *The Trial of the Assassin Guiteau.* Chicago: University of Chicago Press, 1968.

Rosenthal, J. Jail census finds 52% not convicted. *New York Times,* January 7, 1971, 1, 17.

Rougeau, M. *L'Attentat d'Orsini* [Orsini the assassin]. Paris, 1964.

Rusk, H. A. The cause of death. *New York Times,* September 29, 1968, 56.

Salisbury, H. E. Review of *Khrushchev remembers. New York Times Book Review,* January 3, 1971, 1–2.

Sandhu, H. S. Therapy with violent psychopaths in an Indian prison community. *International Journal of Offender Therapy,* 1970, 14, no. 3.

Satten, J., Menninger, K., Rosen, I., and Mayman, M. Murder without apparent motive: A study in personality disorganization. *American Journal of Psychiatry,* 1960, 116, 48–53.

Scheidemandel, P. L., and Kanno, C. K. *The Mentally Ill Offender.* Washington: Joint Information Service, 1969.

Scheidlinger, S., and Holden, M. Group therapy of women with severe character disorders. *International Journal of Group Psychotherapy,* 1966, 16, 174–89.

Scher, J. M. Psychiatrist urges support of nation-wide programs to control drug abuse. *Executives' Club News,* 1970, 47(10), 1–8.

Schlesinger, A., Jr. The dark heart of American history. *Saturday Review,* October 19, 1968, 20–23, 81.

Schmideberg, M. The treatment of criminals. *Psychoanalytic Review,* 1949, 36, 403–10.

Schumacher, M. J., and Molnar, J. "Hate bond" treatment provides delinquent with conscience. *Frontiers of Hospital Psychiatry,* April 15, 1968, 5–6.

Schur, E. M. *Our Criminal Society.* Englewood Cliffs, N.J.: Prentice-Hall, 1969.

Sellin, T. *Culture Conflict and Crime.* New York: Social Science Research Council, 1938.

Shearing, J. *The Angel of the Assassination.* London: Heineman, 1935.

Sheldon, W. H., with Hartl, E. M., and McDermott, E. *Varieties of Delinquent Youth.* New York: Harper, 1950.

Shultz, G. D. *How Many More Victims? Society and the Sex Criminal.* Philadelphia: Lippincott, 1965.

Simmons, L. W. Statistical correlations in the science of society. In Murdock, G. P. (ed.). *Studies in the Science of Society.* New Haven: Yale University Press, 1937.

Sington, D., and Playfair, G. *Crime, Punishment and Cure.* London: Secker and Warburg, 1965.

Smith, D. A doctor and a parole officer remember Manson. *Life,* December 19, 1969, 26.

Smith, T. Woman is sought for questioning in Kennedy assassination. *New York Times,* June 7, 1968, 1, 22.

Snider, A. J. When threats mean murder. *Chicago Daily News,* May 9, 1967.

Sparrow, G. *The Great Assassins.* New York: Arco, 1969.

Speer, A. *Inside the Third Reich.* New York: Macmillan, 1970.

Stafford, J. *A Mother in History.* New York: Bantam, 1966.

Staub, H. *Zum Kampf um die todess trafe* [Concerning the controversy about capital punishment]. *Psychoanalitik Bewegung,* 1931, 3, 448–56.

Stearns, A. W. Murder by adolescents with obscure motivation. *American Journal of Psychiatry,* 1957, 114, 303–5.

Sullivan, H. S. *Conceptions of Modern Psychiatry.* Washington: William Alanson White Foundation, 1947.

Sutherland, E. H., and Cressey, D. R. *Principles of Criminology.* 5th edition. Philadelphia: Lippincott, 1955.

Sykes, G. M., and Matza, D. Techniques of neutralization: A theory of delinquency. *American Sociological Review,* 1957, 22, 664–700.

Tanny, E. Psychiatric study of homicide. *American Journal of Psychiatry,* 1969, 125, 1252–57.

Textor, R. B. *A Cross-Cultural Summary.* New Haven: Human Resources Area Files Press, 1967.

Thayer, W. N. The criminal and the Napanoch plan. *Journal of Criminal Law and Criminology,* 1925, 16, 278–89.

Thornley, K. *Oswald.* Chicago: New Classics House, 1965.

Tompkins, P. *The Murder of Admiral Darlan.* New York: Simon and Schuster, 1965.

Toth, R., and Smith, D. Sirhan Sirhan, Robert Kennedy's accused assassin. *New York Post,* January 6, 1969, 41.

Townshend-Rose, R. U.K.: The case against capital punishment. *The Humanist,* July–August, 1970, 30(4), 36–38.

Trainer, R. *The Lolita Complex.* New York: Citadel, 1966.

Tului, G. *Tra i segregati* [Among the segregated]. *Archivodi Anthropologia,* 1927, 47, 155–84.

Tumlirz, O. *Der Fall Manasse Friedlander* [The cure of Manasse Friedlander]. *Die Jugendlichen und ihre Erzieher, 11, Manas Pad. Mag.,* 1930, No. 1314, 45–69.

Tuteur, W., and Glotzer, J. Murdering mothers. *American Journal of Psychiatry,* 1959, 116, 447–52.

Tyler, V. O., and Brown, G. D. The use of swift, brief isolation as a group control device for institutionalized delinquents. *Behavior Research and Therapy,* 1967, 5, 1–9.

Vollmer, A. The recidivist. *Journal of Delinquency,* 1927, 11, 72–87.

Von-Hammer-Purgstall, V. *The History of the Assassins.* New York: Burt Franklin, 1835, 1968.

Von Hentig, H. *Gangster: A Criminal Psychological Study.* Berlin: Springer-Verlag, 1959.

Voss, H. L., and Hepburn, J. R. Patterns in criminal homicide in Chicago. *Journal of Criminal Law, Criminology and Police Science,* 1968, 59, 99–508.

Waldron, M. Trial is resumed without Manson. *New York Times,* October 3, 1970, 56.

Waldron, M. Manson leaps at judge in the Tate murder trial and declares "someone should cut your head off." *New York Times,* October 6, 1970, 27.

Waldron, M. Manson asserts judge is biased. *New York Times,* October 8, 1970, 93.

Waldron, M. Inmate testifies on Tate killings. *New York Times,* October 10, 1970, 12.

Waldron, M. A Manson motive is heard at trial. *New York Times,* October 18, 1970, 61.

Walford, R. L. The original irreplaceable vision. *Evergreen Review,* March, 1970, No. 76, 47–49, 84–92.

Walker, A. E. Murder and epilepsy. *Journal of Nervous and Mental Disease,* 1961, 133, 430–37.

Walsh, M. N. A contribution to the problem of recurrent mass homicide. *Journal of the Hillside Hospital,* 1966, 15, 84–93.

Warren Commission. *Report of the Warren Commission on the Assassination of President Kennedy.* New York: Bantam, 1965.

Wedge, B. Training for a psychiatry of international relations. *American Journal of Psychiatry,* December 6, 1968, 125, 731–36.

Weinstein, E. A., and Lyerly, O. G. Symbolic aspects of presidential assassination. *Psychiatry,* 1969, 32, 1–11.

Weisz, A. E., and Taylor, R. L. American presidential assassinations. *Diseases of the Nervous System,* 1969, 30, 659–68.

Wertham, F. *Dark Legend: A Study in Murder.* New York: Duell, Sloan and Pearce, 1941.

Wertham, F. The matricidal impulse: Critique of Freudian interpretation of Hamlet. *Journal of Criminal Psychopathology,* 1941b, 2, 455–64.

Wertham, F. *The Show of Violence.* New York: Doubleday, 1949.

Wertham, F. *A Sign for Cain.* New York: Macmillan, 1966.

West, D. J. *Murder Followed by Suicide.* Boston: Harvard University Press, 1966.

Wheaton, E. B. *Prelude to Calamity: The Nazi Revolution 1933–1935.* Garden City, New York: Doubleday, 1968.

Whitaker, K., and Malone, T. *The Roots of Psychotherapy.* New York: McGraw-Hill, 1953.

Whiting, B. B. Paiute sorcery. *Viking Fund Publications in Anthropology,* 1950, No. 15.

Wicker, T. Playboy interview with Ramsey Clark. *Playboy,* August, 1969, 16(8), 53–74.

Wiesenthal, S. *The Murderers Among Us: The Simon Wiesenthal Memoirs.* Edited by Joseph Wechsberg. New York: McGraw-Hill, 1967.

Wilford, J. N. Psychiatrist urges brain tests for suspects in violent crimes. *New York Times,* November 18, 1970, 35.

Wilson, T. Tate killing a thrill, she says. *New York Daily News,* October 14, 1970, 82.

Wilson, T. Link Leslie to LaBianca deaths. *New York Daily News,* November 3, 1970, 10.

Windeler, R. Suspect is a strong nationalist who hoped to return to Jordan. *New York Times,* June 7, 1968, 1, 22.

Wittner, D. Logjam in our courts. *Life,* August 7, 1970, 18–26.

Wolf, M. M., Risley, T., and Mees, H. Application of operant conditioning procedures to the behavior problems of an autistic child. *Behavior Research and Therapy,* 1964, 1, 305–12.

Wolf, R. Editorial. *Rational Living,* 1966, 1(2), 37–38.

Wolfgang, M. *Patterns in Criminal Homicide.* Philadelphia: University of Pennsylvania Press, 1958.

Wolfgang, M., and Ferracuti, F. *The Subculture of Violence on Integrated Theory of Criminality.* London: Tavistock, 1967.

Wolfgang, M., and Strohn, R. B. The relationship between alcohol and criminal homicide. *Quarterly Journal of Studies in Alcoholism,* 1956, 17, 411–25.

Wood, A. L. A socio-structural analysis of murder, suicide and economic crime in Ceylon. *American Sociological Review,* 1961, 26, 744–53.

Yanouskaya, E. U. Catamnestic study of patients suffering from a paranoid form of schizophrenia who had committed dangerous acts for delirious reasons. *Zhurnal Nevropathologii Psikhiatrii,* 1966, 66(9), 1392–97.

Zinberg, N. H., and Fellman, G. A. Violence: Biological need and social control. *Social Forces,* 1967, 45, 533–41.

Author Index

Subject Index

About the Authors

Albert Ellis was born in Pittsburgh and grew up in New York City. He holds a bachelor's degree from the City College of New York; and M.A. and Ph.D. degrees in Clinical Psychology from Columbia University. He has taught at Rutgers University and New York University; has been Chief Psychologist of the New Jersey Department of Institutions and Agencies; was a Consultant in Clinical Psychology to the Veterans Administration and to the Board of Examiners of the New York City Board of Education; is Executive Director of the Institute for Rational Living and Director of Clinical Services of the Institute for the Advanced Study of Rational Psychotherapy; and for almost thirty years has been in the practice of psychotherapy, and marriage and family counseling in New York City.

Dr. Ellis is a Fellow of the American Psychological Association and has been President of its Division of Consulting Psychology, a Member of its Council of Representatives, and a Member of the Executive Board of its Division of Psychotherapy. He is a Fellow (and past-President) of the Society for the Scientific Study of Sex; and a Fellow of the American Orthopsychiatric Association, the American Association of Marriage Counselors, the American Sociological Association, the Association for Applied Anthropology, and the American Association for the Advancement of Science. He has been Vice-President of the American Academy of Psychotherapists; Chairman of the Marriage Counseling Section of the National Council on Family Relations; and a member of the Executive Board of the American Association of Marriage Counselors, Psychologists in Private Practice, and the

New York Society of Clinical Psychologists. He has served as Associate Editor of the *Journal of Marriage and the Family, International Journal of Sexology, Journal of Sex Research, Rational Living, The Journal of Existential Psychiatry,* and *Voices: The Art and Science of Psychotherapy.* He received the Humanist of the Year award of the American Humanist Association in 1971.

Dr. Ellis has published over three hundred and fifty papers in psychological, psychiatric, and sociological journals, periodicals, and anthologies. He has authored or edited twenty-seven books and monographs, including: *The Folklore of Sex, The American Sexual Tragedy, Sex Without Guilt, How to Live with a Neurotic, The Art and Science of Love, The Encyclopedia of Sexual Behavior, Creative Marriage, A Guide to Rational Living, Reason and Emotion in Psychotherapy, Homosexuality: Its Causes and Cure, How to Prevent Your Child from Becoming a Neurotic Adult,* and *Is Objectivism a Religion?*

John M. Gullo, born and raised in Springfield, Illinois, attended the University of Illinois, Springfield Junior College, and MacMurray College, from which he holds the Bachelor of Arts Degree in Chemistry and Psychology. He received his Master of Arts Degree in Clinical Psychology from Bradley University.

Mr. Gullo has been Director of the Jacksonville (Illinois), Chicago, and St. Louis branches of the Institute for Rational Living, and Senior Staff Psychologist and a Training Director of the Jacksonville State Hospital; and Senior Staff Psychologist and a Director of Training and Research of the Chicago State-Read Mental Health Center. He is now Senior Staff Psychologist at the MacFarland Zone State Mental Health Center in Springfield, Illinois, and is in the private practice of Psychotherapy and Marriage and Family Counseling in Springfield.

Mr. Gullo is the author of several articles in professional journals and a member of numerous professional organizations. These include: American Psychological Association and its Divisions of Psychotherapy, Personality and Social Psychology, and General Psychology; Society for the Psychological Study of Social Issues; Illinois Psychological Association; Society for the Scientific Study of Sex; the American Humanist Association; and the Academy of Psychologists in Marital and Family Therapy.